THE CHRISTIAN ART OF DYING

The Christian Art of Dying

LEARNING FROM JESUS

Allen Verhey

WILLIAM B. EERDMANS PUBLISHING COMPANY

GRAND RAPIDS, MICHIGAN / CAMBRIDGE, U.K.

Published 2011 by
Wm. B. Eerdmans Publishing Co.
2140 Oak Industrial Drive N.E., Grand Rapids, Michigan 49505 /
P.O. Box 163, Cambridge CB3 9PU U.K.
www.eerdmans.com

Printed in the United States of America

17 16 15 14 13 12 11   7 6 5 4 3 2 1

Library of Congress Cataloging-in-Publication Data

Verhey, Allen.
    The Christian art of dying : learning from Jesus / Allen Verhey.
        p.   cm.
    Includes bibliographical references and index.
    ISBN 978-0-8028-6672-1 (pbk.: alk. paper)
    1. Death — Religious aspects — Christianity.
    I. Title.

BT825.V47   2011
241'.69709 — dc22

                                        2011015870

Cover and interior illustrations are from *The Ars Moriendi (Editio Princeps, circa 1450)*, edited by W. Harry Rylands (London: The Holbein Society / Wyman & Sons, 1881).

To my many caregivers

Contents

Preface

There are at least two great remedies for the conceit of independence. One is being sick. The other is writing a book. Both are full of reminders that we depend on others, that thanks are due!

When I was first contemplating this book on the art of dying, I was reminded of my own mortality. "Amyloidosis," the doctor said, "and if you leave it untreated, you will die in a couple of years." There were options for treating it, of course, all involving various forms and dosages of chemotherapy. My wife and I, after consulting with specialists and our kids (especially Kate, our daughter who is a physician), decided on an aggressive therapy, a massive dose of chemotherapy followed by a stem cell transplant using stem cells retrieved from my own blood. It was the treatment that promised to do me the most good — if it did not kill me first.

The chemotherapy left me without an effective immune system for about three weeks. There was nausea, of course, and mouth sores. And then the feared fevers came. That sent me back to the hospital, while whatever little infection that had caused the fever raced to kill me before enough white blood cells could arrive to fight it off. We cheered when the lab reports displayed that some white blood cells were finally being produced. And I got well. There are still some imperfect numbers on the lab reports; there are regular visits to the doctors; and there are some other minor residual effects. But I am well — and grateful; reminded of my mortality — and grateful.

The list of those on whom I depended while I was sick is a long one, a humbling one. Thanks are due to Dr. Kovalik, nephrologist at Duke University Medical Center, to Dr. Gaspareto of the Duke University Medical Center Adult Bone Marrow Transplant Center, and to all the skilled doctors and nurses who attended to me, from the internist who made an early diagnosis to the nurse's aide who smiled charitably at me while she cleaned up the results of my nausea. Thanks are due to Dr. Greg Jones, dean of Duke Divinity School, and to all the colleagues who covered for me. Thanks are due to Rev. Joe Harvard, pastor of First Presbyterian Church in Durham, and to all those who visited with and prayed for me. And thanks are due to Phyllis, my wife and nurse, and to the kids. They all cared for me in their own ways, and I am deeply grateful. To them, my many caregivers, I dedicate this book.

But writing a book is another reminder of the fact that we depend upon others. It is frequently a quite solitary task, of course. You have to do it yourself. But you cannot do it without the help of many others. Thanks are due!

Thanks are due to those whose works have formed this one, even when I have disagreed with them. Every time I pulled from the shelf another book to consult, I was reminded of the senile pastor who was given to the use of clichés in his prayers. He intended to make the familiar petition "Make us ever mindful of the needs of others," but he said instead, "Make us ever needful of the minds of others." I have been reminded countless times that I am needful of the minds of others. The footnotes are an effort to say "thanks," but they are a feeble and, I fear, an insufficient effort to acknowledge my indebtedness to others.

Thanks are due also to the Luce Foundation and to Duke Divinity School. The generosity of the Luce Foundation in naming me a Luce Fellow and the kindness of Duke Divinity School in granting me a sabbatical hard on the heels of medical leave allowed me to devote a full academic year to this writing project.

Thanks are due also to the readers of earlier versions of this manuscript. It was very much a first draft when I gave it to them. But they read it carefully, encouraged me kindly, and challenged me to rethink some claims and to rephrase many sentences. Among those readers were three very bright students, Aaron Klink, Brett McCarty, and Bo Helmich. Brett and Bo did me the additional service of attempting to track down many of the references within the *Ars Moriendi* literature. Two colleagues at the Duke Institute for Care at the End of Life, Ray Barfield and Richard Payne, provided thoughtful responses to an early draft. My good friend David H. Smith, currently the director of the Yale Interdisciplinary Center for

Bioethics, read the whole manuscript of the penultimate draft and provided helpful commentary on my presentation at the Luce Conference in 2009. At that conference (and in previous meetings with the other Luce scholars) my work was nurtured and challenged by rich and collegial conversation.

Thanks are due also to other students and colleagues at Duke who listened patiently to some of these ideas in class or in conversation. One of them deserves special mention. It was Daneen Warner who brought one of the wood-block prints from the *Ars Moriendi* to our class at Duke on "Death, Resurrection, and Care at the End of Life." That was the beginning of my consideration of *Ars Moriendi.* Thanks are also due to Hope College and the Religion Department there for inviting a former colleague to give the Danforth Lecture in 2009 and for allowing me to talk about "The Art of Dying." The thoughtful exchanges that followed the lecture and the delightful hospitality of friends were more evidence to me that Hope College is a special place and that I am lucky to have been a part of it for so long.

Thanks, of course, to Jon Pott and to his colleagues at Eerdmans Publishing Company for their interest in my work and for their help in bringing it to publication. Without all these people, and more besides, this book could not have been written.

I fear I am not yet completely cured of my conceit of independence, but I have learned again by my illness and by this project just how deeply indebted I am to others. I thank them all for their care, for their minds, and for their help.

CHAPTER ONE

Introduction

Like the cleaning lady, we all come to dust.

Peter De Vries, *Slouching toward Kalamazoo*[1]

People have been dying for a while now. It started, I guess, with the first human being, and since then the death rate has been right around 100 percent. One might suppose that not much has changed over the years. At the end of life, death; "at the last a little earth is thrown upon our head, and that is the end forever."[2] Much has changed, however, about the ways human beings think about death and about the ways they act in the face of it. The inevitability of death does not make inevitable any particular response to it. Throwing a little dirt on the head of the dead — or burial — is not, after all, a universal practice, and many have challenged the claim that death "is the end forever."

Reflective people have thought about death and dying for as long as there have been reflective people, and the great variety of their thoughts is as plain as the universality of death. Here, in the ancient Babylonian epic

1. Peter De Vries, *Slouching toward Kalamazoo* (New York: Penguin Books, 1984), p. 23. Or, as Shakespeare had put it in *Cymbeline* (4.2.263-264):

Golden lads and girls all must,
As chimney-sweepers, come to dust.

2. Blaise Pascal, *Pascal's Pensées* (New York: Dutton, 1958), 210, p. 61.

of Gilgamesh, Siduri, barmaid to the gods, counsels Gilgamesh to give up his hopeless quest for immortality: "Gilgamesh, where are you hurrying to? You will never find that life for which you are looking. When the gods created man they allotted to him death, but life they retained in their own keeping. As for you, Gilgamesh, fill your belly with good things; day and night, night and day, dance and be merry, feast and rejoice. Let your clothes be fresh, bathe yourself in water, cherish the little child that holds your hand, and make your wife happy in your embrace; for this too is the lot of man."[3] There, in Plato's *Phaedo*, Socrates welcomes his death, insisting confidently that the human soul is immortal and that the death of the body simply frees the soul from its imprisonment in the body. And there he counsels his friends against attachment to the very things Siduri had commended.[4]

Here, in a letter to a friend, Seneca gives good Stoic advice to meet death cheerfully, for "dying well means dying gladly."[5] There, in his famous poem, Dylan Thomas gives quite contrary advice:

> Do not go gentle into that good night,
> Old age should burn and rave at close of day;
> Rage, rage against the dying of the light.[6]

Thinking about death has almost inevitably accompanied reflection about the human condition. Who are we? And where are we going? Is there a life after death? And if there is, how shall we prepare for it? Or, if death is the end forever, how should we live knowing that we shall die? Philosophers and theologians and poets and essayists and social scientists — and almost certainly, you — have thought about these questions. Some have despaired of ever answering them; others have quite confidently not only answered them but also recommended their answers as wisdom for living and, of course, for dying. The answers, however, have been various indeed.

It turns out, then, not only that death has a long history but also that

3. *The Epic of Gilgamesh*, trans. N. K. Sanders, 3rd ed. (New York: Penguin Classics, 1972), p. 102. Siduri's advice is echoed in the advice of the Teacher in Eccles. 9:7-10.

4. See *Phaedo* 64C-67B.

5. Lucius Annaeus Seneca, *Epistle* 61, "On Meeting Death Cheerfully," in Seneca, *Epistles 1–65*, trans. Richard M. Gummere, Loeb Classical Library 75 (Cambridge: Harvard University Press, 1917/2002), pp. 425-27.

6. Dylan Thomas, "Do Not Go Gentle into That Good Night," in *The Poems of Dylan Thomas*, ed. Daniel Jones (New York: New Directions, 2003), p. 239.

that history is marked by a great variety of human responses to death and a great variety of reflective anticipations of death. It is that great variety that makes an effort to write "a brief history of death" imprudent, if not impudent. There is, to be sure, a fine little book by that title by Douglas J. Davies, and there is much to be learned from it, but on one point at least it is quite misleading. Davies claims that "Christianity glorified death."[7] It is true, as we shall note, that "Christianity [sometimes] glorified death." But it was not always so. And it can be argued that it was not so in Scripture. At the very least, there have been a variety of responses to death within the Christian tradition. Indeed, while it is true that "Christianity [sometimes] glorified death," it is also true that Christianity sometimes demonized death. Scripture, after all, can call death "the last enemy," a demonic power whose malicious hold on us is only surrendered when God triumphs over death (1 Cor. 15:26).

The Christian tradition does not speak with one voice about death — nor for that matter does the Christian canon. There is too much variety within the Christian tradition to attempt even "a brief history of Christian death." This book will not undertake anything like a complete and objective history of death. It will not undertake even "a brief history of Christian death." It admits to being partial — and partial in two senses of the word.

It is partial, first, by being quite selective. It will attend to just three episodes in the history of death, the "medicalized" dying of the mid–twentieth century, the "art of dying" in the fifteenth century, and the death of Jesus in the first century.

It will attend to "medicalized" dying because that episode in the recent history of death is often blamed for undercutting "the art of dying." People still die, of course, but the accusation is that in a "medicalized" dying, people frequently do not die well. The first part of the book will join the chorus of voices that have complained that the medicalization of death makes dying well difficult. In a "medicalized" dying death is regarded as the great enemy to be defeated by the greater powers of science and medicine. The death rate remains right around 100 percent, of course, but in a "medicalized" dying there is only one focus: avoiding death. Moreover, the confidence in medicine's great powers and the hope of avoiding death have

7. Douglas J. Davies, *A Brief History of Death* (Oxford: Blackwell, 2005), p. 7. This book is not really a history but something closer to a social anthropology. The title was determined by the Blackwell series to which it belongs.

nurtured a denial that anyone is dying. People may be sick, quite sick, but to admit that they are dying seems a betrayal of the confidence we have in medicine and its technology. The "dying role" is lost; only the "sick role" remains. And the "sick role" requires that we put ourselves in the hands of a competent medical expert and hope for recovery. So a "medicalized" dying usually happens in a hospital, in a sterile environment, and in the company of technology and the medical experts who know how to use it. Little wonder, then, that death has been reduced to a medical event and that the art of dying well has been largely lost.

"Medicalized" dying can be traced to the triumphs and the ambitions of medical science in the mid–twentieth century. We may and should be grateful, of course, for the great advances of medical care in the last century. None of us wants to return to bloodletting and snake oil. We must not neglect the fact that there was a time, not so long ago, when physicians were relatively powerless against the diseases that threaten death and when their ministrations were as likely to kill you as to cure you. The desire of medicine to heal motivated those advances. It is not difficult to understand and to appreciate that desire. It belongs to the long history of medicine and of medical ethics. To understand how that ambition became Promethean, however, it will be necessary to revisit briefly the seventeenth and eighteenth centuries and the Enlightenment's dreams of scientific progress. There has been great scientific progress, but with the great advances in the powers of medicine have come some problems. There have been great successes, but with the great successes of medicine have come the failures of those successes. And among those problems and failures many now count a "medicalized" dying.

We still live in that episode of the human history of dying, but there have been complaints about it and increasingly powerful challenges to it. Complaints about "medicalized death" have echoed in the literature on medical ethics, in the death awareness movement, and in the hospice movement. It is not difficult to understand and to appreciate the complaints either. To the complaints are usually joined some proposals to remedy the problems, and we will attend briefly to the proposals of standard bioethics, of the death awareness movement, and of hospice. These proposals have had some successes, but the successes have been limited, and with the successes have come again some failures of the successes.

Having joined the chorus of voices complaining about a "medicalized" dying but having complained as well that some of the voices in that chorus sound a little off-key, the book begins its search for a better way of dying. One earlier episode in the long history of dying that presents an obvious alternative to "medicalized" death is the "art of dying" in the fifteenth century. That will be the focus of the second part of the book.

In the fifteenth century a little self-help book was published with the title *Ars Moriendi* (the "art of dying"). It gave instructions about how to die well. It was an illustrated and abridged edition of a longer text, the *Tractatis Artis Bene Moriendi*, which was translated into several European languages and provided a model for a number of other works on the theme of the "art of dying." Such works were enormously popular in the late fifteenth century and continued to be written and read for centuries after that. They remained popular to the middle of the nineteenth century.[8] There were works in a variety of languages. There were works by Catholics, Lutherans, Calvinists, Anglicans, and Anabaptists. As popular as such works were in the late medieval and early modern periods, however, they are largely neglected and forgotten today.[9]

We will revisit this neglected tradition in the second part of this book, attempting to understand and appreciate this other way of dying. Again, however, to do that will require that we reach a little further back in the history of dying, back to the Black Death, surely, but also back to the Renaissance philosophers and theologians who retrieved Plato and the consolation literature of the Stoics as resources for a theological response to death. There is much to appreciate in this neglected tradition. Its concern for a faithful dying, its attention to the virtues for dying well, and much else in it may help us to imagine a contemporary alternative to "medicalized death," to begin to construct a contemporary Christian *ars moriendi*. But there are also problems in it, and any effort to retrieve it must also acknowledge those problems. Indeed, any effort to retrieve it must engage in the tasks of assessment, selection, and correction. Because *Ars Moriendi* recognized Scripture as the final source and test for the

8. Jeremy Taylor's *Rule and Exercises of Holy Dying*, first published in 1651, was not the last of the works in this genre, but it was, according to Nancy Lee Beaty, "the artistic climax of the tradition." See Nancy Lee Beaty, *The Craft of Dying: A Study in the Literary Tradition of the* Ars Moriendi *in England* (New Haven: Yale University Press, 1979). Editions of Taylor's *Holy Dying* remained popular through the middle of the nineteenth century.

9. There are many reasons for this, I suppose. In her study of the American Civil War, *This Republic of Suffering: Death and the American Civil War* (New York: Knopf, 2008), Drew Gilpin Faust begins with an account of the popularity of the *ars moriendi* tradition in America at the beginning of the Civil War and argues that the tradition could not finally survive the horrific carnage of the war any more than the 620,000 soldiers who died could.

meaning of a faithful dying, it will not be inappropriate either to it or to my own convictions to test it and qualify it by remembering the story Scripture tells.

Ars Moriendi itself had called attention to that still earlier episode in the history of dying, the death of Jesus. It regarded the death of Jesus as paradigmatic for a Christian's faithful dying. So does the third part of this book. Taking that cue from *Ars Moriendi,* it turns to the story of Jesus. The death of Jesus is hardly what we think of when we think of dying well. He died young and violently, the victim of a judicial murder. He died — according to Mark, at least — abandoned by friends and followers. And he died an excruciatingly painful death. Even so, the story has quite clearly paradigmatic significance for Christians; they are called, after all, to follow him, indeed, to "take up the cross." The story of Jesus is the story Christians remember, the story they love to tell and long to live, even as they are dying. It is the story that is determinative for Christian discernment, and it provides, I think, a corrective both to the tradition of *Ars Moriendi* and to "medicalized" dying. The story does not "glorify" or even commend either death or suffering, but neither does it deny death and suffering or allow us to reduce them to medical events. The story of Jesus may, I hope, provide some clues to the meaning of a faithful dying today, a contemporary Christian *ars moriendi.*

The final part of the book returns to the present, attending to practices of Christian community that bear the promise of helping Christians to die well and faithfully and of forming communities that care well and faithfully for those who are dying. We will attend to some practices central to the common life of the church, to gathering for worship, to reading Scripture and to prayer, to the Eucharist and baptism, and to the ways these practices could form and inform our dying and our care for the dying. And we will attend to some other practices that have a place in Christian community, to practices of mourning and comforting and to funerals and remembering the stories of the saints, of course, but also to the practices of catechesis and communal discernment.

The book, as you have surely noted by now, is also partial in another sense. I have acknowledged that it is hardly comprehensive; it will deal only with these selected episodes in the long history of death. But let me acknowledge also that it is hardly unbiased. I do not pretend to consider death with an impartial objectivity — as if that were possible without reducing death to a crude fact of nature (and that too would be partial). Let me be candid about my perspective. I write as a Christian theologian, as someone who cherishes the gospel and tries to think about all things, including dying, in relation to that gospel. And I write as a mortal, as someone who has been reminded recently of my own mortality. I do not claim to be "impartial," not at least in the sense of being a "disinterested spectator" of human mortality.

A few years ago I was diagnosed as having amyloidosis, a rare blood disorder. I told the story briefly in the preface. But for about six months my own mortality was vivid to me. I wanted to live, and I was grateful for the skillful doctors and sophisticated technology upon which my life depended. But if I was going to die, I wanted it to be my death, the final chapter in my story and not a footnote in a research report some day. I wanted it to be a faithful dying, a dying worthy of one who cherishes the gospel. This book started in conversation with myself, myself as theologian talking with myself as mortal. Sometimes, frankly, the mortal talked back. I think I became a better theologian by listening to my mortal self, and I hope my voice in this book is that of a mortal theologian, a man who knows that he will die and who believes that the last word belongs to God, a man who cherishes both the Christian tradition and life. I also hope that my voice can bring both comfort and courage to other mortal Christians and confidence to the Christian communities who are called to care for them.

This book, however, is not a memoir. When some friends who knew I had been sick asked what I was working on, I told them I was working on a book on dying. And when their reaction displayed some alarm, I thanked them for their concern and assured them that I was not writing a memoir.[10] This book is not a memoir. It is not about me or about my experience of dying. I will, however, tell a story or two from my experience along the way, and one story, a story that celebrates mortal life, seems a fitting way to conclude this introduction.

My wife, Phyllis, is a big fan of Frank Capra's *It's a Wonderful Life*. When the kids were growing up, she would insist that everyone in the family watch it together on the weekend before Christmas. The kids knew all the lines and would sometimes quote a line or two. If there was a crash somewhere in the house, for example, it was not unusual that it would be followed by somebody quoting Uncle Billy, "I'm alright! I'm alright!" Now that the kids are grown, they sometimes give Phyllis gifts related to the

---

10. It may be, however, that memoirs are the *Ars Moriendi* literature for our time. The success of *Tuesdays with Morrie* and *The Last Lecture* is evidence that people are still looking for models and paradigms for dying well.

Capra movie. We have, for example, ornaments for the Christmas tree, one that captures the joyful final scene with George holding Suzi, and another that is an angel bearing the words "Every time a bell rings, an angel gets its wings." We have a (boring) board game based on the movie. For her birthday a few years ago the kids gave Phyllis a wall plaque that simply bore the legend "It's a Wonderful Life." She instructed me to hang it above the back door, so that as we left each day we would be reminded that it is a wonderful life. I did as I was told, but evidently not very well. That was a couple of weeks before I would visit the doctor and be told that I had amyloidosis. A couple of days after that visit, when I left the house and closed that back door, I heard a crash. I wanted to say, "I'm alright! I'm alright!" but the words caught in my throat. When I opened the door, it was as I had feared. "It's a Wonderful Life" had come crashing down. "This is not a good omen," I said to myself. But I examined the broken corner of the fiberboard plaque, and because I knew Phyllis would be disappointed, I did my best to repair it. Then I hung it up more securely. Phyllis noticed the broken corner soon enough, of course. But she did not seem disappointed. Indeed, she seemed touched by the new gift the old gift had become. Now every time we leave the house, even when we go to the hospital or to the clinic, we are reminded that it's still a wonderful life, a little broken now, surely mortal, but still a wonderful life.

PART ONE

Medicalized Dying

We who must die demand a miracle.
How could the Eternal do a temporal act,
The Infinite become a finite fact?
Nothing can save us that is possible:
We who must die demand a miracle.

W. H. Auden, *For the Time Being*[1]

---

1. W. H. Auden, *For the Time Being*, "Advent," III, in W. H. Auden, *Collected Poems*, ed. Edward Mendelson (London: Faber and Faber, 2007), p. 353.

CHAPTER TWO

From "Tame Death" to "Medicalized Death"

Tame Death

Philippe Aries began his classic study of death with the stories of the deaths of Roland and the Knights of the Round Table.[1] The stories, he said, displayed deaths that not only were typical of death in the early Middle Ages but also expressed traditions surrounding dying that were already centuries old. Death then was simple and public. "Tame death," he called it. It was regarded as an evil, to be sure, but it could be rendered meaningful by the rituals that surrounded it and by the companions who attended it. The rituals and the community gave human meaning to death, rendered it something more and other than a crude fact of nature (p. 604).

The rituals were simple enough. After acknowledging the imminence of death with a certain ambivalence, expressive at once of regret and resignation, the dying person said good-by to his family and friends, forgiving them and asking forgiveness, blessing them and instructing them, and commending them to God's care and protection. Having said his farewells, the dying person would pray, confessing his sins and commending his soul to God (pp. 14-18).

These familiar rituals of death themselves testified to the importance of the community. Attended by family and friends, the dying person was the center of attention. Even strangers would sometimes fill the room, fol-

---

1. Philippe Aries, *The Hour of Our Death*, trans. Helen Weaver (New York: Knopf, 1981). The page references in the following text are to this work.

Death happened in and to the community

lowing the priest who brought the sacrament. Death was not a solitary event. Like life, it happened in community. And death happened not only in community but also *to* the community. It was a communal loss, and both grief and comfort were communal tasks. Together they held tight to their humanity in the face of the sad truths of suffering and death. Suffering and death were regarded as the common lot of humanity, the effect of sin, and they required solemn and communal recognition (p. 605). Death was not "tame" because nature was benevolent, but because God was. With hope in God the dead could rest in peace, awaiting the resurrection of the dead,[2] and the community could go on.

A sudden or unexpected death was hard, of course, to "tame." A sudden death was regarded as a bad death, as somehow a little shameful, as if the wrath of God had struck.

"Tame death" survived for centuries, and it still survives here and there. But Aries' study also tells the story of challenges and changes to this way of dying. It would be challenged and modified first by the "scholarly cultures" of the later Middle Ages and the Renaissance, when the *contemptus mundi* of medieval spirituality and the recovery of Platonic and Stoic philosophy sacrificed something of the ambivalence toward death that had characterized the "tame death" (p. 15). It would face a different challenge in the early modern period, when extravagant hopes in scientific progress suggested human control over nature and relief from human mortality. In that early modern period, Aries said, "tame death" began to be "savage" (p. 608). Death was regarded as a part of nature, but nature was regarded as what threatened human well-being. Nature brought plague and misery and death. The human response to death began to rely less on ritual and community and more on the promise of human mastery over nature, on the progress of science and technology. Ro-

transition

---

2. Aries points out that the image of "sleep" is typical of early medieval accounts of the state of the dead (pp. 22-23). He calls attention to the popularity of the story "The Seven Sleepers of Ephesus." They were martyred during the reign of Decius (249-251 C.E.) and laid to rest in a sealed grotto. Two hundred years later, when a heresy began to circulate during the reign of Theodosius II denying the resurrection of the dead, God raised them up. A crowd gathered, of course, to see and to hear these martyrs raised from the dead. The message was that God had awakened them from their sleep to show his power to raise the dead. Then the Seven Sleepers laid on the ground and went back to sleep, to rest, and to wait for the general resurrection. For a thirteenth-century account of the legend, see Jacobus De Voragine, *The Golden Legend*, trans. William Granger Ryan (Princeton: Princeton University Press, 1993), pp. 15-18.

manticism would make an effort to revive a "tame death," but its affection for "untamed nature" and its suspicion of the tradition's claim that evil had a hold on nature and on human nature also profoundly modified it. "Death was no longer familiar and tame, as it had been in traditional societies, but neither was it absolutely wild. It had become something moving and beautiful like nature, like the immensity of nature, the sea or the moors" (p. 610). By 1977, however, when Aries first published the original French version of *The Hour of Our Death*, the "tame death," he said, had all but disappeared. In its place there was "denied death," "excluded death," "invisible death." In its place was "wild death," untamed by ritual or community. In its place was "medicalized death" (p. 585).

Medicalized Dying

Aries traced "the triumph of medicalization" (p. 583) to the end of World War II and to the advances in medical and surgical techniques in the third quarter of the twentieth century. The techniques required not only skilled personnel but also auxiliary services like laboratories and pharmacies and, of course, the technologies themselves. All these were found concentrated in a hospital. And a first characterization of "medicalized death" is that it happens in a hospital. In a swift but almost imperceptible transition, dying was transferred from the home to the hospital. At the end of the war in 1945, 40 percent of deaths happened in the hospital; in 1995, 90 percent did.

When people became seriously ill, they would go to the hospital. They entered it with considerable anxiety, of course, but also with great expectations. Something like Auden's line was written on their hearts, "We who must die demand a miracle." Auden's line is from an advent prayer, a petition for the miracle of God's sharing our human flesh. But we have grown accustomed to the rhetoric of "the miracles of modern science," and when we are sick, we look for one, plead for one to be performed with technological grace. Perhaps it will be simply the old "miracle drug," penicillin, or maybe the miracle of stem cell therapy. At any rate, we know that in the hospital great things can be attempted and sometimes accomplished. Sometimes the sad stories that patients tell with their bodies and about their bodies will be given a happy ending after all. But other times those sad stories still end with death, and sometimes with a lingering dying, in a hospital or in a nursing home, in a coma or in pain, hooked up to a respirator or to a feeding tube or to both. Reports of such lingering

13

deaths can prompt us to say, "I'd rather die suddenly, with a heart attack or in a car wreck." Suddenly the sort of death most lamented when death was "tame" seems preferable.

When dying was moved to the hospital — to be accompanied there by technology and by those who knew how to use it, accompanied also by great expectations of that technology and of those experts — there were some profound, if unintended, consequences for the dying role. Most notably, it was simply undercut, replaced by the "sick role." In a transition as swift and imperceptible as the transfer of dying to the hospital (and, of course, related to it), the dying were no longer treated as if they were dying; they were treated like anyone else who was recovering from major surgery or a serious disease. You do not go to the hospital, after all, to die. You go there to get better. You are expected to admit that you are sick, but you are also expected to share the hospital's goal, to avoid death. So, suddenly no one was "dying" any more. They were just "sick." That spelled the end of "the dying role" with its rituals and community. All that was left was "the sick role" and, of course, death itself.

There were still rituals — like putting on the hospital gown, like waiting patiently for the visit of the doctor in the white coat, like having vital signs and a little blood taken. And there were still companions; they were called "Nurse." But these are rituals and companions for the sick, not for the dying. In "tame" death the companions were family and friends and priest, not medical experts. In "tame" death the dying were the primary actors, expected to perform some of the rituals of the "dying role." In "medicalized" death, the dying have no role to play except the "sick role," and that is quite a passive role. According to Talcott Parsons, at least, the "sick role" requires that the sick be exempted from ordinary responsibilities and exempted as well from any blame for their condition, but it also requires that they seek competent medical help and cooperate in the process of getting well.[3]

People still died, of course, but until they did, they were just sick and, therefore, still expected to seek competent medical help and to cooperate in the process of getting well. It required of the dying — pardon me, of "the sick" — a slightly revised version of Auden's petition, "We who must *not* die demand a miracle." A medicalized dying is characterized by the effort to avoid death.

3. Talcott Parsons described the sick role first in 1951 in *The Social System* (Glencoe, Ill.: Free Press, 1951). He revisited the notion in Talcott Parsons, "The Sick Role and the Role of the Physician Reconsidered," *Milbank Memorial Fund Quarterly* 53 (Summer 1975): 257-78.

The effort to avoid death in the hospital was accompanied by an effort to avoid mentioning it. A heavy silence surrounded death. In the middle of the twentieth century many doctors refused to tell patients they were dying, and many families and friends cooperated in the deception.[4] When dying was moved to the hospital, it was accompanied not only by great expectations of the "miracles of modern science" but also by silence about death. The doctors and families who conspired in silence and deception might justify their conduct by saying that the patient must not be allowed to "give up hope," but their silence and denial also reflected the uneasy silence of the culture concerning death.

In a stunning essay called "The Pornography of Death," the sociologist Geoffrey Gorer noted that in the middle of the twentieth century our culture seemed both obsessed with death and unwilling to mention it.[5] He compared the culture's attitude to death to the Victorian attitude toward sex. Death, he said, had become the new taboo subject, not to be discussed, unmentionable. Gorer noted especially the change in mourning customs. When his father died in 1915, the public mourning rituals were still intact. Less than half a century later, however, they had all but disappeared. In the absence of those public mourning rituals, the widow of a friend of Gorer reported to him that, although many had given her good professional advice, she felt abandoned by her friends. They evidently regarded grief as a private matter, not to be mentioned or displayed publicly. If one must weep, one should weep in private, as if it were, Gorer says strikingly, "an analogue of masturbation." The Victorian prudery about sex only increased the fascination with the forbidden, and it is not shocking perhaps that the silence and denial around death in the mid–twentieth century evidently only in-

4. See Donald Oken, "What to Tell Cancer Patients," *Journal of the American Medical Association* 175 (1961): 1120-28, reprinted in Stanley Reiser, Arthur Dyck, and William Curran, eds., *Ethics in Medicine: Historical Perspectives and Contemporary Concerns*, 2nd ed. (Cambridge: MIT Press, 1977), pp. 224-32. Oken's 1961 study found that 88 percent of physicians reported that their "usual policy" was not to tell patients that they had cancer. "The physician's lie" was hardly the invention of mid-twentieth-century America, however. Plato mentioned it — and approved of it (*Republic* 389b) — and the Hippocratic treatise *Decorum* commended the practice of deception lest the patient give up hope (*Decorum* 16, in *Hippocrates*, vol. 2, trans. W. H. S. Jones [Cambridge: Harvard University Press, 1925], pp. 296-99). Nevertheless, the practice of deception was quite at home in the culture of silence and denial in mid-twentieth-century America.

5. Geoffrey Gorer, "The Pornography of Death," first published in 1955, reprinted as an appendix to his book *Death, Grief, and Mourning* (Garden City, N.Y.: Doubleday, 1965), pp. 192-99.

creased the culture's fascination with death. Images of death, especially violent death, began to fill the screens of movie theaters and television sets and the pages of novels. Unmentionable, death became titillating. More to the point, where death is unmentionable, it is difficult to learn to die well. It's like trying to learn to love one's spouse well by watching pornographic sex.

Another feature of "medicalized" dying is that it is a "depersonalized" dying. When death was "medicalized," it became a medical event. Death itself, for a patient hooked up to machines that pump blood and move breath, required expert diagnosis. Death became a flat line on an electroencephalogram. And dying was no less "depersonalized." It is not hard to understand. In diagnosis, medicine fixes its objective gaze on the body and sees the body as an object. In therapy, medicine treats the body as a manipulable object. The "person" sometimes gets lost — and so indeed does the body. At least the patient's relation to her own body as "me" can be displaced by the physician's diagnostic and therapeutic (and "scientific") relationship to the body as "it." It became a familiar complaint that medicine treats "me" like an "it."[6]

The body of the dying person became the battlefield where heroic doctors and nurses waged their war against death. The lab reports and body scans provided surveillance and dictated strategy, but the doctors remained in charge, even in the face of almost certain defeat. Death's triumph could be marked — diagnosed — by that flat line on an electroencephalogram, but it required some medical explanation, the identification of some medical "cause of death." Death and dying had been taken over by medicine. Death became medicine's agony of defeat. "Tame death" was given a "do not resuscitate" order.

Death, of course, cannot finally be avoided. And it cannot finally be reduced to a merely medical event. Indeed, the medical efforts to avoid it display not only the remarkable human powers to intervene sometimes against it but also the pathos of human powerlessness against it. Death is inalienably a human event, reaching into life, taking hold of human hopes and worries, loves and fears, long before the end itself. When it is "medicalized," it grows "wild" and threatening, untamed. Then, if we must die, we long for the sudden death, the unexpected death, the death that comes suddenly in our sleep, the death that comes without our knowledge, the very sort of death regarded as a bad death in the twelfth century.

6. See Michel Foucault, *The Birth of the Clinic: An Archaeology of Medical Perception*, trans. A. M. Sheridan Smith (New York: Vintage, 1994); see footnote 44.

It's a long story Aries told, this story of death from the twelfth century to the twentieth, from "tame death" to "wild death." But the story continued, of course, and it still continues. In the twenty-first century, people still live — and die — in that episode of the human history of death Aries called "wild." And where death is "wild," or medicalized, it is difficult to die well. Indeed, where dying is medicalized, it is sometimes death, not life, that makes its power felt in a hospital. That is the sad irony of medicalized death, that in our very resistance to death, death can make its power felt before the end of a person's life, before that line on the electroencephalogram goes flat. That sad irony requires some explanation, and the rest of this chapter hopes to provide an account of it.

The Triumph of Death in the Medicalization of It

Death threatens to alienate us from our own flesh, from our communities, and from God.[7] Those threats are real and horrible — and uttered menacingly already by sickness, that "forerunner and messenger of death."[8] Medicine is right to resist such threats, to resist both sickness and death. But the sad irony is this, that the resistance to death in medicalized dying sometimes allows death a premature triumph. It is not, of course, that patients die sooner rather than later. It is that in a medicalized dying death seems to make good on its threats before death itself. Patients are sometimes prematurely alienated from their own bodies, from their communities, and from God — and for the sake of their survival.

Death and Our Flesh

Death threatens, first, to alienate us from our own flesh. The threat is real and terrible, for we are embodied selves, not ghosts. Sickness, that forerunner and messenger of death, reminds us that we *are* our bodies, that our

7. See William F. May, "The Sacral Power of Death in Contemporary Experience," in *On Moral Medicine: Theological Perspectives in Medical Ethics*, ed. Stephen E. Lammers and Allen Verhey, 2nd ed. (Grand Rapids: Eerdmans, 1998), pp. 197-208, especially pp. 181-84, and William F. May, *The Patient's Ordeal* (Bloomington: Indiana University Press, 1991), pp. 9-14, 200-206.

8. Karl Barth, *Church Dogmatics* III/4, trans. A. T. Mackay et al. (London: T. & T. Clark, 1961), p. 366.

"selves" depend on the integrity of the bodies we otherwise take for granted, that our health and our lives, our "selves," are radically contingent.[9] This reminder, however, does not come gently; it is not like listening to some friendly preacher read from the Psalms. In sickness this *identification* with the body is experienced at the same time as *alienation* from the body.[10]

Death makes its power felt in serious or chronic illness and in severe pain, when the body is experienced not only as "me," but also as "the enemy."[11] It makes its power felt in the weakness that robs the sick of the capacity to exercise responsible control of themselves and of their world. Death makes its power felt when the wonderful variety of God's creation is reduced to something barren and sterile or to something putrid and foul. It makes its power felt when the body no longer opens up into a larger and sharable world, when the body — and the world — of the sick shrinks to that place "a bandage hides."[12] Death makes its power felt in the sense of a betrayal of that fundamental trust we have in our bodies. (And when such a fundamental trust is broken, all trust can become suspect — more important, to be sure, but more questionable, too.)

To its great credit medicine resists death — and its resistance is sometimes heroic. However, unless there is some other (nonmedical) response to this threat of death, medicine's resistance to death can sometimes grow presumptuous, pretending to rescue human beings from their mortality and their vulnerability to suffering. Unless there is some confidence that death will not have the last word, its resistance is frequently desperate, laboring under the tyranny of survival or ease. Unless there is some other basis for hope than medicine, sometimes — ironically and tragically — death can make its power felt in a hospital and in the sort of medicine that is technologically oriented to biological survival.

9. Arthur Kleinman, *The Illness Narratives: Suffering, Healing, and the Human Condition* (New York: Basic Books, 1988), p. 45.

10. Kleinman, *The Illness Narratives*, p. 45.

11. Kleinman, *The Illness Narratives*, p. 45; Elaine Scarry, *The Body in Pain: The Making and Unmaking of the World* (New York: Oxford University Press, 1985), p. 47; M. Therese Lysaught, "Suffering, Ethics, and the Body of Christ: Anointing as a Strategic Alternative Practice," *Christian Bioethics* 2, no. 2 (1996): 172-201, p. 177.

12. The phrase is from another of W. H. Auden's poems, "Surgical Ward," in *Selected Poems of W. H. Auden* (New York: Random House, Modern Library, 1958), pp. 45-46, also entitled "Sonnets from China XIV," in Auden, *Collected Poems*, ed. Edward Mendelson (London: Faber and Faber, 2007), p. 190.

When the sick, at once identified with their bodies and alienated from them, seek medical care, they sometimes find this self-understanding reinforced;[13] they are sometimes reduced to their pathology, and the body is treated as "the enemy," as that manipulable and untrustworthy "nature" that must, for the sake of my self, be overpowered, but that remains, willy-nilly, my self. Patients suffer then not only from the disease but also from the treatment of it — and death makes its power felt not only in sickness but also in medicine. The alienation from our bodies comes prematurely, and for the sake of our survival. That's the sad irony of medicalized death.

Death and Our Communities

Death threatens also to separate people from their communities. The threat is real and horrible, for we are communal selves, not isolated individuals. Our lives are lives lived with others, and death threatens separation and removal, exclusion and abandonment.

Sickness comes as the forerunner and messenger of this alienation, too. Death makes its power felt when the sick or dying are removed and separated from those with whom they share a common life. It makes its power felt when their environment is inhospitable to family and friends. It makes its power felt when disease so monopolizes attention that there is no space for the tasks of reconciliation, forgiveness, and community. It makes its power felt when the fear of being abandoned is not met by the presence of others who care.

Sickness, with its pain and weakness, pushes people to the margins of public life, forces a withdrawal from the public activities of working and shopping, attending a concert or a ball game.[14] And those of us who are "well" provide some of the leverage that moves the sick to the margins, for we are not hospitable to reminders of our own vulnerability and contingency.[15] We are autonomous, in control, in charge, productive; they are not. We have been successful against the powerful threats of nature; they have not. They have been captured by the power of death, by the forces of chaos, by the nature that threatens us all, by the nature against which our

13. Lysaught, "Suffering," p. 177.

14. Kleinman, *The Illness Narratives*, p. 44; Bradley Hanson, "School of Suffering," in *On Moral Medicine*, pp. 249-55; Lysaught, "Suffering," p. 176.

15. Lysaught, "Suffering," pp. 176-77.

best hope is technology, the power knowledge gives, the knowledge most of us do not have. They belong, therefore, in a hospital and under the care of a physician, not in public spaces reserved for strength and beauty, for efficiency and productivity, for life. They belong — "elsewhere."[16]

Even within their own spaces, moreover, those who suffer can be further isolated and alienated, for suffering can rob the sick of their voice. In W. H. Auden's wonderful and painful line, "Truth in their sense is how much they can bear; / It is not talk like ours but groans they smother."[17] The point is not just that those who suffer are sometimes driven back to the sounds and cries human beings make before they learn a language. The point is rather that there are no words. The person in pain knows it, knows it with a certainty that Descartes might envy, but the one suffering it cannot make sense of it, cannot tell it, cannot communicate it or "share" it.[18] And the silence of death makes its power felt in the lonely dumbness of the sick and the helpless deafness of those who would care!

Medicine resists death, and can sometimes identify the pain, can "objectify" it, make sense of it, and manage it by creating a language for it. But sometimes that language is not the language of the patient; and where that language is the "official" language, there patients find themselves aliens, not knowing the language, "speechless," and with little hope for making their pain — or themselves — known.

Medicine resists death, to its credit, but again, unless there is some other (nonmedical) way of responding to this threat, sometimes — ironically and tragically — death makes its power felt in a hospital. It makes its power felt, first, when a community abandons the sick to medicine, and then, in a hospital when medicine neglects the community and the voice of the patient. The alienation from our communities comes prematurely, and for the sake of our survival. That's the sad irony of medicalized death.

Death and God

Death threatens people, finally, in their relationship with God. The threat is real and terrible, for human beings are religious creatures, in spite of the

16. Auden, "Surgical Ward," or "Sonnets from China XIV."

17. Auden, "Surgical Ward," or "Sonnets from China XIV."

18. This loss of voice is confirmed by the words of a patient (Kleinman, *The Illness Narratives*, p. 68): "That's the worst thing about pain. You can't see it. You can't know what it's like unless, God help you, you suffer from it."

denials of secularism. Death threatens any sense that the One who bears down on us and sustains us is dependable and caring. It threatens abandonment by God and separation from God. It threatens human beings in their identity as cherished children of God. Death makes its power felt whenever the sick and dying, or those who would care for them, are not assured of the presence of a loving God who cares. Death makes its power felt not only in the sense of betrayal by our bodies and by our communities, but also in the sense of betrayal by God.

Such at least was the experience of Stein, a character in Peter De Vries' *Blood of the Lamb*.[19] He described his daughter's leukemia as a "sluggishly multiplying anarchy . . . a souvenir from the primordial ooze. The original Chaos, without form and void. In de beginning was de void, and de void was vit God. Mustn't say de naughty void" (p. 177). "God," Stein said, "is a word banging around in the human nervous system." And when he was reminded of the martyrs and of their courage, he called it "Part of the horror. It's all a fantasy. It's all for nothing. A martyr giving his life, a criminal taking one. It's all the same to the All" (p. 178). Then medicine is just, as Stein said, "the art of prolonging disease . . . in order to postpone grief" (p. 179).

To its great credit medicine resists death. But unless there is some other (nonmedical) response to this threat of death, unless there is some confidence that death will not have the last word, unless there is some basis for hope in God, we are finally abandoned to death and all its threats are made good. That's the sad irony of medicalized death. And that's the reason W. H. Auden said, "Nothing can save us that is possible." The miracle we need finally is not to be numbered among "the miracles of modern science." The miracle we need is "a temporal act" of the eternal God. The miracle we need is advent, "the Infinite become a finite fact," God sharing human flesh and its vulnerability to death, and God winning a victory over death.

the miracle we need

However many changes have taken place between the first century and the twenty-first, whatever differences mark human beings and cultures around the world, they are alike in this: people die. That seems scientific enough for most of us. That scientific prognosis puts the question to all of us whether a despairing defiance of death is the best we can do. If so, then a medicalized death is probably also the best we can do.

19. Peter De Vries, *The Blood of the Lamb* (New York: Little, Brown, Popular Library Edition, 1961). The citations in parentheses are from this edition. In the reprint by University of Chicago Press, 2005, the citations are from pp. 181, 182, and 183.

The last word, it seems, belongs to death, and the horror of it is not simply the termination of existence, but the unraveling of meaning, the destruction of relationships, the lordship of chaos. The light seems ephemeral; it is the darkness that seems to surround and to "overcome" the light and life. Then we are right to be fearful of death, to tremble in the face of darkness and chaos.[20]

The science that makes the prognosis, however, cannot answer the question that it puts. It can say death is real, but it cannot say death has the last word. It can say death is no illusion, but it cannot say death has the power ultimately to make good on its threats. Auden's advent petition had it right. "We who must die demand a miracle." And the Christian church has it right, I think. There has been a miracle.

That miracle does not deny the reality or the power of death in the world. Jesus, after all, the eternal Word made flesh, died a real death; he was buried. Death is real — and it is a real evil! But death did not have the last word. Jesus was, so the story of this miracle goes, "the firstborn from the dead" (Col. 1:18; Rev. 1:5). The resurrection does not require — and will not permit — a denial of the reality of death, but it does give us some confidence that death will not have the last word. It does give us some other (nonmedical) basis for hope. And it should form other (nonmedical) responses to the threats of death. It is the burden of this book to try to articulate something of that confidence and to suggest some of those responses, to imagine a better way of dying.

Medicalized death gained its powerful hold on us and on our culture in part because — in spite of our denials — we knew that death is real, because we knew that its threats are terrible, and because our expectations of medicine had grown Promethean. But we are not fated to a medicalized dying. There have been plenty of complaints about it and increasingly powerful challenges to it. Complaints about "medicalization" became commonplace in the last third of the twentieth century. People did not want to die in the hospital, although most did — and do. They did not want to die hooked up to machinery, surrounded by strangers, expert though they may be. Frankly, they did not want to die at all, but if they must, they wanted it to be their death, the end of their story, and not a footnote in some doctor's story.

Powerful challenges to "medicalization" were mounted within the literature on medical ethics, in the literature on death and dying, and in

---

20. Nicholas Lash, *Theology on the Way to Emmaus* (London: SCM, 1986), p. 174.

the literature of the hospice movement. The literature on medical ethics complained primarily about decisions being made about a patient's care without the "informed consent" of the patient. The literature on death and dying complained about the silence and denial of death in the culture. And the literature of the hospice movement complained about the lack of care for the whole person, the whole embodied and communal and spiritual person who was dying, when death was medicalized. Commonplace complaints became movements, the movement for patient rights, the death awareness movement, and the hospice movement. We will turn to those movements and to their challenges to "medicalization" soon enough, but before we do, we should pause to acknowledge and to admire both the achievements of medicine and the long tradition of medical ethics.

CHAPTER THREE

In Praise of Medicine — and What Went Wrong on the Way to "Medicalization"

Honor physicians for their services,
  for the Lord created them;
for their gift of healing comes from the Most High.

Sirach 38:1-2[1]

Aries had traced "the triumph of medicalization" to the advances of medical science in the mid–twentieth century. There is some truth in that claim, as we have seen, but it risks making science and medicine the scapegoats when we look for something to blame for the way we die. There is plenty of blame to go around, but against the temptation to make medicine the scapegoat, it is important to begin with a word of gratitude to medicine and with what is, I hope, a more nuanced account of what went wrong on the way to the medicalization of death.

In Praise of Medicine

The gratitude is personal. I would probably be dead today if I had not had the benefit of remarkable medical technology and remarkably skilled phy-

---

1. Quotations from the Bible and the Apocrypha in this book are taken from the New Revised Standard Version, unless otherwise indicated.

sicians. A little gratitude is only becoming. I am grateful to those doctors and nurses who cared for me, and grateful to God for their knowledge and skill. So, let me spend a moment in praise of medicine and its resistance to death.

The gratitude is personal, but my voice merely joins some ancient voices in praise of the physician. There is, for example, the sage and lovely voice of Jesus ben Sirach. "Honor physicians for their services," he said, "for the Lord created them; / for their gift of healing comes from the Most High" (Sirach 38:1-2).[2] This "gift of healing" was and is ordinary enough; it is the learned skills of making and applying medicines.

> The Lord created medicines out of the earth,
>   and the sensible will not despise them. . . .
> By them the physician heals and takes away pain;
>   the pharmacist makes a mixture from them.
> God's works will never be finished;
>   and from him health [*shalom*] spreads over all the earth.
>
> (38:4, 7-8)

It is not "faith healing," but it is nevertheless fair to call it "miracle," for it is finally the work of God and displays God's intention to bring *shalom*. God "gave skill to human beings / that he might be glorified in his marvelous works" (38:6). The sick, says Sirach, should pray to God, amend their lives, and offer sacrifice to God, but they should also "give the physician his place" (38:12). The physician prays for "success in diagnosis / and in healing, for the sake of preserving life" (38:14). This is wisdom: life is a great gift of God, and so are those with the skill to preserve it.

Jesus ben Sirach praised physicians for their skill in restoring

---

2. The book of wisdom attributed to Jesus ben Sira, called variously the Wisdom of Jesus Son of Sira, or simply Sirach, or Ecclesiasticus, was probably written in Jerusalem around 180 B.C.E. It was translated into Greek by his grandson in Egypt sometime after 132 B.C.E. The Hebrew text was not included in the canon established by Jewish rabbis around 100 C.E., and Hebrew manuscripts of the text were lost until the twentieth century. The grandson's translation, however, was included in the Septuagint and, therefore, in the Bible read by most of the early church. When the Protestant Reformation adopted the Jewish canon, Sirach was assigned to a secondary status as "apocryphal." On Sirach see further the commentary of P. A. Skehan and A. A. DiLella, *The Wisdom of Ben Sira,* Anchor Bible 39 (New York: Doubleday, 1987). And on this passage "in praise of the physician" (Sirach 38:1-15), see especially Daniel Sulmasy, *The Rebirth of the Clinic: An Introduction to Spirituality in Health Care* (Washington, D.C.: Georgetown University Press, 2006), pp. 44-59.

health and relieving pain but also notably for their skill in "preserving life." In all this they are the ministers of God. God remains the ultimate healer (cf. Exod. 15:26), but God gives and uses physicians and their medicines to bring healing and to preserve life. God intends life, not death. So we toast and celebrate life, and praise those with the knowledge and skill that can help to preserve it. God intends human flourishing, including the flourishing we call "health." So we give thanks for health and strength and for those who help to restore it. It is altogether appropriate, the way of wisdom, both to pray to God and to "honor physicians for their services."

To its great credit, medicine resists death. It is part of its service to God and to human beings. That resistance to death led finally to a "medicalized" dying, and it is the burden of this book to resist a "medicalized" dying, to look for an alternative way of dying, a way of faithful dying. Even so, any challenge to "medicalization" that celebrates death rather than life will not be trusted, and any alternative that commends death will be regarded with suspicion. I share the view of Jesus ben Sirach — and of most of the biblical tradition — that embodied life in this world is a great good gift of God. There are better and worse ways of dying, and there are some things worse than death, but I will hesitate to call any death "good." (I will accordingly talk of "dying well" rather than of a "good death.") Any challenge to "medicalization" should be joined to thanks to God for the gifts of God, including the gifts of life and strength — and the skill and knowledge of physicians who help us to preserve them.

Also, any challenge to "medicalization" that makes physicians into "scapegoats," laying all the blame on them, misses the mark. It is not that physicians have been altogether innocent in the "medicalization" of death, but rather that the rest of us are not free from blame. Because the rest of us are unprepared to die, because no one has taught us what dying well might mean, because we are unsure of ourselves in the face of death, we retreat and turn things over to the "experts," to the professionals, to doctors. When under the care of those professionals we do not die well, we can blame *them*. But whose responsibility is it to teach people to die?

There are various answers to that question, of course, and all of them run the risk of creating a new class of "experts." Perhaps the best answer — at least one obvious answer — is that the dying bear a responsibility to teach the rest of us how to die well. But in the context of "medicalization," who will have taught them? I think communities of faith bear a responsibility to teach their members how to die well. If that is so, and if communities of faith have neglected that responsibility, then they share the blame for the "medicalization" of death.

We will turn to the responsibility of the churches soon enough. Here we want to understand a little better what went wrong within the medicine we have praised, what went wrong in the culture that supported and sustained the project of medicine, what went wrong on the way to the "medicalization" of death. That will require that we attend briefly to the long history of medical ethics and especially to that early modern period when Aries said "tame death" began to be "savage" again.

From Hippocrates to Bacon to Medicalization

Medical ethics is hardly a new discipline. It is at least as old as Hippocrates. His oath was the first of a long succession of oaths and codes by which physicians have regulated the conduct and formed the character of other physicians. Medical ethics has a long tradition — and not a static one. It is no more plausible or prudent to attempt a "brief history" of medical ethics than to attempt a brief history of death. From the beginning, however, medical ethics has been concerned with the relationship of doctors to dying patients.

The Hippocratic Oath: Forswearing Poisons

The Hippocratic oath was already the expression of a reform movement within medicine. In ancient Greece physicians had defined their role in terms of restoring health and easing pain. They saw the good of health and their powerlessness against death. When patients were mortally ill, "overmastered by their diseases,"[3] these physicians would refrain from efforts to cure them, and sometimes in order to relieve the suffering of the dying they would kill them. They counted poisons and other techniques to produce a painless death among the tools of their trade. Against such a practice the Hippocratic oath famously swore, "I will neither give a deadly drug to anybody if asked for it, nor will I make a suggestion to this effect."[4]

---

3. As the Hippocratic treatise "The Art" would put it somewhat later; in Stanley Reiser, Arthur Dyck, and William Curran, eds., *Ethics and Medicine: Historical Perspectives and Contemporary Concerns* (Cambridge: MIT Press, 1977), p. 6.

4. Ludwig Edelstein's translation, in Ludwig Edelstein, "The Hippocratic Oath: Text,

The oath was originally a minority report, but this effort to reform the practice of medicine was remarkably successful and would shape the ethos of physicians for centuries. When the Christian church, another minority community originally, turned its attention to medicine, it supported and nurtured that ethos. The Christian physician would not, of course, take an oath "by Apollo Physician and Asclepius and Hygeia and Panacea and all the gods and goddesses." But there was an "Oath According to Hippocrates In So Far as a Christian May Swear It," and it contained the same forswearing of poison, set now in the context of faithfulness to God and to God's work in Christ.[5] The Hippocratic physicians refused to use the skills of medicine to serve ends alien to medicine, and they regarded the destruction of human life as an alien, indeed conflicting, end. But while the Hippocratic physicians would not kill, there was not yet any sense of an obligation to prolong the life of those "overmastered by their diseases."

Francis Bacon: Knowledge, Power, and the Search for a Cure

Medical ethics was to shift again, however, with the development of a new vision and new powers. In the seventeenth century, at the beginning of modernity, Francis Bacon suggested a "third end" for medicine, the preservation of life, which he regarded as the "most noble of all." That suggestion by itself was not all that novel. As we have seen, Jesus ben Sirach had praised both God and the physician for the skills exercised "for the sake of preserving life" (Sirach 38:14). What was novel, however, was Bacon's rejection of that traditional category of those "overmastered by their diseases" and the traditional resignation in the face of such a diagnosis. He complained that "the pronouncing of these diseases incurable gives a legal

---

Translation and Interpretation," in Oswei Temkin and C. Lillian Temkin, *Ancient Medicine* (Baltimore: Johns Hopkins University Press, 1967), pp. 3-63.

5. It began with a *berakoth*, "Blessed be God the Father of our Lord Jesus Christ, Who is blessed for ever and ever; I lie not." Some copies of the Christian oath were written in the shape of a cross. (See facsimiles in W. H. S. Jones, *The Doctor's Oath: An Essay in the History of Medicine* [New York: Cambridge University Press, 1924], frontispiece and p. 26.) On the Hippocratic oath and its Christian version, see further Allen Verhey, "The Doctor's Oath and a Christian's Swearing It," in *On Moral Medicine: Theological Perspectives in Medical Ethics,* ed. Stephen Lammers and Allen Verhey, 2nd ed. (Grand Rapids: Eerdmans, 1998), pp. 108-19.

sanction, as it were, to neglect and inattention and exempts ignorance from discredit."[6] That was innovative! And it set medicine on the course of seeking a cure for all manner of human diseases.

Joined to that complaint concerning the medicine of his time was his call for the reform of learning, his advocacy of inductive learning and "practical knowledge." He derided the speculative learning of Aristotle as "the boyhood of science" and as "barren in works,"[7] and he proposed the scientific method for "the advancement of learning." Bacon, no less than the Hippocratic oath, called for the reform of medicine. And Bacon, no less than the "Oath Insofar as a Christian May Swear It," set this reform in the context of the Christian story. He was, after all, a Puritan (however impatient he may have been with theological quarrels).

A number of historians of science have noted that the scientific revolution of the seventeenth century followed in the wake of the Protestant Reformation of the sixteenth century.[8] The "new learning" flourished especially in countries influenced by Calvinism. The causes for the advances of science and medicine during this time are complicated, of course, and the new research was hardly the monopoly of Protestantism. Nevertheless, Bacon's Puritanism did provide a context for his call to reform and contributed to it. There was the affirmation of God's sovereignty, the celebration of a worldly "vocation," and the Protestant readiness to question authority.[9]

6. Francis Bacon, *De Augmentis Scientiarum: The Philosophical Works of Francis Bacon*, ed. J. M. Robertson (New York: Books for Libraries Press, 1970), pp. 487-89. *De Augmentis Scientiarum* will be included in volume 9 of the Oxford Francis Bacon series (forthcoming).

7. Francis Bacon, *The Great Instauration*, in *The Instauratio magna Part II: Novum Organum and Associated Texts*, ed. Graham Rees and Maria Wakely, Oxford Francis Bacon, vol. 11 (Oxford: Clarendon, 2004), p. 11.

8. A connection, or at least a congruity, of Calvinism and the rise of science has been observed by a number of historians of science. Thomas Sprat's 1667 *History of the Royal Society* would be the first of them. Robert Merton, *Science, Technology, and Society in Seventeenth Century England* (New York: Harper and Row, 1970 [a reprint of Merton's 1938 edition]) would be the classic statement. See also I. Bernard Cohen, ed., *Puritanism and the Rise of Modern Science: The Merton Thesis* (New Brunswick, N.J.: Rutgers University Press, 1990); Reijer Hooykaas, *Religion and the Rise of Modern Science* (Grand Rapids: Eerdmans, 1972); Charles Webster, *The Great Instauration: Science, Medicine, and Reform, 1626-1660* (New York: Holmes and Meier, 1976); and recently and perceptively, Peter Harrison, *The Bible, Protestantism, and the Rise of Natural Science* (Cambridge: Cambridge University Press, 1998).

9. That the affirmation of God's sovereignty played a role is widely recognized. Some have suggested that the Calvinist doctrines of predestination and providence were the theo-

For Bacon science and medicine were Christian vocations; they were ways to serve God's cause in the world and the neighbor's good. Bacon wanted this "advancement of learning" to bring about "the great instauration," the restoration of humanity to the "dominion" over nature that it had before the Fall, the renewal of "that pure and unstained knowledge of nature . . . by which Adam gave names to things according to their kind."[10]

His sense of Christian vocation was on display when he set this prayer at the beginning of *The Great Instauration*:

> I pour forth most humble and hearty prayers to God the Father, God the Word, and God the Holy Ghost, that having in mind the afflictions of the human race and the pilgrimage of this our life wherein we wear out days short and evil, they will think fit through my hands to endow the human family with new mercies. I also humbly pray that things human stand not in the way of things divine; and that with the pathways of the sense made accessible, and the natural light burning brighter, nothing of the night or of unbelief arises in our souls respecting the divine mysteries, but rather that, from a clear intellect, stripped of fantasies and vanity but still subject and wholly dedicated to divine oracles, we give to faith that which is faith's. Lastly I pray that, with the sciences discharged of the serpent's poison which swells and puffs up the human soul, we do not aspire to know what is too exalted or beyond the bounds of discretion, but cultivate the truth in charity.[11]

---

logical precursors for the mechanistic determinism of the scientists (e.g., Stephen F. Mason, *A History of the Sciences,* new rev. ed. [New York: Collier, 1962]). Abraham Kuyper, too, in his Stone Lectures in 1898 had called attention to "the Calvinist dogma of predestination as the strongest motive in those days for the cultivation of science" (Kuyper, *Lectures in Calvinism* [Grand Rapids: Eerdmans, 1931], p. 112), but for Kuyper the emphasis fell on the order and stability of God's rule. Order comes from the gracious hand of God no less than extraordinary events; "nature," no less than "miracle." The order of the universe and of the body is simply the way God ordinarily works, and the study of God's work — as by medicine — simply provides evidence of the "wonderful wisdom" of God (John Calvin, *Institutes of the Christian Religion,* ed. John T. McNeill [Philadelphia: Westminster, 1960], 1.5.2).

The other side of the Reformers' appreciation for God's work in the order of things was their suspicion of extravagant claims made for the miraculous effects of relics and shrines. It was not science but Protestantism that first challenged the magical account of diseases and cures prevalent in the late medieval fascination with relics. Protestants repudiated the popular and magical understanding of the use of relics, the invocation of saints, the pilgrimages to shrines, and the use of holy water (see Thomas).

10. Bacon, *The Great Instauration,* p. 23.

11. Bacon, *The Great Instauration,* pp. 21-23.

Moreover, he admonished his readers quite explicitly to set the knowledge and power of science in the context of human responsibility to God. He warned them that "the sense (like the Sun) illuminates the face of the terrestrial globe but blots out and closes up the face of celestial." He told them not to think that "any aspect of the inquiry into nature" is forbidden, but he admonished them to remember "the true ends of knowledge." It was not contemplation that was that true end of knowledge, but neither surely was it contention or pride or profit or power; the true end of knowledge, he said, is "for the benefit and use of life." Then it may be "perfected and regulated in charity."[12]

Bacon's call for the scientific advancement of learning, his advocacy for the preservation of life, and his suspicion of the category of those "overmastered by their disease" were no less innovative for his time than the oath had been for its. And Bacon's project would shape the ethos of medicine no less powerfully than the once innovative oath had. Physicians were enlisted on the side of life, fighting a messy but heroic battle against death. Their courage was their refusal to call any disease incurable. Their weapons were forged in scientific study and research. Their allies were the university and its laboratories. This Baconian shift would lead to great advancements in science and in medicine, and finally, three centuries later, to the ability, indeed, to cure a number of diseases that had once "overmastered" the sick. It was a great accomplishment, and I am — as we all are — surely in Bacon's debt.

The Baconian Project and the "Medicalization" of Death

But this Baconian shift also led to what has been called "the Baconian project"[13] and to the "medicalization" of death. "The Baconian project" names the Promethean modern effort to eliminate human mortality and vulnerability to suffering by means of technology. It is aptly named, for its advocacy of science and technology, its celebration of human mastery over nature, and its confidence that technology could finally deliver human beings from the death and misery to which nature seems to condemn them, all find a seed in Bacon.

12. Bacon, *The Great Instauration*, p. 23.
13. See Gerald McKenny, *To Relieve the Human Condition: Bioethics, Technology, and the Body* (Albany: State University of New York Press, 1997).

Still, the hubris of the "Baconian project" should not simply be identified with Francis Bacon even if it can be traced to him. His attention to God provided a context for his advocacy of "the new learning," and a limit as well as a motive for its ambitions. But it is as if Bacon's heirs forgot his prayer — or forgot to pray it.

In Bacon, or at least in Bacon's time, the Christian tradition could still simply be assumed — and it was assumed. Indeed, the Christian tradition provided the warrants for the celebration of embodied life — and for much else in Bacon.[14] But whatever resources there may have been in Bacon himself to resist the presumption of the Baconian project, they were largely neglected in the "enlightenment" of the eighteenth century that followed hard on the heels of the scientific revolution that Bacon had helped to inaugurate.

In that "enlightenment," Bacon's conviction of the harmony of science and religion remained, but the control shifted to science. Attention to God as the one to whom we are finally and ultimately responsible was neglected. Bacon himself, as we noted, had admonished his readers to set the advancement of scientific learning in the context of an understanding of the human responsibility to God. He had regarded his "great instauration" as a form of obedience to God and as a way to honor God's intentions of life and flourishing. He had hoped for the restoration of the creation, and he thought humanity could in a measure respond to that hope and participate in it. His Puritan friends had heard his call for knowledge to be practical, tested by experience and experiment, and apt for the restoration of "dominion" over nature to human hands, as a religious vocation that God would bless by progress toward human well-being. Bacon and the Puritans of the Royal Society may be faulted for their eschatological — indeed millennial — hope that "the great instauration" would be finally the work of human hands and minds,[15] but they never quite forgot that they worked in response to God and in loyalty to the cause of God. Such hope — with the

14. See, for example, the work of Peter Harrison, *The Bible, Protestantism, and the Rise of Natural Science.* It is not unusual to trace modernity (and medicalization) to Bacon and Descartes, but it is often overlooked that they were attempting to give words to Christian convictions and flesh to Christian hopes. Their accounts of anthropology and "dominion" and eschatology were deeply flawed — and those flaws nurtured medicalization — but the resistance to death was theologically grounded.

15. The Social Gospel would make the similar mistake when it construed "the kingdom of heaven" as an ideal social order that human beings could initiate as if it were a simple historical possibility.

help of a little success in science and technology — turned Promethean in the imagination of a mundane "heavenly city" by the eighteenth-century philosophers.[16]

Bacon had warned, moreover, that as the sun that lights the world makes it hard to see the stars, so the new light of science might make it hard to see God. And indeed, the scientific gaze upon the world led histori-cally to a different conception of God, to the conception of God as a de-signer God who, having fashioned a world, politely withdrew, leaving the world to the masterful hands of human freedom and reason. If the Puritan had concluded that nature must have an order because God's rule is or-derly rather than capricious, the Deist concluded that God must be a de-signer because the universe is a machine. That different conception of God led inevitably to a certain indifference to the God so conceived.[17] Only a few were prepared to dispense with God altogether, but the god of the De-ists was hardly personal and never inconvenient. When science assumed hegemony over all knowledge, "God" became an object of "scientific" in-quiry, no longer the subject who addresses us.[18] Worse than that, "God" was reduced to a hypothesis that may or may not be useful to human proj-ects, including the project of understanding the world scientifically.[19] And when "God" became an unnecessary hypothesis for understanding the world scientifically, "God" — or at least human talk of God — could not even find a home in the gaps of human knowledge. Then "God" — or hu-man talk of God — was reduced to "an instrumentalized deity," possessing still, perhaps, some therapeutic utility.[20] But that, too, would have to be

16. See Carl L. Becker, *The Heavenly City of the Eighteenth Century Philosophers* (New Haven: Yale University Press, 1959; original 1932).

17. See Becker, *The Heavenly City*, p. 49; also Webster, *The Great Instauration*, pp. 246-92.

18. See Nicholas Lash, *The Beginning and the End of "Religion"* (New York: Cambridge University Press, 1996). Lash tells the story of the invention of "religion" in the seventeenth century as an alternative to faith in a particular God made known in a particular revelation.

19. See Michael Buckley, *At the Origins of Modern Atheism* (New Haven: Yale Univer-sity Press, 1987). Buckley tells the story of theology's abandonment of its traditional position that God is known in God's revelation, of the effort to find reasons for believing in God in nature, and of how that effort failed. Describing the position of Diderot in the eighteenth century, Buckley says, "The great argument, the only evidence for theism, is design, and ex-perimental physics reveals that design" (p. 217). But the notion of design in the Newtonian physics on which Diderot relied turned out to be unnecessary. Mathematical probability and "chance" would replace it, and God became an unnecessary hypothesis.

20. See Joel James Shuman and Keith Meador, *Heal Thyself: Spirituality, Medicine,*

tested like any hypothesis. God became "it." God as "thou" was eclipsed. Bacon's hope turned to the fatuous optimism of the Baconian project and to a faith and confidence not so much in God as in scientific and technological progress. Pride, "that serpent's poison that swells and puffs up the human soul," was not so easily cured; to cure pride evidently requires a mastery of human nature that technology does not provide.

Bacon might have also warned that science and its tools could hide not just God but humanity; at least he should have. In subsequent centuries, when in scientific diagnosis medicine fixed its objective gaze on the body, it saw the body as an object, as an "it." And when in therapy scientific medicine treated the body, it treated the body as manipulable nature, as "it." The "person" got lost. Indeed, ironically, so did the body. At least, the physician's diagnostic and therapeutic relationship to the body as "it" displaced the patient's relationship to her body as "me." The irony is captured nicely in the story of the physician carefully listening to a patient's chest with his stethoscope. The patient tried to ask the physician a question, but the physician said, "Quiet. I can't hear you while I'm listening."[21] Similarly, when physicians turned their clinical gaze upon the body as object, they lost sight of the person and of the body as "me." The "clinical gaze" gave birth to a "biomedical view" of the body as object to be measured and calculated, managed and controlled, manipulated and corrected.[22] According to Peter Freund and Meredith McGuire, the "biomedical view" makes five assumptions for knowing the human body scientifically: a dualism of

and the Distortion of Christianity (New York: Oxford University Press, 2003), pp. 44-70. Making good use of Lash and Buckley, they tell the story that ended with an "instrumentalized deity."

21. Richard Baron, "An Introduction to Medical Phenomenology: I Can't Hear You While I'm Listening," Annals of Internal Medicine 103 (1985): 606-11, p. 606, cited by Warren Thomas Reich, "A New Era for Bioethics: The Search for Meaning in Moral Experience," in Religion and Medical Ethics: Looking Back, Looking Forward, ed. Allen Verhey (Grand Rapids: Eerdmans, 1996), pp. 96-119, p. 97.

22. See Michel Foucault, The Birth of the Clinic: An Archaeology of Medical Perception, trans. A. M. Sheridan Smith (New York: Vintage, 1994). Foucault traced the beginnings of this "medical perception," this "gaze" (or in Foucault's language, this "regard"), to the development of a "scientific" medicine in the eighteenth and nineteenth centuries — and especially to the significance that the corpse assumed in such medicine. Science made an object of the body, and when physicians turned their clinical gaze upon the body, they lost sight of the person and of the body as "me" (very much like a corpse). The French original was first published in 1963, and although Foucault denied writing the book "against medicine" (p. xix), it provided a historical explanation of the "depersonalization" that was the refrain of many complaints concerning "medicalization" in the sixties.

mind and body, the reduction of the body to the material, the doctrine of specific etiology (i.e., that each disease is caused by a specific and identifiable agent), the metaphor of the machine, and the assumption that the body is an object subject to rational regimen and control. In the "biomedical view" the body becomes an object to be measured, managed, and corrected.[23] With this model for "knowing" the patient, however, one can fail to see the patient as a person.

If the "clinical gaze" gave birth to a "biomedical view" of the body as object to be measured and manipulated, one might regard René Descartes as the philosophical midwife at its birth. Indeed, often called "the father of modern philosophy," he might also be regarded as the father of this view of the body. Everything can be doubted, he famously insisted, but this is certain: *cogito, ergo sum.* I think; therefore I am. Because I think, I cannot doubt my existence as a thinking thing. This thinking thing, this *res cogitans,* this mind, was the essential self, the soul, in Descartes's view, and it was immortal, rational, and free, quite independent of the body and its mortality, transcending any particular social location and its limits. Descartes assigned the body to the realm of matter, to *res extensa,* to be measured and mastered. The body was a fragile machine, an animated corpse, which the soul mysteriously inhabits for a time. As if to stake a claim to his paternity of the biomedical view of the body, Descartes concluded his *Discourse on Method* by calling for the development of a knowledge of nature, or the body, that would master nature and free human beings from disease and from the withering of old age. Cartesian dualism gave medicine permission to see and to treat the body as manipulable matter, as *res extensa,* and it would permit nothing else![24]

23. Peter E. S. Freund and Meredith B. McGuire, *Health, Illness, and the Social Body: A Critical Sociology* (Englewood Cliffs, N.J.: Prentice-Hall, 1991).

24. More than one account of medicine has traced its problematic way of regarding the body to Cartesian dualism. See especially Drew Leder, *The Absent Body* (Chicago: University of Chicago Press, 1960). Richard Zaner, *Ethics and the Clinical Encounter* (Englewood Cliffs, N.J.: Prentice-Hall, 1988), also traces the biomedical view of the body to Descartes, but he focuses on Descartes's medical writings. He finds there not the famous dualism of the *Discourse on Method* but a dualism between nature, or body, as understood in ordinary experience and nature, or body, as an object understood in science. Moreover, Descartes's medical advice would seem to suggest that proper treatment of patients may not be reduced to the treatment of objects. See further the thoughtful account of Leder, Zaner, and Foucault in McKenny, *To Relieve,* pp. 184-210. Descartes was hardly the first to advocate an anthropological dualism. Plato was, of course, the most famous of ancient advocates of an anthropological dualism, and the notion that we are immortal souls inhabiting for a time these mor-

Bacon had also admonished his readers to remember "the true ends of knowledge": that it might be "perfected and regulated in charity."[25] Bacon advocated the advancement of all learning, divine and human,[26] but his suspicion of "speculative" knowledge prepared the way for the hegemony of the empirical sciences among human ways of knowing. The empirical sciences, however, can give no knowledge of ends, not even the ends of knowledge, only of means. The empirical sciences cannot tell people what to do with the great powers they provide. They cannot tell them how to use those great powers without violating the human material upon which they work. They cannot tell people what ends to seek or what limits to observe in seeking them. As Bacon saw, something like charity is required to perfect and govern knowledge, but science is not "self-sufficiently the source of that human quality that makes it beneficial."[27] There remained charity, of course, or something like it. There remained that human and visceral response to the suffering of another that we call compassion. But that visceral response only demands *that* something be done; it does not tell people *what* thing to do. It is always formed by the assumptions we make, by the stories we tell about our world. The Baconian project's confidence in technology as the source of human well-being formed a modern compassion; it told people what thing to do, namely, to pick up the latest tools and to use them. An ancient compassion had included the readiness simply to be present to the sufferer, the readiness to "suffer with" another. The modern compassion, in contrast, is formed not to share suffering but to put a stop to it by means of technology. The confident enthusiasm for technology suggests that we need not either endure it or be present to it. Thus, the one who would care for another who suffers learned to send him or her to the technical expert, to the person who knows the tools and how to use them, to the doctor if the person is sick or dying. And the compassionate doctor would simply pick and use the best instruments. If and when the technology failed, then there was nothing more the doctor — or anyone — could do. So, people would die in the hospital, surrounded by technology rather than accompanied by friends. Science would arm compassion with artifice but not with wisdom.

tal bodies marked (and marred) a good deal of late medieval theology, including, as we shall see, the *Ars Moriendi*.

25. Bacon, *The Great Instauration*, p. 23.

26. The full title of *The Advancement of Learning* (1605) was *The Proficience and Advancement of Learning, Divine and Human*.

27. Hans Jonas, *Phenomenon of Life* (New York: Harper and Row, 1966), p. 195.

Another feature of the Baconian project is its distrust of nature. It can surely be traced to Bacon's account of knowledge as power over nature and to his confidence that such knowledge, or technology, will bring human well-being in its train. In the view of Bacon and his heirs, nature and natural processes do not serve humanity "naturally." Nature threatens to rule and to ruin humanity. It threatens death and misery. It must be mastered — and for that our best hope is technology, the power knowledge gives. Thus would nature with its mortality come to be regarded as the enemy and technology as the faithful savior.

Bacon had envisioned a "great instauration" in which human life would be healthier, longer, and happier, and he had insisted that science and technology could help set things right. Scientific discoveries and medical advances nurtured that hope[28] while the Enlightenment dimmed the significance of its Christian context and assumptions. To use the metaphor of Martin Buber, God was "eclipsed" in the Baconian project. And it was not just the progress of medicine, not just Bacon's effort to reform learning, in which the project went wrong, but rather by eclipsing God. Buber put it quite eloquently in the middle of the twentieth century:

> In our age the I-It relation, gigantically swollen, has usurped practically uncontested, the mastery and the rule. The I of this relation, an I that possesses all, makes all, succeeds with all, this I that is unable to say Thou, unable to meet a being essentially, is the lord of the hour. This selfhood that has become omnipotent, with all the It around it, can naturally acknowledge neither God nor any genuine absolute which manifests itself to men as of non-human origin. It steps in between and shuts off from us the light of heaven.
>
> Such is the nature of this hour. But what of the next? It is a modern superstition that the character of an age acts as fate for the next. One lets it prescribe what is possible to do and hence what is permitted. One surely cannot swim against the stream, one says. But perhaps one can swim with a new stream whose source is still hidden? In another image the I-Thou relation has gone into the catacombs — who can say with how much greater power it will step forth! Who

---

28. Harvey's discovery of the circulation of blood, for example, prompted great hope. It led to experiments concerning rejuvenation by transfusion. Experiments transfusing the blood of young dogs to old suggested rejuvenating results. When it was then tried in human beings (without knowledge of blood types), soon enough, of course, someone died, which led to a moratorium on such experimentation until the early nineteenth century.

> can say when the I-It relation will be directed anew to its assisting place and activity! . . .
>
> Something is taking place in the depths that as yet needs no name. To-morrow even it may happen that it will be beckoned to from the heights, across the heads of the earthly archons. The eclipse of the light of God is no extinction; even to-morrow that which has stepped in between may give way.[29]

The mental landscape changed dramatically after Bacon. Medical realities changed more slowly; medicine in the nineteenth century still probably killed more people than it cured. But by the mid–twentieth century the powers of secularism and the powers of medicine had conspired to medicalize death.

I do not claim that all physicians in the middle of the twentieth century shared this vision or this project. Many celebrated the scientific and medical advances while remaining ready to acknowledge what experience taught, that some are indeed "overmastered by their diseases." And many shared Bacon's vision but also shared his prayer and remained humble enough to recognize that the final victory over death would be a divine triumph, not a technological one. Nevertheless, I do claim that, with the eclipse of Bacon's God, the Baconian project shaped the practice of medicine in the twentieth century and into the twenty-first. The "most noble" end of medicine was regarded as the preservation of life. In pursuit of that end, no patient would be regarded as "overmastered" by disease. The limits of medicine, if acknowledged at all, were relegated to the shadowy background of the physician's vision. Death was the great enemy to be defeated by the greater powers of medicine. The best hope against suffering, disease, and death was thought to be scientific knowledge and technology. To know the patient was to know the patient's body as "it," to know the pathology. It was to know the sum total of the physical and chemical mechanisms that operated on the patient (and in him or her) according to scientific laws. I do not claim that every hospital adopted the policy described by a resident: "As a university teaching service, we tend to attempt resuscitation of all patients, particularly at the beginning of the semester."[30] But I do claim that

29. Martin Buber, *Eclipse of God: Studies in the Relation between Religion and Philosophy*, Harper Torchbook (New York: Harper and Row, 1957), p. 129.

30. Diana Crane, *The Sanctity of Social Life: Physicians' Treatment of Critically Ill Patients* (New York: Russell Sage Foundation, 1975), cited in William F. May, "The Right to Die and the Obligation to Care: Allowing to Die, Killing for Mercy, and Suicide," in *No Rush to*

such a statement and such a policy only made sense where the Baconian project had shaped medicine. I do not claim that every doctor would repeatedly resuscitate a patient with an advanced stage of cancer who had insisted that nothing more be done to preserve his life since the pain of his cancer was more than he would needlessly endure.[31] But I do claim that such behavior is quite unintelligible apart from the formation of medicine by the Baconian project. I do claim that the Baconian project set the stage for the medicalization of death in the mid–twentieth century.

The Baconian project for science and medicine had great success, but the limits of that success were finally told in sad stories of a lingering dying, tragic stories of physicians who saw only diseases and lost sight of the human realities of their patients, sad stories of patients suffering not only from certain pathologies but also from the treatments for them, stories of "medicalized" death.

Ironically, Bacon's complaints about the "neglect" and "inattention" and "ignorance" that were sanctioned by an earlier medicine were widely echoed in the complaints of many patients against the medicine Bacon inspired. Bacon had identified "neglect" with a decision no longer to attempt to cure, but in the face of medicalized dying some patients complained that medical care had been reduced to the effort to cure and that medicine neglected patients and their suffering. Where "attention" to patients was reduced to attentiveness to their pathologies, patients complained about medicine's "inattention" to their particular stories and desires. Where the "clinical gaze" monopolized efforts to know the patient, another kind of "ignorance" was sanctioned, ignorance of the identities of patients, of their stories, of the aims they cherished, and of their communities. And when such ignorance was sanctioned, then physicians would be ill prepared to recognize or to respond to the particular ways in which patients suffered, the particular ways in which they experienced their condition as a threat to their embodied integrity.[32]

It was care that motivated the search for a cure, of course, but the search for a cure pushed care to the margins in the "medicalization" of

---

Judgment: Essays on Medical Ethics, ed. David H. Smith and Linda Bernstein (Bloomington, Ind.: Poynter Center, 1978), p. 154.

31. W. St. C. Symmers Sr., "Not Allowed to Die," *British Medical Journal* 1 (1968): 422; Tom Beauchamp and James F. Childress, *Principles of Biomedical Ethics* (New York: Oxford University Press, 1979), case 14, pp. 263-64.

32. See Eric Cassell's lament about the inattentiveness of medicine to suffering; Eric J. Cassell, "Recognizing Suffering," *Hastings Center Report* 21 (May-June 1991): 24-31.

39

death. Where knowledge was reduced to power over nature and celebrated as the key to human well-being, there the medical imperative became "Cure!," the means became the latest technology, and patients were reduced to manipulable nature in the effort to cure them.

CHAPTER FOUR

Challenging "Medicalization": Patient Rights, "Natural Death," and Hospice

Despite 30 years of litigation, laws and efforts by a range of groups to improve treatment for those near death, too many Americans still receive poor care at life's end and are dying "bad" deaths without adequate palliative care or dignity.[1]

That is from the summary of a special report by the Hastings Center in 2005 entitled "Improving End of Life Care: Why Has It Been So Difficult?" The "30 years" was counted from the case of Karen Ann Quinlan in 1975, when her parents won the court battle that allowed them to remove Karen from a respirator. The Quinlan case was hardly the beginning of complaints about the "medicalization" of death, but it was the first of many court cases that attempted to take death back from the control of medicine. Nevertheless, as the report makes clear, neither the legal victory of the Quinlans nor the "30 years of litigation, laws and efforts by a range of groups to improve treatment for those near death" that followed it have put an end to the complaints.

Complaints about "medicalization" became commonplace in the last

1. "Improving End of Life Care: Why Has It Been So Difficult? — a Summary of a Special Report Produced for the *Hastings Center Report*," available at http://www.deathwithdignity .org/resources/articles.asp. The report itself, *Improving End of Life Care: Why Has It Been So Difficult?* is found in *Hastings Center Report Special Report* 35, no. 6 (2005).

third of the twentieth century. As we have observed, people began to report that they did not want to die in the hospital, although most did (and do); that they did not want to die hooked up to machinery, surrounded by strangers, expert though they may be; that they did not want their death, the end of their story, to be a mere footnote in some doctor's story. The commonplace complaints grew into increasingly powerful challenges to "medicalization." The challenges were mounted not only in court cases like the Quinlans' but also within the literature of the time. The challenges grew into movements, the movement for patient rights, the death awareness movement, and the hospice movement. The literature on medical ethics complained primarily about decisions being made about a patient's care without the "informed consent" of the patient and nurtured the movement for patient rights. The literature on death and dying complained about the silence about and denial of death in the culture, called for the recognition of death as "natural," and nurtured the death awareness movement. And the literature that nurtured the hospice movement complained about the lack of care for the whole person, the whole embodied and communal and spiritual person who was dying, when death was medicalized.

We may applaud these movements for their opposition to a "medicalized" dying, and each of them has had some significant success. But they have also failed in some significant ways. As the Hastings Center special report made clear, medicalization still has a firm grip on our dying: "too many Americans still receive poor care at life's end and are dying 'bad' deaths." Sometimes, as with medicalization itself, the failures are ironically the failures of their successes. So, while we commend and applaud certain features of these movements, we should also temper our enthusiasm with attention to their weaknesses. The movement for patient rights has successfully insisted that any medical treatment — especially at the end of life — should be the choice of the patient, but it has failed to help the patients making decisions to envision a better way of dying. The death awareness movement has helped our culture to move beyond its silence concerning death and its denial, but its mantra that death is "natural" is not, in the end, particularly helpful. The third movement, the hospice movement, has had, I think, the greatest success, and it holds the greatest promise of providing an alternative to a medicalized dying. This movement had its beginnings within medicine and within the Christian tradition with Cicely Saunders, a Christian physician in England. She complained that in the medicalization of death the therapeutic imperative, the commitment to cure, had undercut the duty to care for the dying, and she began the hospice movement as a way to fulfill again that duty to care for dying patients. The hospice movement has been quite successful, even if it has not had quite the success one might have hoped for it. My worries concerning it focus on the possible failures of its success. Nevertheless, it serves as a reminder that there are resources in the Christian tradition that may help us both to resist the "medicalization" of death and to fashion a more faithful dying. My hope in this book is to nurture and sustain the Christian imagination that originally inspired Dame Saunders and the hospice movement. Each of these three movements deserves some brief attention.

Bioethics and the Movement for Patient Rights

Medical ethics is hardly a new discipline. It may be traced all the way back to Hippocrates and his famous oath, but in the mid–twentieth century it was reborn. The renaissance of medical ethics was prompted by developments in medical science and technology that gave physicians new powers to intervene in the processes of human procreation, sickness, and dying. These new powers seemed to raise some novel moral problems, problems not encountered previously, at least not in the same way or with the same frequency. There were questions at the beginning of life with the development of assisted reproductive technologies (like in vitro fertilization) and the power to make a genetic diagnosis of the fetus. There were questions about access to medical care, including access to scarce new lifesaving technologies (like kidney dialysis). There were questions about the use of human subjects in the medical research and experimentation that led to these new powers. And there were questions at the end of life, questions prompted by the new powers to intervene against death and to preserve life, questions prompted by the success of these powers and the medicalization of death. Among the questions that demanded an answer was this one: Now that we can keep a person alive with technologies that keep the blood flowing and the lungs pumping, must we?

The Hippocratic oath had called for the reform of a medicine that had counted poisons among the tools of the craft. Bacon had called for the reform of a medicine that had counted any as "overmastered" by disease. And now a new reform of medicine was called for. In this reform "medical ethics" would become "bioethics." The change in terminology seemed required by the broader set of questions addressed, but it also marked a different set of practitioners and different moral assumptions. It was no longer the special province of physicians, and it no longer assumed that medicine was a practice with its own standards of moral excellence. Early in the renaissance Robert Veatch wrote a classic essay against "the generalization of expertise."[2] The burden of that essay was to insist that physicians, while indeed experts about the workings of the body, should not be regarded as experts about everything. They should not be regarded as experts about ethics, and surely not as experts about what it might mean for a particular patient to live well or to die well. Another — and different — reform of medicine was called for. This reform of medicine would give power to the patients. It would wrestle back to patients the control physicians had conscientiously assumed. It would take back dying from medicine and from medicalization. Medical ethics, or bioethics, was born again as a discipline by which people and patients could restrain the powerful scientists and physicians with their experimental and therapeutic agendas.

The language of rights was the preferred language for much of the literature on bioethics. That was no accident. The language of rights had historically been the language of protest against the arbitrary power of absolute monarchs and holy priests. The liberal political theorists of the eighteenth century intended to limit the domineering power of king and nobility and clergy. All persons have dignity, they insisted, and must be respected. They asserted a social contract at the foundations of society, a contract that guaranteed certain rights to every member of society. And first among those rights was the right to liberty, or freedom, or autonomy. The freedom of any was to be limited by the equal freedom of all others, but the freedom of each was to be protected. The language of rights had been the most compelling language available to restrain the powerful for centuries,[3] and it was not surprising that it was adopted in the reform called for by bioethics. Advances in medicine had made the doctor a powerful figure, generally benevolent, to be sure, but still threatening the same arbitrary dominance as the benevolent despot of the eighteenth century. Bioethics noted and regretted the transfer of authority over one's life when one entered a hospital and the powerlessness of the patient that was gestured in countless rituals. Against the powerful the language of rights and the stress on autonomy looked like a promising way to restrain also the

2. Robert M. Veatch, "Generalization of Expertise," *Hastings Center Studies* 1, no. 2 (1973): 29-40.

3. In the previous decade, moreover, the language of rights had been used with considerable success by the civil rights movement to challenge the power and authority of those who would enforce segregation and disenfranchisement.

power of that new despot of dying, the physician. Against the powerful it waved its flag, "Don't tread on me!"

The language of rights was important already in 1954 with Joseph Fletcher's groundbreaking book *Morals and Medicine,* and in much of the literature that followed. Such language characteristically set aside the substantive moral question about what should be decided in favor of the procedural question about who should decide. And it answered that procedural question by rejecting the paternalism of the doctors and by insisting on the moral principle of respect for the patient as a person, that is to say, respect for a patient's autonomy. It is the patient's life, the patient's body, and decisions about treatment should be the patient's decisions. It is the patient's right to refuse medical treatment, even lifesaving medical treatment, if the patient judges the treatment too burdensome. It was not such an innovative point. Pope Pius XII, speaking quite self-consciously from within the Roman Catholic tradition, also defended the right of patients to refuse "extraordinary treatment."[4] But the emphasis on "patient rights" surely sounded innovative against the background of the assumptions about physician authority and control in a "medicalized" dying.

The language of rights was accompanied from the beginning by talk of "persons." Indeed, the complaint that medicine and medicalization had "depersonalized" the patient was something of a refrain.[5] The influential Belmont Report (1978) set "respect for persons" first in the list of principles to guide medical research.[6] From the beginnings, of course, there were

4. Pope Pius XII, "Address on the Question of Reanimation," November 24, 1957, in *The Pope Speaks,* vol. 4, 1958, pp. 393-98.

5. If one dates the "birth of bioethics" to this complaint, then bioethics is at least as old as 1936 and may have hospital chaplaincy as a sibling. In 1936 Richard Cabot, a physician at Massachusetts General Hospital, and Russell Dicks, a minister who served as chaplain there, published *The Art of Ministering to the Sick* (New York: Macmillan, 1936). In it they called attention to the "whole person" and insisted that healing is not simply a matter of curing the body by scientific medicine; they called for cooperation between the physician and the minister. By 1940 the American Protestant Hospital Association adopted a set of standards for hospital chaplaincy. One might also mention the extraordinary Swiss physician Paul Tournier, whose call for a medicine attentive to the "whole person" was quite self-consciously oriented by a reading of the Bible. See Paul Tournier, *A Doctor's Casebook in the Light of the Bible,* trans. Edwin Hudson (London: SCM, 1954).

6. The Belmont Report is the short name for the 1978 report of the U.S. Department of Health, Education, and Welfare, "Ethical Principles and Guidelines for the Protection of Human Subjects of Research" (Washington, D.C., 1978). It identified three principles: respect for persons, justice, and beneficence.

important disagreements about what it means to *be* a person — and about whether the fact that human persons have (or *are*) bodies is relevant to the meaning of their being "persons." Those disagreements were on display early in the debates between Joseph Fletcher and Paul Ramsey, who agreed that the patient was a person but differed as to what that meant. The disagreements remain — and they remain important, reflected in other disagreements about who counts as a person and about what it means to be counted as a person, about the meaning, that is, of the moral requirement of "respect for persons." We need not consider those differences here.[7] Here it is enough, first, to appreciate this challenge to medicalization and, then, to attend to its shortcomings.

It was indeed an important challenge to the medicalization of death. From the perspective of this reform, medicalization was a violation of the rights of patients, a violation of their dignity, a violation of their person. The principle of respect for autonomy demanded the "informed consent" of the patient (or the patient's agent). And there could be no genuinely *informed* consent, of course, unless the patient were told the truth about his or her condition. The truth was to be told. Respect for the patient's autonomy demanded it. That demand by itself was an important corrective to the denial and deception that surrounded medicalized dying. Armed with the truth about their condition and with the authority to make decisions about their own dying, patients could take back dying from medicine. That at least was the hope. Bioethics and its advocacy of autonomy would protect the right of patients to die their own deaths. And court case after court case following the final decision concerning Karen Ann Quinlan gave evidence of the persuasive power of appeals to autonomy — and of the success of the movement for patient rights.

It is a story frequently told in the literature on bioethics. That story goes something like this: Sometime around 1975 people became aware of two facts about dying: first, that dying was often a horrible experience for the dying individual, and for his or her family and caregivers, and second, that medical experts frequently made dying worse rather than better. But then Karen Quinlan's parents won their legal battle for the right to remove Karen from the respirator that was keeping her alive with no prospect of recovery. Subsequent court cases reiterated and reinforced this right to re-

7. See Allen Verhey, *Reading the Bible in the Strange World of Medicine* (Grand Rapids: Eerdmans, 2003), pp. 68-98, where those differences are reported and considered.

fuse treatment. Those victories prompted a reform of end-of-life care as patients wrestled control over their dying away from the doctors. Court decisions and then public policy authorized advance directives in order to give decisions back to the patients or their representatives. These refusals of treatment prompted medicine to improve care at the end of life. By the last decade of the twentieth century the needed reform was accomplished, signaled by the Supreme Court's decision concerning Nancy Cruzan, which reaffirmed the right to refuse life-sustaining treatment, including artificial nutrition and hydration, and by the national Patient Self-Determination Act. Now people were able to die well. It is, so the story goes, one of the great accomplishments of bioethics.

There is some truth in the story, of course, but not enough to allow us to be satisfied with it. It is true that the courts and public policy have underscored the rights of patients to refuse life-sustaining treatments and have allocated choice-making power decisively to patients and their delegated agents. But one may ask whether this emphasis on autonomy, on control, has really helped people to die well.

There are reasons to be a little suspicious of the familiar story. Stories of aunts and uncles and parents who did not die well, in spite of this acknowledgment of the rights of patients, may be enough to make one suspicious. But in addition to such anecdotal evidence, there was a careful study in the 1990s called "The Study to Understand Prognoses and Preferences for Outcomes and Risks of Treatments," or SUPPORT. It found that aggressive medical treatments to preserve life were still being used even when the treatments were futile and even when the patients or families did not want them. It showed, moreover, that many patients had suffered their way to their deaths with unrelieved pain.[8]

One response to the SUPPORT study, a response characteristic of standard bioethics, was simply to call ethicists to work harder to promote autonomous decisions, to get people to create advance directives, to assert their rights. But another — and, in my view, better — response would be to acknowledge that the emphasis on autonomous choice in standard bioethics is insufficient. One need not — and should not — assert that the rights of patients are insignificant. One should not — and cannot — deny that neglect of the rights of patients had sometimes been a regrettable (and unjustifiable) feature of medical research and treatment and surely a

8. See *Dying Well in the Hospital: The Lessons of SUPPORT, Hastings Center Report* 25, no. 6 (1995): S1-S36.

feature of medicalization. Still, it is time to acknowledge the weaknesses of this emphasis on rights and this stress on autonomy.

The fundamental weakness of this stress on autonomy is its minimalism. But its minimalism shows up in a variety of ways. First, by attending to the procedural question about who should decide, it allows us to ignore the substantive moral questions about what should be decided and about the virtues that should mark the one who decides. Indeed, it can deliberately adopt a kind of agnosticism about what should be decided, treating a decision as right simply because it is freely made. Second, its minimalism is displayed in its negativism. The most compelling rights, after all, are the so-called negative rights, the rights not to be interfered with. The emphasis falls, therefore, on not interfering with another's liberty rather than on meeting another's needs. The emphasis falls on what we should not do to people rather than on what we should do for them. Moreover, its minimalism is displayed in the reduction of relationships of covenant to contracts between independent and autonomous individuals.

It is little wonder, then, that this emphasis on rights and this stress on autonomy have not been altogether successful against the medicalization of death. To be sure, it has provided an effective constraint against the physician who would run roughshod over a patient's rights, but it has not provided — and cannot provide — any vision of an alternative to a medicalized dying.

While it celebrates freedom, it does not nurture the virtues of character necessary to face death honestly or to die well and faithfully. The stress on the freedom of independent individuals and the reduction of relationships of covenant to contractual arrangements cannot nurture community; indeed, it puts community at risk. Because "patient autonomy" allows the question of who should decide to monopolize our moral imagination, it has also failed to nurture a conversation about what should be decided. Indeed, it can put a stop to important conversations about death and dying well as decisively as "physician authority" once did. Moreover, this emphasis on freedom and independence and control of one's own life and body displays to all who face death just how much our society despises the weakness and withering, the dependence and lack of control, that frequently accompany death. It makes us loath to die — and loath to face our own dying. Death must be opposed by the great powers of medicine. And so patients fall back to the perspective of the Baconian project, now adopting as their own the very perspective that had led to the medicalization of death. In the Quinlan case and in most of the cases that followed it, it was the doctors who insisted on keeping the patient alive. But it is no longer always the doctors who insist on doing "everything possible" to resist death; it is now frequently the patients or their agents. Moreover, given the sad history of the lack of access to medical care in the United States, it is understandable that some patients are more interested in access to health care at the end of their lives than in limiting it. Finally, the ironic result of the procedural protections of patient autonomy in living will legislation and advance directives is that they can make it harder to die. Medicalized death remains the default position, and if someone has no advance directive, the assumption is too often that everything and anything medical is authorized.

This emphasis on patient rights is not so much wrong as minimal, and when its minimalism is not acknowledged, it subverts a moral life — and dying well, too. It was adopted by standard bioethics in no small measure because of distrust of physicians. Physicians were regarded as hopelessly captive to the Baconian project, treating their patients as manipulable nature and ignoring their wishes, refusing to acknowledge that one might be "overmastered" by disease and using painful and aggressive treatments with no realistic hope for their success, and finally neglecting and abandoning the patient who could not be cured. The emphasis on the autonomy of patients was successful in limiting the power of the crusading physicians, but it could not nurture trust in the physician who had learned by experience some wisdom about life and death in a mortal body. Instead, it left patients to their own resources, and it has put on display too frequently the poverty of those resources and the reluctance of many to consider their condition honestly or to have the conversation about their own dying.

But perhaps that reluctance is simply part of our culture's "denial of death." Perhaps we simply need to work harder not only to get people to create advance directives but also to end the silence that surrounds death. Perhaps we need to see death as "natural." Perhaps then we could make progress against medicalization. Such was the hope of the death awareness literature.

The Death Awareness Movement and "Natural" Death

The work of Elisabeth Kübler-Ross was another powerful challenge to the medicalization of death. Her book *On Death and Dying*[9] was published in

9. Elisabeth Kübler-Ross, *On Death and Dying* (New York: Macmillan, 1969).

1969 and was widely read. It was not the first book to be published in the middle of the twentieth century with the aim of increasing public awareness and acceptance of death. That distinction may belong to Herman Feifel, who a decade earlier had edited an anthology, *The Meaning of Death*.[10] Indeed, by the time Elisabeth Kübler-Ross's work was published there was already a considerable literature on death and dying.[11] Nevertheless, because the work of Kübler-Ross was so remarkably successful in reaching a broad audience, she may be said to have started the death awareness movement.[12] Following the publication of *On Death and Dying*, workshops for both the interested public and professional caregivers were given "on death and dying." It was a staple of these workshops to lament the conspiracies of silence and deception that surrounded death in the middle of the twentieth century and to insist that death was "natural."

The popularity of the movement may be related to what Gorer called "the pornography of death." There was something slightly exciting about talking about a forbidden subject, something mildly countercultural about defying a cultural taboo. But there can be no question that Kübler-Ross and the movement she helped to start rejected the reduction of dying to a medical event and initiated nonmedical conversations about death. The very fact that her list of the five "stages" of dying (denial, anger, bargaining, depression, and acceptance) became part of popular culture is evidence of the impact she and the movement had.

The death awareness movement has no particular orthodoxy. There is no central organization, surely no magisterium. There is not even any particular disciplinary commitment (although sociologists, psychologists, and psychiatrists probably outnumber the rest). It is, therefore, dangerous to generalize about the movement. Still, from the beginning, it has challenged the medicalization of death. It has insisted that death cannot be avoided. It has demanded that death not be denied. The mantra has been that death is "natural."

Philippe Aries mentioned Feifel and Kübler-Ross at the end of his book as "pioneers" in a movement to resist the medicalization of death.

10. Herman Feifel, ed., *The Meaning of Death* (New York: McGraw-Hill, 1959).

11. See Orville G. Brim Jr. et al., eds., *The Dying Patient* (New York: Russell Sage Foundation, 1970), with its bibliography of over 300 works on the subject of dying published between 1955 and 1970.

12. I have found Lucy Bregman, *Beyond Silence and Denial: Death and Dying Reconsidered* (Louisville: Westminster John Knox, 1994), a helpful account of the death awareness movement.

And he reports that each had encountered initial resistance from doctors and hospital authorities. When Feifel wanted to interview dying patients about their dying, hospital authorities were incensed. They regarded the proposal as "cruel," "sadistic," and "traumatic." And when Kübler-Ross asked permission to interview dying patients, the response of the hospital authorities was, "Dying? But there are no dying here!"[13] It was precisely such resistance to the acknowledgment of death and to conversation about death that the death awareness movement set out to overcome.

And to some extent it has succeeded. For that we are all, I think, in the debt of the death awareness movement. Still, the success has been limited, so limited that the movement must still inveigh against silence and denial. It remains the case that, while images of death fill our televisions, many remain reluctant to discuss their own death. That reluctance might prompt not just a continuing lament about silence and denial but also a consideration of the weaknesses of the movement and especially of its mantra that death is "natural."

One weakness of the mantra is simply that "natural" is such a slippery word. It means different things to different people in different contexts.[14] I suspect it means different things to different people who adopt the slogan. But as the different meanings are sorted out, a variety of other weaknesses become apparent.

Sometimes "death is natural" seems to mean nothing more than that death is inevitable. At the end of life, people die. What could be more "natural" than that? The death rate is finally 100 percent. It is simply "a part of life," to use another mantra of the death awareness movement. (One might, of course, wonder how the absence of life can be a part of life, but leave that quibble aside.) Death is, on this reading of the slogan, merely a biological event that is predictably and universally the end of any organism's life. Dogs, dinosaurs, plants, and people die. It is hard to disagree with that, of course. But it has little, if any, power against the denial of death. People are less tempted to deny death as a biological event than as an autobiographical event. They are unlikely to deny that death is universal, but they remain reticent to acknowledge their own death. It is not

13. Philippe Aries, *The Hour of Our Death,* trans. Helen Weaver (New York: Knopf, 1981), p. 589.

14. In *Nature and Altering It* (Grand Rapids: Eerdmans, 2010), I began by sorting out sixteen different senses of "nature" and "natural." See also C. S. Lewis, *Studies in Words,* 2nd ed. (London: Cambridge University Press, 1967), pp. 24-74.

death-in-general that we have trouble comprehending and facing but death as self-involving (and self-destroying).

Leo Tolstoy made this point long ago in *The Death of Ivan Ilych*. Ivan Ilych could grasp the syllogism that he had learned in logic class, "Caius is a man, men are mortal, therefore Caius is mortal," but it "had always seemed to him correct as applied to Caius, but certainly not as applied to himself." He was not Caius, "not an abstract man, but a creature quite, quite separate from all others. He had been little Vanya, with a mama and a papa" and with a story that was his own. So, in spite of the acknowledgment in the abstract that death is universal and inevitable, Ivan resists the acknowledgment that he is dying. "It cannot be that I ought to die. That would be too terrible."[15] Tolstoy's story is surely a favorite of the death awareness movement for its depiction of the silence and denial surrounding death, but the mantra of the death awareness movement, at least this particular reading of it, would have had little, if any, power against Ivan's denial of death.

Moreover, if this is what the mantra means, that death is merely a biological event, then it would seem a cousin to the reduction of death to a medical event that the death awareness movement rightly finds objectionable. Medicalization has turned death into a medical event, as if we could give an adequate account of death if we could attribute it, for example, to congestive heart failure. But to regard death merely as a biological event is correlative to regarding death as a medical event. Then dying is a biological process, traced in lab reports and electrocardiograms, all measurable and, one hopes, manageable. Then we can define death as a flat line on the EEG. But the meaning of death and of dying resists reduction to the medical chart, resists reduction to either a medical or a biological account of it. People are organisms, of course, but not simply organisms. And the death of a person is always something more than either a medical event or a biological event. Indeed, the death awareness movement has insisted on that point. The mantra must, therefore, mean something more and something other than that death is predictably and universally the end of any organism's life. But what?

Fairly early in the movement, "death is natural" was taken to mean not simply that death is a biological event but that its meaning could be found in the natural process of growth. In 1975 Kübler-Ross edited a book

15. Leo Tolstoy, *The Death of Ivan Ilych and Other Stories*, trans. Aylmer Maude and J. D. Duff (New York: Penguin Books, Signet Classic, 2003), p. 129.

entitled *Death: The Final Stage of Growth.*[16] To say "death is natural" is here to invoke an organic metaphor to make some sense of it. Death is natural because it is, or can be, growth. I admit that I do not find much sense in this metaphor. One problem here is surely and simply that the claim is so counterintuitive. Death is not growth; it is the end of growing. The proper organic metaphor would seem to be that death is decay rather than growth. (There is here the same problem as with that other mantra. Death is not "a part of life"; it is the end of life, the absence of life.) It does make some sense, of course, to say that dying is a part of life and that dying can be a time of growth.

But even if we take "death is natural" as a way to invoke the biological metaphor to characterize dying as a time for growth, the growth metaphor in this context still seems to rely on the model of self-realization at work in so much popular psychology. In this model growth is not just a biological process; it is a moral ideal. Human beings should "grow"; they should realize their biological and personal potential.

One problem here, of course, is that every person has a great variety of potentialities. We cannot realize them all. We need to make decisions about which to attempt to realize — and which to attempt to stunt! It is clear, for example, that we have the potential to die, sometimes even perhaps an urge to die, but is that a potential we should make actual? The death awareness movement says no such thing, of course, but it cannot be the notion of realizing one's potential that keeps them from saying such a thing. Human potentialities and the possibilities of actualizing them are not an answer to our moral questions; they are among the reasons we ask moral questions. You do not have to be an ascetic to be a little suspicious of the advice "Follow your bliss." Moreover, once we have made some decisions about which potential to attempt to realize, it will require some discipline, some sacrifice of other potentialities in order to actualize it.

But the problem is not just that every person has a great variety of potentialities but also that there are a great variety of persons. And just as there is conflict between the potentialities of one person, so there is sometimes conflict between one person actualizing her potential and other persons actualizing theirs. The doctor may have the potential to keep me alive while I have the potential to die. "Self-realization" or "growth" does not help much in such contexts. Whose potential is to be realized? Against

16. Elisabeth Kübler-Ross, ed., *Death: The Final Stage of Growth* (Englewood Cliffs, N.J.: Prentice-Hall, 1975).

medicalization the language is used to assert that one should be allowed to die one's own death. But if the language simply translates into the emphasis on choice and autonomy so important to standard bioethics, then all the problems identified above are revisited.

The notion of self-realization is part of the culture of "expressive individualism" that Robert Bellah described and criticized in *Habits of the Heart*.[17] The criticism there is on the mark: the metaphor of "growth" and the valorization of "self-realization" is too frequently a cover for doing whatever one wants to do at the moment. It is too often an excuse for ignoring the effect of one's conduct on others and for neglecting consideration of what conduct and character are morally appropriate and binding. The only significant obligation is finally the duty of self-realization. If dying is "growth" in this sense, the only advice one can give the dying is to die the way they want to die. A curious consequence for the death awareness movement is that if you want to die unaware that you are dying, that too has to be accepted. Even "acceptance" of death, the final stage of Kübler-Ross's "stages of dying," cannot be said to be an obligation.

But sometimes the mantra evidently means something else, something more. Sometimes "death is natural" is a way of setting death in the context of the ecology of nature, of construing it as part of a natural rhythm of birth and death, the natural progress from spring to winter and back again. Then death is not just a biological event but a biological event that is part of a larger whole, part of a harmonious ecology. Then death is not just an individual's "growth," the realization of individual whims under cover of that metaphor from nature. Here there is rather an acknowledgment that the individual is part of a larger whole. And in this larger whole, in the ecology of nature, death plays a significant role; it has a place. Little wonder, then, that the death awareness literature and many of the memoirs influenced by this literature often invoke images from nature to cope with death. Streams rush to disappear in the lake. Birds return to the wetlands. Habitat is restored by decay. Eagles fly. And people find some transcendence over death by participation in this vast and quite glorious nature.

People do evidently find some comfort and consolation in nature. But we should not exaggerate the power of the natural rhythm of birth and death, the natural progress from spring to winter and back again, to overcome resistance to the consideration of one's own death. Death remains an

---

17. Robert N. Bellah et al., *Habits of the Heart: Individualism and Commitment in American Life* (Berkeley: University of California Press, 1985).

autobiographical event, a self-involving event, a self-destroying event. Winter leads back to spring, back to life, to be sure, but the death of a person does not lead back to the life of *that* person. *That* person is simply dead, gone. *That* story is over. Ivan Ilych's line, "It cannot be that I ought to die. That would be too terrible," still echoes from the horizon of both the sunrise and sunset of the days of our dying. And the hole in a life left by the death of one loved is not filled by the "larger whole" of nature. That loved person is not replaceable. Eagles and streams are no substitute for that particular person.

If the death awareness movement were to become more explicit about some return of particular persons to life, about an afterlife for particular persons, then that presumably, rather than the claim that "death is natural," would be the basis for courage and consolation in the face of death. Elisabeth Kübler-Ross did in fact move in the direction of an affirmation of life after death. In *On Death and Dying* she had dismissed religious confidence in a life after death as a form of denial.[18] She was, to be sure, a little more appreciative of religious forms of the denial of death than she was of the forms of denial she discerned in the medicalization of death. Religious belief offered hope and a sense of purpose in the face of death, but it was still dismissed as denial. By 1983, however, when she published *On Children and Death*, she had adopted the image of a caterpillar turning into a butterfly in order to comfort parents.[19] The image is "natural" enough, I suppose, but the shift in images both acknowledges that there is no substitute for this beloved child, no consolation in the ecology of nature, and suggests that the child still lives on in some other form. "Death" seems to have disappeared from the mantra. It is not death now that is natural but life. This is not death comprehended as a part of a larger whole, not death set in the context of the rhythms of a natural ecology. That whole material world, along with the body, is simply left behind in a Platonic transcendence. There is only continuing life, life transitioned into another reality, a disembodied reality. This shift in Kübler-Ross's perspective was not based on the beliefs of any particular community of faith nor on any philosophical argument for immortality. It was based, rather, on reports of near-death experiences. But it looks no less like a denial of death than the religious beliefs that she had earlier dismissed. It looks like a de-

18. Kübler-Ross, *On Death and Dying,* p. 15.
19. Elisabeth Kübler-Ross, *On Children and Death* (New York: Macmillan, 1983), p. 141.

nial of the hard reality of the death of a child. The transition from "death is natural" to "life is unending" is curious, and the book is more than a little muddled. But the poverty of the mantra that "death is natural" as a resource to deal with the death of a beloved child is surely on display.

The death awareness movement may most plausibly be regarded as a retrieval of Romanticism in protest against medicalized death. The Romantic movement, which began toward the end of the eighteenth century, was a reaction to the Enlightenment's emphasis on unqualified reason and its confidence in science as a way to manage nature. It was an important challenge to the mastery of nature sponsored by the Baconian project. It emphasized feelings and the imagination, and it rejected both the image of nature as an enemy to be mastered and the image of nature as a mechanism that had grown up in the scientific revolution. Rousseau first uttered the slogan "Back to nature," but the Romantics made it popular. The universe was not mechanical but organic, one living world spirit. Indeed, there was the old apotheosis of nature. Nature was, as Marcus Aurelius had said long before, "the eldest of deities."[20] Nature was "Mother Nature," and "It's not nice to fool with Mother Nature." Many of them were pantheists, attending to the absolute spirit that was immanent in everything. The ways of God and the ways of nature were thought to be the same ways. And ancient people were thought to be more in tune with those ways than the people of their own century were. Nostalgia for the life of those "good old days" marked Romanticism.

Theoretically nature was seen as a whole, but Romanticism was largely an urban movement, and "nature" usually meant the countryside as opposed to the city. It meant green landscapes in a swirling mist. Wordsworth congratulated Coleridge, for example, on the fact that, although he had been "reared in the great city," he had "long desired to serve in Nature's temple."[21] But the apotheosis of nature was a creed that could not abide the city — and that the city could not abide, however attractive it may have been to discontented city dwellers. Romanticism finally and despairingly had to accept a compartmentalization of life. There is the life of the city, where nature is mastered and altered, and there is the wilderness, where Nature's altar stands.

Romanticism rejected the emphasis on reason in the Enlightenment,

20. *Meditations* 9.1.
21. William Wordsworth, *The Prelude*, ed. J. C. Maxwell (New Haven: Yale University Press, 1981), book II, lines 452-53, 463-64; quoted as cited in Lewis, *Studies in Words*, p. 72.

but many Romantics nevertheless saw themselves as standing in the line of Kant. Kant had shown that the knowing self contributes to cognition, to knowledge. The Romantics took the point to insist on the freedom to interpret reality in their own ways. They emphasized both the value of experience and the significance of the artistic genius. Byron (1788-1824), for example, whose "Byronic hero" was a moody and rebellious soul (as was Byron evidently), was regarded as such an artistic genius. The consequence was a celebration of the self, the ego. Romanticism honored expressive individualism and self-realization.

The death awareness movement echoes much of Romanticism. It is all there: the suspicion of the Baconian project as that came to expression in the medicalization of death, the celebration of Nature, the nostalgia for premedicalized death, the appeal to experience, the expressive individualism. To be sure, not everyone who uses the mantra assumes the pantheism of the Romantics. But there is surely a spirituality assumed and nurtured in the death awareness movement. For all the pretense of secularity, there is a spirituality here that trusts and celebrates the harmony of nature and that finds human meaning by participation in that harmony. "Death is natural" finally invokes "Mother Nature" to make meaning of death. As Romanticism was a reaction against what we have called the Baconian project, so the death awareness movement was a reaction against the medicalization of death.

But there are problems with Romanticism, and those problems, too, find an echo in the death awareness movement. We have already attended to the problems of expressive individualism and self-realization. Nostalgia for the past is problematic simply because we do not live in it. But the compartmentalization of life and of dying is also problematic. We are double-minded and conflicted about whether to live and die in the city or in the country, whether to live with the alterations of nature in a city and in a hospital or whether to seek the altar of "Nature" by refusing interventions and dying "naturally." The hard division of "nature" and "mastering it" into separate compartments does not help us draw a fine line between using medicine when appropriate and refusing it when it is not. Reaction is itself a problem, for every reaction is unstable. It is almost certain to prompt a subsequent reaction. The reaction to Romanticism, after all, was the positivism of Comte, which set aside theology and metaphysics as childish things for the sake of scientific understanding.[22]

22. We have already noted that contemporary medicine has been formed by the story told within the Baconian project, that knowledge as power over nature brings human well-

But all these problems pale before the fundamental problem. Nature has a dark side. It brings both weal and woe. And it seems indifferent to the suffering of any particular creature that it spawns. Francis Bacon could agree that "death is natural" — and then insist that we master nature in order to achieve human well-being. Nature, Bacon had insisted, does not serve human well-being naturally. One may accuse Bacon and the Baconian project of rendering nature as the enemy that must be mastered by human reason and technology. But the reaction of Romanticism and of the death awareness movement celebrates nature without sufficient attention to the ways in which it can in fact threaten particular creatures. If the Baconian project seems always to force resistance to death, the Romantic movement — and the death awareness movement with its mantra — seems seldom to acknowledge that death is a threat to particular creatures. Neither helps us much with decisions about when to resist death and when to accept it. Neither helps us much with discernment concerning what dy-

---

being. But it is worth noting the family resemblance between that story and the narrative told by August Comte. Comte's story of "progress" in human knowledge is a triumphalist tale of science. Progress in the quest for human knowledge has proceeded, Comte said, through three stages, and progress requires that each stage leave behind the previous stage as ignorance. The first stage, the most primitive stage, Comte called "theological." That was superstition, and humanity, at least the enlightened ones within humanity, have transcended it, leaving it behind as myth and legend. The second stage Comte named "metaphysical." It was progress, to be sure, but not yet real knowledge, more like guesswork. And it is left behind as ignorance in the final stage, the "scientific" stage. Finally human beings truly know, and this knowledge gives them great power to make further progress. Medicine has made also this story its own. It acknowledges, to be sure, that health care may have had its beginnings in religion and philosophy, but in the story it frequently tells of itself it has transcended that past, making "progress" by science. It prides itself on being a scientific discipline. When medicine and the culture celebrate medicine as "scientific," however, the celebration itself is hardly a matter of "science." The celebration puts medicine at risk of forgetting, of neglecting, and of distorting the human context of care for the suffering. There is always some context, of course, some narrative that orients and locates us, some *mythos* that shapes an *ethos*, even if the myth is that we can do without myth, even if the story is that we have no story. Some narrative context seems inescapable, however, even for science, even for those who would use science to debunk myths. See Joel Shuman, *The Body of Compassion: Ethics, Medicine, and the Church* (Boulder, Colo.: Westview, 1999), pp. 11-12. At the end of the story, even as we continue to tell it, we know better. Human progress cannot be reduced to scientific progress. Knowing a patient cannot be reduced to scientific knowing. Indeed, the scientific "view," if the complaints are to be credited, can distort our vision and blind us to persons and to the body as "me." But if religion and philosophy have been left behind as "theological" and "metaphysical" ways of knowing, then where shall we look for corrective vision?

ing well would look like. Neither helps Christians much to discern what a faithful dying would be.

The problem with the death awareness movement is not any denial of death (except in Kübler-Ross's work on the death of children). The problem is rather the denial of the threat of death to particular embodied and communal selves. The problem with its mantra that "death is natural" is its denial not of death but of the wrongness of death. The sense of the wrongness of death is hard to repress. Ivan Ilych's judgment still echoes in the thoughts of many: "It cannot be that I ought to die. That would be too terrible." And neither the conscious repetition of the mantra that "death is natural" nor any feigned indifference has finally much power against medicalized death. The promise of the death awareness movement, that if we just learned to regard death as "natural" we could avoid a medicalized death, is unfulfilled.

The Hospice Movement

Both standard bioethics and the death awareness movement give truncated accounts of the problems with medicalized death. The problems are not just the violation of patient control or simply silence and denial but the alienation from our bodies, the separation from our communities, and the eclipse of God. That is what death threatens, and in a medicalized death — in the very resistance to death — death makes good on those threats before the end of our lives and for the sake of our survival. We are not fated to a medicalized dying, but it has a strong hold on us precisely because we recognize that life is a great good and that the threats of death are real and terrible. Resistance to medicalized death need not deny the sadness of death. Indeed, it must recognize the threats of death and meet those threats with attention to the dying person as an embodied and communal and spiritual being.

That recognition and a commitment to such attention gave birth to a third challenge to medicalized death, a challenge that had its roots in the deep Christian faith of Cicely Saunders, the founder of the modern hospice movement. She was a British physician who had trained first as a nurse. It was her vision of a home for the dying that led to the establishment in 1967 of St. Christopher's Hospice in London. In the late 1940s she had met a young Jewish patient dying of cancer on a forty-bed ward in a London hospital. He had no family and no home in England. When she told him of her vision of a home where patients like him, dying and unable to be in their own home, would be welcome to stay and would be provided with help for their pain, he told her, "I'll be a window in your home."[23] Nearly twenty years later the vision had bricks and mortar — and windows — at St. Christopher's Hospice.

A home for the dying was an innovative challenge to the medicalization of death. But Cicely Saunders was herself a physician, and her vision was a challenge not to medicine itself but to the narrowing of its ministry to the effort to cure. Her vision incorporated medicine and its authority, joining it to care for the dying. She insisted that research-based medical treatment for pain relief should accompany attention to the psychological, social, and spiritual needs of dying patients. St. Christopher's provided not just care for dying patients but also training and research facilities for nurses and medical students (and for people preparing for social work and for ministry).

However innovative the challenge to medicalization, Cicely Saunders regarded her vision as solidly within the Christian tradition of care for the sick. She acknowledged her indebtedness to two religious institutions for her vision, St. Joseph's and St. Luke's. St. Joseph's was a Roman Catholic program; St. Luke's was a Methodist foundation; both were begun in the early twentieth century, and both were committed to the care of the sick and poor of London. She acknowledged as well the longer history of Christian care for the sick and dying. As she said, "For a thousand years, Christian charitable institutions carried the burden of the sick and the poor — the indigent, orphans and others — amounting almost to a general national health and welfare service."[24]

The Aim and Basis Statement of St. Christopher's gave words to Saunders's vision and made explicit its foundation in the Christian faith.

> St. Christopher's Hospice is a religious foundation, based on the full Christian faith in God, through Christ. Its aim is to express the love of

23. Cicely Saunders, "The Modern Hospice," in *In Quest of the Spiritual Component of Care for the Terminally Ill*, ed. Florence Wald (New Haven: Yale University School of Nursing, 1986), p. 42. Ann Bradshaw, "The Spiritual Dimension of Hospice: The Secularization of an Ideal," *Social Science and Medicine* 43, no. 3 (1996): 409-19, cited this passage and alerted me to the existence of this volume of the proceedings from a conference at Yale University School of Nursing in 1986. Bradshaw's article is an instructive account of the "secularization" of the hospice movement.

24. Saunders, "The Modern Hospice," p. 41.

God to all who come, in every possible way; in skilled nursing and medical care, in the use of every scientific means of relieving suffering and distress, in understanding personal sympathy, with respect for the dignity of each patient as a human being, precious to God and man. It is planned that the staff should form a community, united by a strong sense of vocation with a great diversity of outlook in a spirit of freedom.[25]

Clearly Cicely Saunders did not regard science and religion, or medicine and Christian faith, as contradictory. As in the case of Francis Bacon, Christian convictions had been presupposed by many at the beginnings of the scientific revolution, notably, the conviction that because the creation is the work of God, it must be orderly and intelligible. And as also in the case of Bacon, Christian care had motivated the search for a cure, had prompted the complaints about the neglect of those regarded as "overmastered by their disease." With Cicely Saunders in the last half of the twentieth century, the Christian tradition prompted a retrieval of care for those whom medicine, in spite of the successes of the Baconian project, could not cure.

The key concept was not the rights of patients but the care of patients. To be sure, the dignity of each patient was explicitly recognized (and proselytizing forbidden).[26] But the model was not a contract between self-interested individuals but a covenant and a community. And the mantra, if there was one, was not "death is natural," but Matthew 25:40, "just as you did it to one of the least of these . . . you did it to me."[27]

The vision of Cicely Saunders was carried to the United States soon after St. Christopher's was established. Less than a decade later, in 1975, a hospice modeled on St. Christopher's opened in Connecticut. And across the country volunteers and nurses and doctors who shared something of Saunders's vision initiated programs to care for dying persons in their homes.

Those programs operated outside the traditional hospital-based

25. Saunders, "The Modern Hospice," p. 45. Dr. Saunders acknowledged the help of the theologian Olive Wyon in drafting the Aim and Basis Statement.

26. One of the five principles enunciated by Saunders at the beginning was "that dying people must find peace and be found by God, quietly, in their own way, without being in any way subjected to pressure from others, however well-meant." Saunders, "The Modern Hospice," p. 45.

27. Saunders, "The Modern Hospice," pp. 41, 46-47.

health care system, but in 1982 the United States Congress passed the Medicare Hospice Benefit. The Medicare benefit provided payment for hospice services to patients older than sixty-five who had a prognosis of less than six months to live and who agreed to forgo therapies intended to provide a cure for their disease. Patients were entitled to the care and support of a hospice team, supervised by a physician, who would attempt to relieve pain, manage symptoms, and alleviate psychological, social, and spiritual stress. Gradually private insurance programs and Medicaid began to include some coverage for hospice. By 2004 there were more than 3,200 hospice programs in the United States, caring for more than 900,000 people. About half of these people have a diagnosis of cancer, and the rest have a variety of diseases that include a period of debilitation and dependency before death. Depending on the locale, between 50 and 90 percent of cancer patients receive hospice care before their deaths.

The quite remarkable development of hospice care nurtured equally remarkable developments in palliative care as a medical specialty. Cicely Saunders had utilized what research-based treatments for pain there were in the 1960s, and she had called for further research. The "hospice cocktail" and other interventions for pain relief developed in hospice care were further developed in palliative medicine. The story of hospice is a quite remarkable story, full of successes and much to be commended as institutional support for dying well. But there are problems even here.

In the first place, hospice remains an underutilized resource. Many physicians and others remain unwilling or unable to tell patients that they are dying, and many patients remain unwilling or unable to hear the prognosis that could lead to the utilization of hospice. Silence and denial are still realities, as is medicalized death. Even those who do utilize hospice frequently enter late in the process; one-third die within seven days of admission to a hospice program. Hospice remains underutilized for other reasons as well. Minority populations who have suffered injustices concerning access to medical care in the past can interpret the suggestion of hospice care as one more way to deny them appropriate medical services. And some religious people have refused to shift the emphasis from cure to care because it seems to them a denial of God's power to do a miracle. But the reticence to acknowledge that one (or a loved one) is dying remains the most significant reason that hospice is underutilized.

The underutilization prompted by silence and denial is, however, not the only problem. Ironically, there is a risk of medicalization in the hospice movement itself, not the medicalization of death, which Cicely Saunders had challenged, but the medicalization of suffering. It is another instance of the old problem of the failure of our successes — or the vices of our virtues. As the success of the Baconian project led both to cures for many who had been "overmastered by disease" and to medicalized death, so the success of palliative medicine has led both to great advances in pain management and also to the risks of reducing suffering to pain and reducing care for the dying to the management of their pain. Again, as one may and must celebrate the advances in medicine that allowed it to cure many of those with diseases once regarded as incurable, so one may and must celebrate the developments in palliative medicine that have made possible the relief of pain. But again, as one may and must rue medicalized death, so again one should worry a little about the medicalization of the suffering that can attend dying. Dying without pain is important, and effective pain relief makes an important contribution to the possibilities of dying well, but dying well and faithfully cannot and should not be reduced to a death without pain.

Indeed, drugs can be an instrument by which professionals (and families) can manage a dying patient, can make the patient's dying a little easier for themselves. When a dying patient is distressed, drugs may not address the real cause of the distress but may simply mask it. Indeed, if the patient is rendered too drowsy to talk or think, the drug may make dealing with the real cause of the distress more difficult. The danger of being misunderstood is great here, so I repeat, the problem is not drugs but the reduction of the suffering that can attend dying to pain, and then managing the pain — and the patient — by medication. Cicely Saunders's vision surely included the management of pain, but to reduce care for the dying to pain management puts at risk the very values and traditions with which and for which she had challenged the medicalization of death.

The risk of medicalization here has grown with the success of the hospice movement. The great advance of the inclusion of hospice care with health care coverage has risked subsuming hospice care under health care, risked once more, if differently, rendering death and dying medical events rather than human events. The growing professionalism of palliative care, which can be and should be celebrated, has been attended by the risk of breaking community with the dying. The expertise involved in hospice and palliative care is worthy of our praise and gratitude, but it can form relations of "expert" and needy beneficiaries. Worse, those of us who are not "expert" but have "compassion" may exercise it by sending the one suffering or dying away, surrendering her care into the hands of the expert stranger. This "compassion" is a compassion formed by the Baconian project, a compassion reduced to eliminating suffering by means of technology administered by people who know how to use it. It is not a compassion that is formed by the Christian tradition of a readiness to suffer with another, a readiness to share the suffering. And such compassion can be experienced by the suffering and dying as abandonment and make dying worse rather than better. Cicely Saunders had insisted that hospice care utilize the best practices of pain relief and symptom management, but she also insisted on a relationship with the suffering and dying that was not simply a relation of professional and client but a relationship Martin Buber had described as an I-Thou relationship, a genuine meeting of two persons in a covenantal relationship.[28] She had envisioned a "home," a building, to be sure, but also a place of warmth and welcome, a place to get comfortable with family and friends, a place to be yourself. Compassion required access to the best palliative care possible, but it also required just being there with and for the suffering. Keeping company was no less a component of care, no less a key to dying well, than pain management.

But there is another problem. A generic spirituality has replaced Saunders's commitment to the Christian faith. Some, of course, regard this not as a problem but as an advance, as a necessary adjustment to the religious pluralism of American society (and, perhaps, as a requirement of government funding). Religious differences are a significant issue for hospice. And to its credit, it did not deliberately adopt a perspective that set aside a person's faith (or religious beliefs or spirituality) in favor of scientific objectivity. It recognized that in dying, as in living, we are surrounded not only by puzzles but also by mystery. And at the depths and heights of our lives, and at the ends of them, there is the Ultimate Mystery, whom many call God. There is no escaping this mystery.

Little wonder, then, that human beings are so incorrigibly religious, that spirituality is as natural to human beings as breathing. We live and die in God's world, and we encounter mystery. Mystery evokes among us a sense of dependence upon some dimly known but reliable order. It evokes a sense of gratitude for the givenness (the gifts) of life and health. It evokes a sad sense of a tragic flaw that runs through our lives and through our world. It evokes a hopeful sense of new possibilities just over the horizon. And it evokes a keen sense of responsibility to the inscrutable Mystery who

28. See Cicely Saunders, "I Was Sick and You Visited Me," *Christian Nurse International* 3, no. 4 (1987); cited by Bradshaw.

sustains the order, gives the gifts, judges the flaw, and promises hope. To its credit, hospice did not attempt to empty the world, or dying, of mystery.

The obvious problem, of course, is the problem of difference. The world is full not only of mystery but also of different ways of naming it. But name it we must if we are to begin to interpret its presence and to orient those senses of dependence and gratitude and remorse and hope and responsibility. Of course, we always experience those senses already oriented in one way or another toward someone or something, toward mothers or friends or nature or technology. One way or another we learn to name the Mystery, and the way we live and die is a response to the Mystery, so named. There is no purely rational foundation for talking about the Mystery any more than there are purely rational ways for talking about morality. There is no religious Esperanto any more than there is a moral Esperanto, no universal language for talking about either the Mystery or morality. That's the first problem with the sort of generic spirituality adopted by hospice.

Hospice has adopted this generic spirituality that refuses to name the Mystery because it wanted to respect religious and spiritual diversity, but generic spirituality can have an ironic result; it is not finally hospitable to difference. When "spirituality" is reduced to some lowest common denominator, to something like "the Ultimate Mystery," then the ways in which it is named can be trivialized. Or worse, "spirituality" can be reduced to an internal and individual search for meaning. Then particular religious communities and their practices can be regarded as less relevant to the dying than this individual quest for meaning.

I am a Christian. I know of no other way to talk faithfully about the Mystery at the heart of our world than as a Christian. I know of no other way faithfully to make sense of these senses than as a Christian. Of course, it is easy to be presumptuous here, easy to claim to know too much. Even so, as a Christian, I dare to claim that all our responses to Mystery are in fact responses to the God whose story is told in Scripture.

One can do worse, I think, than to name the Mystery wrongly. One can respond to the Mystery — even if it is named rightly — by ignoring it. One can deny or suppress the senses evoked by it. Even those who can name the Mystery rightly can still be guilty of refusing to trust and to honor God. They can — and sometimes do — regard God as the enemy of God's own work. More often, they turn the Mystery into a giant puzzle. And more often still, they domesticate the Mystery, rendering the inscrutable not only scrutable but also serviceable to their own projects, to their

65

own communal or individual causes. Those who know enough to say, "Lord, Lord," can still be guilty of domesticating God, drafting God into the service of this army or that one, into the service of this ecclesiastical organization or that one, or into their own service. But the Mystery resists, and a commandment prohibits, the effort to domesticate God. And the domestication of the Mystery is the second problem with the sort of generic spirituality adopted by hospice. It virtually sponsors the domestication of the Mystery, regarding it as "helpful," even if it is a helpful fiction. It is rendered another opiate.

Cicely Saunders had set care for the dying in the context of the Christian faith. The Mystery known and named by the Christian community in the light of Scripture called her to the service of God's cause, and that cause in the light of Scripture included care for any who suffer. Now the hospice movement, with its generic spirituality, is at risk not only of losing its sense of vocation but also of domesticating spirituality, of rendering it useful to the task that they have undertaken, making it another tool in their palliative arsenal.

It is worth remembering that a Jewish man dying from cancer became a "window" in Saunders's home for the dying. Her response to religious difference was not to proselytize. And it was not to water down anyone's faith to a lowest common denominator. Her response was to practice hospitality to one who is different.

Emphasizing the individual's internal quest for meaning and undercutting the role of particular religious communities, this generic spirituality is too easily co-opted by notions of individual autonomy advanced by the patient rights movement. But it can also be co-opted by the death awareness movement when the spirituality assumed by its mantra that "death is natural" is regarded as somehow transcending religious differences.

At the beginnings of hospice a list of the stakeholders in hospice would have included the Christian church. Now it is less than clear that the Christian church would be included in that list. Nevertheless, the Christian community does have a stake in the care for the dying. Cicely Saunders's vision should be enough to remind us of that. Hospice remains a movement in which many Christian doctors and nurses and social workers and chaplains and volunteers can and do fulfill their vocations. And many Christians die well and faithfully with the help of hospice. The Christian community's stake in the care of the dying may also suggest, however, both support for new hospice programs, self-consciously and deliberately formed in accord with Saunders's originating vision, and (more importantly) a refusal simply to leave the task of ministry to the dying to hospice.

Conclusion

I do not deny that some progress has been made against the medicalization of death since the Quinlans had to fight to take their daughter off the respirator. I do not deny that progress has been made since Geoffrey Gorer wrote about the "pornography of death." Conventional bioethics and the death awareness movement have both issued important challenges to medicalized death. But their challenges have not been joined to credible alternatives. The single-minded focus of conventional bioethics on the rights of individual patients has emphasized the question of who should decide, but it has been unable or unwilling to present an alternative or to give advice about what should be decided. It has turned out that many patients are as deeply formed by the Baconian project and the denial of death as many doctors have been. The advice of the death awareness movement, insofar as it is summarized by its mantra that "death is natural," seems to be a retrieval of Romanticism's suspicion of technology. But it also shares with Romanticism a celebration of the solitary individual, nostalgia, a spirituality that celebrates nature and the natural, and a compartmentalization that leaves us double-minded. The death of a particular human creature is, after all, a matter of indifference to nature. Neither of these movements seems to have had much impact on the way we die. Hospice not only challenged medicalization; it provided an alternative. The alternative was founded on the vision and faith of Cicely Saunders. Hospice — and the palliative care medicine with which it is allied (although these two are also sometimes in competition) — now helps hundreds of thousands of people each year to die with less pain. But its very success in alleviating pain has created the danger that it may medicalize the suffering that attends death, reducing it to the pain that drugs can manage. It is included now in the health care delivery system, but that very success can put at risk the sense of vocation that inspired Cicely Saunders. It has become increasingly professionalized, but that success can risk substituting contractual relationships of expert and client for the relationships of community and covenant that Saunders regarded as critically important. And in response to American pluralism it seems to have adopted a generic spirituality as a substitute for the robust Christian faith of its founding.

CHAPTER FIVE

The Silence and Surrender of the Church

Save me, O God,
   for the waters have come up to my neck.
I sink in deep mire,
   where there is no foothold. . . .
I looked for pity, but there was none;
   and for comforters, but I found none.
They gave me poison for food,
   and for my thirst they gave me vinegar to drink.

                                         Psalm 69:1-2, 20-21

We said from the beginning that any challenge to "medicalization" that makes physicians into "scapegoats," laying all the blame on them, misses the mark. It is not that physicians have been altogether innocent in the medicalization of death, but that the rest of us are not free from blame. There is plenty of blame to go around, of course. Doctors sometimes blame the lawyers whose litigation for malpractice cases not only costs them time and money but also forces them to practice "defensive medicine" and to regard their relationship with patients as contractual. Perhaps we could blame the policy makers who write the laws that make malpractice litigation so profitable for some lawyers and create the policies that encourage medical specialization and do not reward the primary care physicians who spend time with patients getting to know them and their suffering. There is, as I said, plenty of blame to go around.

I am not a doctor or a lawyer or a public policy maker. I am a Christian theologian and a member of the Christian community. And instead of pointing the finger at others, the church should acknowledge its own silence about death and its surrender of dying to medicalization. Let judgment "begin," as Peter said, "with the household of God" (1 Pet. 4:17).

The church, no less than medicine, has a long and worthy tradition of moral reflection about the human events of suffering and dying and caring for those who are suffering or dying. How could it have been otherwise where Jesus is remembered? Jesus himself healed the sick, displaying in his works of healing the good future of God. In that healing ministry he made real and present God's power to make alive and to make well. And he charged his disciples not only to preach but to heal (Matt. 10:7-8; Luke 9:2). In that ministry it was made clear that embodied life and the flourishing we call health are great goods, part of the creative and redemptive cause of God. In memory of Jesus Christian churches have sponsored hospitals and regarded the profession of physicians and nurses as a "calling," indeed, as a "holy" calling.[1]

Still, this same Jesus walked steadily and courageously a path that led to his death. He suffered under Pontius Pilate, was crucified, was dead and buried. It was his faithfulness to God and his readiness to serve others that led to that Roman cross. And he charged his disciples to take up the cross and follow him (Mark 8:34; Matt. 10:38; 16:24; Luke 9:23; 14:27). In that cross and in that command it was made clear that, although life and its flourishing are great goods, they are not the greatest goods. Jesus counted some duties as more compelling than his own survival and ease, and so, he said, must his disciples. Sometimes death must be risked. Sometimes suffering must be endured. Sometimes death and suffering must be accepted. In memory of this Jesus Christian churches have celebrated the martyrs and acknowledged the limits of human powers to remedy our human vulnerability to death and suffering.

This same Jesus was raised from the dead by the power of God. Death did not have the last word with Jesus, and in memory of this Jesus Christian churches learned to hope that death would not have the last

---

1. See Walter Rauschenbusch, *Prayers of the Social Awakening* (Boston: Pilgrim Press, 1925), pp. 81-82, reprinted in Stephen E. Lammers and Allen Verhey, eds., *On Moral Medicine: Theological Perspectives in Medical Ethics,* 2nd ed. (Grand Rapids: Eerdmans, 1998), p. 5.

word in God's good creation. They learned to say, "I believe . . . in the resurrection of the dead." That hope has been their comfort and their courage
in the face of death.

The story of Jesus shapes not only attitudes toward life and death but
also attitudes toward those who are suffering and dying. In memory of his
solidarity with the suffering and dying, Christians learned to care for those
in need. They learned to count care for those in need, including the sick
and dying, as care rendered to Christ in his absence. Jesus said as much, of
course, when he told the parable of the last judgment (Matt. 25:31-46); to
care for "the least of these," including the sick and suffering, is to care for
him. By tradition and vocation Christian churches have a responsibility to
care for the sick and dying, to teach them to live well and to die faithfully,
to care for those who suffer their way to death.

That tradition and vocation have not been altogether forgotten, but
the churches have grown too often silent about death. When Christians
have spoken, they have too often participated in the denial of the hard reality of death, serving up warmed-over Platonic platitudes as if they were
genuine consolation. And the churches have been too often silent about
the medicalization of death, in effect surrendering death — or at least dying — to medicine and to the hospitals they helped to establish. Many
Christian patients seem more under the spell of the Baconian project than
many doctors. A study of patients with advanced cancer determined that
those patients who identified themselves as people of religious faith (most
of them Christians) were more likely to opt for aggressive medical treatment, including mechanical ventilation, at the end of their lives, more
likely not to prepare an advance directive for end-of-life care, and more
likely not to die well.[2] Perhaps they thought that God could use the aggressive treatment to work a miracle. Perhaps they thought their prayers would
supplement the medical technology and make it successful. These are issues to which we must return. For now it is enough to let the finding stand
as a confirmation that the churches have not taught us to die well.

To be sure, Christians have sometimes joined their voices to the
complaints about medicalization, but when they have, they have too often

---

2. Andrea C. Phelps et al., "Religious Coping and Use of Intensive Life-Prolonging
Care Near Death in Patients with Advanced Cancer," *Journal of the American Medical Association* 301, no. 11 (2009): 1140-47. Good and honest physicians may lead the way to a recognition of the limits of their good art and to the recognition of the need to develop alternative
ways of dying. It is sometimes patients who still demand the miracle that good and honest
physicians know they do not have the power to provide.

surrendered the language of their own tradition for the language of the death awareness movement or standard bioethics. They have sometimes sounded more like followers of Elisabeth Kübler-Ross or like followers of Kant than like followers of Jesus. They have sometimes adopted the mantra that "death is natural" without sufficient critical reflection. They have sometimes adopted the universal moral language favored by standard bioethics rather than a language formed in Christian community in remembrance of Jesus.

Robert Coles, the eminent Harvard psychiatrist, tells the story of a friend of his who complained about the visit of a priest who was, in his estimation, more clearly a follower of Elisabeth Kübler-Ross than of Jesus.[3] Coles's friend was a physician who knew that his cancer was not likely to be beaten back and a Christian who knew that death would not have the last word. When Coles visited him in the hospital, his friend was angry. He was not angry because of his cancer; he was angry because he had just been visited by a priest who displayed in his visit more confidence in the "stages of dying" than in the story of Jesus. Coles's friend had wanted to talk about God and about the ways of God, about Jesus and about his life and death, about his own dying and destiny. But the chaplain was eager to talk about his psychological state, about his "coping," about his "managing" the stress he must feel. He was, Coles's friend said, a psychobabbling fool, who had emptied his role of the practices of the faith, like reading Scripture and praying, and had filled it instead with the words and phrases of popular psychology. What Coles's friend needed and wanted, as Coles said in another essay, was some good "hard praying."[4] What he got instead was the priest's attention to the "stages of dying" as if they were the Stations of the Cross.

Coles's friend said he was eager for this priest to return. He was ready for him. He would, he said, "wait for him to do his little song and dance about my 'feelings.'" And then he would interrupt the priest, hand him the Bible, and ask him to read it. The bookmark would be set at Psalm 69, the psalm set at the beginning of this chapter. Coles quotes the opening words of the psalm, "Save me, O God, for the waters have come up to my neck." It is a lament, one of the great cries of anguish that one finds in Psalms, a call for help in times of trouble. But if the priest had read on, he would have discovered what Coles failed to mention, that Psalm 69 is an imprecatory

3. Robert Coles, "Psychiatric Stations of the Cross," in his *Harvard Diary* (New York: Crossroad, 1990), pp. 10-12.

4. Coles, *Harvard Diary*, p. 94.

psalm, one of those cries of anguish that vents its anger in curses upon those who fail to help. That anger and its curses may have been no small part of the reason Coles's friend chose Psalm 69 for that particular representative of the church.

> I looked for pity, but there was none;
>> and for comforters, but I found none.
> They gave me poison for food,
>> and for my thirst they gave me vinegar to drink.
> Let their table be a trap for them.

Coles's friend, of course, was not complaining about hospital food. He was complaining about a priest who had surrendered his vocation for that of a psychological counselor, who was silent about the story and the faith that might provide courage and comfort in the face of death. The curse was not intended to disparage the skills and language of psychology — surely not in Coles's report, at any rate. Rather, it was to remind the priest that we may eat and drink judgment to ourselves if we neglect the gifts of God for the people of God. And those gifts include not just a little bread and wine but also prayer and Scripture, the presence of a suffering and risen Christ, and the presence of the community that is Christ's "body."

This priest was silent about the story, surrendering both it and his vocation in his conversation with Coles's friend, because he had a little training in Kübler-Ross's "stages of dying." But it is not just this priest who has been guilty of silence and surrender. It is not hard to imagine another representative of the church, a chaplain perhaps, who had conscientiously volunteered to serve on the hospital's ethics committee. There he had received a little training in standard bioethics. There he had learned, perhaps, a little Kant and a little John Stuart Mill. There he had learned to respect and protect a patient's autonomy and to regard human relationships as contracts between self-interested and autonomous individuals. If that chaplain were to visit Coles's friend, he might be anxious not so much about psychological states and stages as about not interfering with the rights of the patient, including the right to be left alone. Enthusiasm for generic moral principles learned from standard bioethics might make this chaplain no less hesitant to speak in a distinctively Christian voice than the priest who visited Coles's friend. He, too, might hesitate to offer the gifts of prayer and Scripture, and he, too, might be guilty of silence about the story and the surrender of his vocation. And Coles's friend might once more mark his Bible to Psalm 69. Again, the point would not be that philosophical skills or the generic moral principles favored by standard bioethics are useless. But Coles's friend needs and wants not just to have his autonomy respected. He needs and wants someone to talk of God and of the ways of God. He needs and wants to attend to God. He does not need or want a conversation in moral Esperanto, that universal moral language that few besides "bioethicists" speak, a language that he little understands and does not really care to learn, not now as he lies dying, at any rate. He may indeed have some hard decisions to make, but he wants to make them prayerfully, in ways that are attentive to God and to the cause of God, and not just with impartial rationality.

I am no more interested in blaming particular clergy or churches than I am in blaming doctors, but I am interested in calling the church to take seriously its responsibilities to teach people to die well and faithfully and to care well and faithfully for the dying. It needs to recover its own voice concerning death and dying and to nurture practices of dying well and caring well for the dying. The Christian community once did take responsibility for teaching people how to die well; the *Ars Moriendi* of the fifteenth century, to which we will turn in the next part of this book, is one stunning example of instruction concerning "the art of dying." But the Christian community does not always get its own story straight. Sometimes, perhaps always, the cultural context distorts the way the story is told. And the *Ars Moriendi* of the fifteenth century may also be an example of that. Nevertheless, the church can recover its voice — and check its voice — by retrieving again and again the story told in Scripture and by setting it alongside all the stories of our dying and our care for the dying so that they may be challenged and made new by it. By retrieving its own story, perhaps the Christian community can take death back from medicine without denying that medicine is a gift of God and a "holy calling." Medicine needs the church not only to limit and challenge the Promethean triumphalism of the Baconian project but also to sustain its vocation not only to preserve life but also to care for the dying.[5] By retrieving its own story, the Christian community may be able to imagine a contemporary *ars moriendi*. Mortal members of the Christian community, like Coles's friend, need the church to take that possibility — and responsibility — seriously.

It is ironic that the community that has a story of a death at the cen-

---

5. Stanley Hauerwas, "Salvation and Health: Why Medicine Needs the Church," in *Suffering Presence* (Notre Dame, Ind.: University of Notre Dame Press, 1986), pp. 63-83.

ter of its Scripture and at the center of its practices of baptism and Eucharist should fall so often silent about death and about the practices of dying well and faithfully and of caring well and faithfully for the dying. The contemporary church, too, of course, has been formed by the culture in which it lives, but it has the resources to resist it and its medicalization of death. It has the presence and power of the Spirit to nurture and sustain faithfulness in the face of death. And it has, by the same Spirit, the power to challenge, qualify, and transform the culture.

That power is on display often enough to give us hope. When family members and friends die well and faithfully, those who keep company with the dying learn how to face death faithfully. Sometimes the faithful dying find a voice of their own, but sometimes others must tell their stories. My friend Neil Houk had a voice of his own. His cancer would not be fought back, and he died on September 2, 2007. He lived with honesty, courage, and grace while he was dying, and he taught his friends at First Presbyterian in Durham something of the same virtues. He wrote poems. This one he called "Light in Darkness."[6]

> At the doctor's words,
> "Cancer . . . progressing,"
> shouldn't time
> at least have hiccupped,
> keeping cadence with
> the lurch in my heart?
>
> Now I brood fear and anger,
> like a mother hen, her chicks,
> grudgingly watching
> daylight dissolve,
> the sun sagging silently,
> unawares of me.
>
> Overhead pink clouds
> rush to possess the horizon
> with brilliant hues of rose.
> Leaning toward the window
> I will the colors tarry, yet darkness deepens.

6. Neil's poems were published posthumously in Neil Houk, *Skipping Stones.* St. Andrews College Press, 2008. Reprinted with permission.

Across our little lake,
apartment lights blink on
in the rhythm of the city,
squares of hope,
as if signaling me,
shining in the cold.

So must I shine, I know.
Because I am.
Because you are near.
Because I saw a child's face today.
Because grace surprises.
Because night is.

Still, sometimes, I cry.

Neil was a light to me in my own encounter with my mortality. He was a light to Linda Postema, who would also die from her cancer and who displayed in her own gentle way honesty and courage and grace. He was a light to us all. We all cried at his death. Still, we knew we had learned from him, and we celebrated his dying life. There are other stories to be told in families and congregations that can form the virtues to die well and faithfully. But the story that Neil and Linda participated in needs also to be told again and again, the story of Jesus' death and resurrection.

Then we might learn what it is to die well and faithfully. Then we might be a little less unsure of ourselves in the face of death, even if we still sometimes cry. Then we might be able to resist the medicalization of death. Then the church might take back death from medicine, setting medicine in the context of the gospel (instead of letting the medicalization of death and suffering provide the context for "spirituality").

PART TWO

Ars Moriendi

I have a sinne of feare, that when I have spunne
  My last thred, I shall perish on the shore;
Sweare by thy selfe, that at my death thy Sunne
  Shall shine as it shines now, and heretofore;
  And, having done that, Thou hast done,
  I feare no more.

John Donne, "A Hymne to God the Father"[1]

We began with Aries' story of the transition from "tame death" to "wild death," to medicalized death. We paused to praise physicians and their medicine. We attended briefly to the long story of medical ethics. We noted the challenges to medicalization in the movement for patient rights, in the death awareness movement, and in the hospice movement. We noted as well certain weaknesses of each. And we called for the church to renew its vocation and to fulfill its responsibility to teach people how to die well and how to care well for the dying, to take death back. We turn now to that fifteenth-century effort to teach people an art of dying well, the *Ars Moriendi.*

---

1. John Donne, "A Hymne to God the Father," in *Donne,* Laurel Poetry Series (New York: Dell, 1962), p. 175. The poem was probably written during the sickness of 1623 that nearly took his life. This is the last of three stanzas, and it makes use, of course, of the puns on "done" and "Donne" and on "sun" and "son."

CHAPTER SIX

Death and the Art of Dying in the Fifteenth Century

Ars Moriendi ("The Art of Dying") names both a particular work from the fifteenth century and the genre of literature to which it belongs. Both the particular work and the genre are decidedly nonelitist, the late medieval equivalent of the self-help literature you can find at your local bookstore. Today the title would probably be something like *Dying Well for Dummies.*

Self-help literature, or conduct literature, as it was called then, was popular in the late medieval period. It included topics like courtship, courtesy, education, games, and warfare, but no topic was more popular than "the art of dying." This is not surprising. Death haunted the imagination of the fifteenth century. And little wonder. They had seen too much of it. A series of ruthless plagues, beginning with the Black Death of 1348-50, pandemic warfare, and recurrent famines had been messengers of death, death, and more death. As Johan Huizenga has said, "No other age has so forcefully and continuously impressed the idea of death on the whole population as did the fifteenth century."[1]

It was a fearful time. The messengers of death seemed everywhere, and an awareness that one's own life was a fragile thing was unavoidable. Moreover, in the face of that fear the one institution that had for centuries promised and provided security seemed broken by schism and corrup-

---

1. Johan Huizenga, *The Autumn of the Middle Ages,* trans. Rodney J. Payton and U. Mammitzsch (Chicago: University of Chicago Press, 1996), p. 156.

tion.[2] It was a century lived in the shadows of the Black Death and the "Great Schism" of the Western church.

The Black Death and Plague

In 1348-49 the Black Death ravaged Europe, killing more than a quarter of Europe's population. Endemic following the initial outbreak, plague remained a threatening presence throughout the fifteenth century (and into subsequent centuries; there was, for example, another serious plague in London in 1666). The "pest," as it was called, was an unwelcome guest in the homes of rich and poor. It claimed alike village priest, nobleman, rural housewife. No one was safe from it.[3]

The "pest" was regarded as extremely contagious. Fear of contagion and death prompted parents to abandon their dying children, children to flee from their dying parents, spouses to leave their husbands or wives alone to die. Magistrates and merchants fled the cities for healthier regions. Physicians fled, and so did clergy. Stories of abandonment are commonplace in the literature of the Black Death, most famously in Boccaccio's "Preface to the Ladies," in his *Decameron*. But there are also stories of heroic and faithful caregivers.[4]

2. See, for example, Alberto Tenenti, *La vie et la mort à travers l'art du XVe siècle* (Paris: Colin, 1952); Jean Delumeau, *La peur en Occident: XIVe-XVIIIe siècles, une cité assiégée* (Paris: Fayard, 1978); and Daniel Schafer, *Texte vom Tod. Zur Darstellung und Sinngebung des Tods im Spatmittelalter* (Göppingen: Kummerle, 1995). Delumeau asserted that the role of fear in history had been overlooked; he defined fear as a "shock-emotion" prompted by an awareness of a danger that threatens one's survival (pp. 11-13), and he argued that the centuries following the Black Death were a particularly fearful period. Daniel Schafer, after examining a number of German texts, argued that there was a shift in attitude from the fourteenth to the fifteenth century. It was a shift from confidence to uncertainty in the face of death and from confidence to suspicion of the church, a shift due in large part, he argued, to two events, the Black Death and the Great Schism.

3. Colin Platt, *King Death: The Black Death and Its Aftermath in Late-Medieval England* (Toronto: University of Toronto Press, 1996), provides a powerfully written account of the plague in England.

4. Darrel W. Amundsen, *Medicine, Society, and Faith in the Ancient and Modern Worlds* (Baltimore: Johns Hopkins University Press, 1996), p. 290: "For every account of a magistrate fleeing his office, of a physician hiding in terror, and of a priest refusing to tend to the spiritual needs of his suffering parishioners, there are descriptions of magistrates seeking to do all in their power to serve the public good, of physicians trying desperately to help their patients, and of priests administering the sacraments to the dying."

We have noted Johan Huizenga's claim that the fifteenth century "forcefully and continuously impressed the idea of death on the whole population." He goes on to say that the fifteenth century was morbidly obsessed with death and that its "macabre vision of death lacked everything elegiac as well as everything tender." The fifteenth-century attitude to death was, he said, "self-preoccupied": "It does not deal with sadness over the loss of those beloved, but rather with regret about one's own approaching death, which can be seen only as misfortune and terror. There is no thought given to death as consolation, to the end of suffering, eternal rest, the task completed or broken off, no tender memories, no surrender."[5] There is plenty of evidence for the accuracy of Huizenga's judgment. In much medieval art the skeletal figures of the "Dances of Death" snatched the living and dragged them to their own deaths. Much poetry of the time exhibited a certain macabre realism, fixated on the stench, the rot, and the worms of the corpses we are all — whether kings or clerics or commoners — destined to become. Even so, in the midst of the fifteenth century, the *Ars Moriendi* attempted to show Christians the way toward a good death. It may be regarded as "self-preoccupied," but it otherwise is an exception to Huizenga's judgment that the century was empty of thoughts of consolation and relief from suffering, eternal rest and surrender. It was an effort not to instill terror at the prospect of death but to meet that fear and to overcome it.

The subject of death has always been present in literature, and it was never a more popular topic than in the late Middle Ages. But the *Ars Moriendi* was not a literary treatment of a theme. It was not a reminder of death that we may live well. It did not dwell on death in order to commend a virtuous life. It was not an *Ars Vivendi,* although the genre would eventually move in that direction. It was a self-help manual for the person who was dying. In times of plague one could not always count on a visit by the priest. It was to be read (and perhaps memorized) while one was still in good health, but it was to be kept and used in the days and hours of dying. It was a set of instructions for dying well.

The plague prompted some bizarre responses not only in the macabre images to be found in the art and literature of the time but also in both medicine and religion. It is no surprise that quacks flourished during plague, greedily promising cures to the anxious and gullible sick ready to try anything. But the physicians who urged prophylactic measures frequently recommended some odd behaviors, including carrying various precious

5. Huizenga, *Autumn,* pp. 170-71.

stones.[6] Religious responses were sometimes no less odd. They included, for example, self-flagellation. To be sure, the flagellant movement did not begin in response to the plague; the order of the Penitents, whose members whipped themselves in an effort to identify with the suffering of Christ and to appease God's wrath against the sins of humanity, had been founded already in the thirteenth century. But it became a popular movement during the Black Death. Because the plague was widely regarded as God's punishment for sin, groups of people would engage in self-flagellation as a way to appease God's wrath, cleanse themselves from sin, and end the plague.

There were also, of course, less bizarre responses. The plague prompted many physicians to question more openly the authority of the medical tradition and to rely more on experience and experiment.[7] And it prompted many churchmen to question more openly the authority of the church's hierarchy, especially the cult of relics and practice of indulgences. And although it was a time when physicians and priests who abandoned their patients and parishioners during plague brought themselves and their vocations into disrepute, it was also a time when faithful physicians and priests won the admiration and affection of the population for their courage and fidelity.[8]

In general the church and medicine cooperated in their efforts to meet the challenge of the plague. When the Black Death came to Avignon, which was then the seat of the papacy, Clement VI took measures to try to limit the spread of the disease. He hired physicians to care for the sick and provided a mass to petition for a quick end to the plague. He also gave special indulgences to priests who would minister to the sick and dying, less time in purgatory in exchange for enduring the risks of ministry. Some

6. Amundsen, *Medicine, Society, and Faith*, p. 298.

7. Amundsen, *Medicine, Society, and Faith*, p. 300. This new attitude, suspicious of ancient "authorities" and eager for knowledge tested by experience (and experiment), prepared the way for Francis Bacon's suspicion of "speculative" knowledge and his celebration of "practical knowledge."

8. The accounts of mass hysteria and panic may be exaggerated; so, at least, Richard W. Emery suggested (Emery, "The Black Death of 1348 in Perpignan," *Speculum* 42 [1967]: 620-21, cited by Amundsen, *Medicine, Society, and Faith*, p. 290). Amundsen's account of the plague tractates is itself an important piece of evidence for courage and compassion in the face of the plague. There is no doubt, however, that the Black Death prompted considerable fear and anxiety both about death and about an uncertain eschatological future. But whether because many brave clergy died or because a fearful clergy could not be counted on to minister to the victims of the plague, the church would before long provide the self-help literature of the *Ars Moriendi*.

theologians argued against the use of physicians, either on the grounds that the plague was God's punishment and should be simply endured with repentance or on the grounds that the efforts of physicians were obviously not effective. And there were physicians — and others — who lost confidence in the church and its hierarchy because of the ineffectiveness of relics and special masses and processionals against the plague (and because the church seemed unwilling to heed physicians' concerns about contagion at massive processionals).[9]

It was not just some physicians, however, who had lost confidence in the church. In a century of fear and anxiety prompted by the plague, the one institution that had for centuries promised and provided security seemed broken by schism and corruption.

The "Great Schism" in the Western Church

The uncertainty of many in the face of death had been exacerbated by a loss of confidence in the church and especially in the papacy. At the time of the Black Death the papacy had been transferred from Rome to Avignon, a tiny principality in the south of France. The departure of the papacy from Peter's see was widely regarded as a scandal, and the scandal diminished the authority of the papacy in the minds of many, especially those who lived outside France.[10]

Pressure grew to return the papacy to Rome. Lest the papacy risk losing all authority in other countries, Gregory XI recognized that the papacy

---

9. Amundsen, *Medicine, Society, and Faith,* p. 208.

10. Since the residence of the pope in Avignon lasted from 1305 to 1378, or approximately seventy years, the period would come to be called the Babylonian captivity of the papacy in memory of the captivity of the Jews. The popes, of course, were in Avignon voluntarily. The causes of this Avignon "captivity" were largely political. With the rise of nations the nascent states of France, England, and Spain challenged the power of the papacy, which had once provided unity and solidarity to the West. The kings defied papal authority when it served their national interests. And the church, which had exercised political and financial power for centuries, was loath to give it up. Pope Boniface was almost unavoidably enmeshed in political intrigue, and although he asserted papal power quite successfully for a time, when he died in 1304 the cardinals were split into a pro-French and an anti-French faction. The pro-French faction succeeded in electing a French cardinal, who became Clement V. He never left France to go to Rome; instead, he became the first pope to reside at Avignon. A succession of French popes favored France, supporting the French cause against England in the Hundred Years' War, which began during this time. And they lived lavishly, spending exorbitant funds on the construction of a papal palace at Avignon and on pomp and ceremony.

would have to leave Avignon and return to Rome. In 1377 he did return to Rome. His French cardinals, however, stayed in Avignon. At his death in Rome in 1387, angry Roman crowds demanded an Italian pope. Urban VI was elected, but some French cardinals, citing the civil disorder at the election of Urban VI, elected another pope, Clement VII, who returned to Avignon after an armed battle for the control of Rome. Now there were two popes. The church was divided, and all Europe along with it. The French supported Clement VII and Avignon, while England, Germany, and many others sided with Urban VI and Rome. Rival bishops in each country supported the rival popes. If Avignon was a scandal, the Great Schism was a disgrace.

In an effort to remedy the schism, some pious and thoughtful leaders on both sides called for the revival of the Conciliar Movement, in which the great ecumenical councils had decided the great doctrinal questions from the fourth through the eighth century. But never had the councils deposed or elected popes. It was a radical innovation that would place authority in the church under Christ in a representative assembly. Cardinals on both sides of the schism called for a council at Pisa in 1409. The rival popes refused to attend. With disgust the Council of Pisa deposed them both and elected Alexander V in their place. Neither Rome nor Avignon, however, recognized this new pope or, when he died a year later, his successor, John XXIII.[11] Now there were not two but three popes. If Avignon was a scandal and the schism a disgrace, this was a farce.

But the reform movement was not done. It was decided that a pope, not cardinals, must call the council, and John XXIII, unwelcome at either Rome or Avignon, had nothing to lose, so he was persuaded to convene a council in 1414, the Council of Constance, in what is now Switzerland. The council tried and deposed John. The Roman pope Gregory XII resigned in 1415. The Avignon pope Benedict XIII was tried and deposed in 1417. When it elected a new pope, Martin V, there was finally an end to the Great Schism.[12]

---

11. Perhaps that is just as well. John XXIII so disgraced the name that no subsequent pope took the name until the beloved pope of the twentieth century took again the name of John XXIII.

12. The Council of Constance had other things on its agenda as well, of course, notably responses to the movements initiated by John Wycliffe in England and by Jan Huss in Bohemia. Given a safe-conduct that presumably guaranteed his safe return home, Huss welcomed the summons to Constance to be examined. But the safe-conduct was revoked, and when the council declared him guilty of heresy, he was burned at the stake. It was a shameful episode in an otherwise commendable council.

The Council of Constance did not end the threat of the plague, of course, or suddenly restore confidence in the church or the papacy during the anxious times of the fifteenth century. But it did put an end to the Great Schism. And it may have played a small role in the development of the *Ars Moriendi*.

Jean Charlier Gerson and His Pastoral Handbook at Constance

Jean Charlier Gerson (1363-1429), the chancellor of the University of Paris, had been one of the earliest champions of the Conciliar Movement and played a leading role at the Council of Constance. He knew, however, that the reform of the church required not just an end to schism but the renewal of parish ministry. Toward that end he had written a little pastoral handbook called *Opusculum Tripertitum*, whose purpose was to instruct both clergy and laity engaged in Christian service. It was the precursor to the *Ars Moriendi* literature.

Chancellor of the university, highly regarded among his peers, he was an advocate of the contemplative life, the author of *De Mystica Theologia*, among other works, but he was no elitist. He did not want mystical theology to be the sole possession of a favored few. Mystical theology is, he said, an "experiential knowledge of God attained through the union of spiritual affection with Him."[13] That mystical union is not an "essential union" or "equality with God" but "that which unites the one who loves with the beloved." To clarify the meaning of this union Gerson quoted Aristotle's notion of friendship: "'Among friends there is a conformity of will.' Thus, when our spirit clings to God through the most intimate love it is one spirit with Him through conformity of will (1 Cor. 6:17)."[14] This mystical knowledge, Gerson insisted, is accessible to any faithful Christian, regardless of status, sex, or education. He regarded it as the calling of the pastor to nurture that knowledge in the laity. And he regarded faithfulness and competence in that vocation as no less important to the renewal of the church than the efforts of the council to end the schism.

Gerson's pastoral handbook *Opusculum Tripertitum* had three parts: the first part treated the Ten Commandments; the second, confession; and

---

13. Jean Gerson, *Selections from "A Deo exivit," "Contra curiositate studentium," and "De mystica theologia speculativa,"* ed. and trans. Stephen E. Ozment (Leiden: Brill, 1969), p. 64.

14. Gerson, *Selections*, pp. 48-49.

the third, ministry to the dying, entitled *Scientia Mortis*. The work was composed in Latin and then translated by Gerson himself into French in an effort to broaden its audience and its influence.[15] It is likely that he took copies to the Council of Constance for the same purpose. Gerson's handbook did come to have a wide audience and it did prove influential. The French clerical hierarchy, for example, requested that the pastorate deliver this work orally to their congregations.[16] But no part of it proved more influential than its third section on ministry to the dying. The plague was the spur for the development of the *Ars Moriendi* manuals for self-help, and Gerson's handbook was the model.

Ars Moriendi

Soon after the Council of Constance, treatises on the art of dying began to appear, frequently entitled *Speculum Artis Bene Moriendi* or *Tractatis Artis Bene Moriendi*, incorporating material from Gerson's final section.[17] Such treatises became popular and influential in the fifteenth century. They characteristically bore the marks of Gerson's nonelitist mystical theology, nurturing the union of the dying person with God in spiritual affection for God and conformity of the will to God's will, emphasizing experiential knowledge without demeaning a cognitive element,[18] and emphasizing the relation of affection between the believer and God without denying the necessity of the church's doctrine and sacraments.[19]

15. The Latin text may be found in Johannes Gerson, *Opera Omnia*, ed. Louis Ellier Du Pin (Hildesheim: George Olms Verlag, 1987 [a reprint of Antwerp 1706]), 1:425-50; the French text, in *Oeuvres complètes*, ed. Mgr. Glorieux (Paris: Desclée, 1960-73), 7:404-7.

16. Scott L. Taylor, "'L'age plus fort ennaye': *Scienta Mortis, Ars Moriendi* and Jean Gerson's Advice to an Old Man," in *Old Age in the Middle Ages and Renaissance*, ed. Albrecht Classen (Berlin: Walter de Gruyter, 2007), p. 408 n. 2. When the work was translated into Dutch in 1512, the Dutch hierarchy did the same.

17. Taylor, "L'age plus fort ennaye," p. 408. According to Mary Catherine O'Connor, the original work in the genre was an anonymous text from the early fifteenth century, *Tractatis Artis Bene Moriendi*. Mary Catherine O'Connor, *The Art of Dying Well: The Development of the* Ars Moriendi (New York: Columbia University Press, 1942), p. 1.

18. Steven E. Ozment, *Homo Spiritualis: A Comparative Study of Johannes Tauler, Jean Gerson, and Martin Luther in the Context of Their Theological Thought* (Leiden: Brill, 1969), p. 71, says that for Gerson mystical theology is "in an experiential mode *(experimentalis)* but it will also be knowledge *(cognitio)*."

19. See Ozment, *Homo Spiritualis*, pp. 76-77.

Variations on the theme of *ars moriendi* were soon published in every major European language. The popularity of the genre is attested by the fact that there are at least three hundred manuscripts in both Latin and the vernacular languages. Editions made from engraved wood blocks and from movable type were published well over a hundred times before 1500. Works in the genre continued to be produced during the sixteenth century, and the genre influenced books on dying well into the eighteenth century.[20] Roman Catholics, Lutherans, Calvinists, and Anglicans all provided works within the genre.

One early variation was a much abridged version accompanied by striking wood-block prints. It made the older treatises on the art of dying available to a wide audience. It was this extraordinarily popular[21] shorter and illustrated version, a fifteenth-century equivalent of a *Reader's Digest* edition, that was entitled *Ars Moriendi.*

The *Tractatus Artis Bene Moriendi* and its early variations and translations[22] contain six parts. The first part is a commendation of death. The second part warns the dying person of the temptations confronted by the dying and gives advice about how to resist them. The third part provides a short catechism with questions and answers concerning repentance and the assurance of God's pardon. The fourth part offers instructions on the imitation of the dying Christ and suggests prayers for use by the dying. The fifth part counsels persons, both the sick and those who care for them, to attend to these matters as matters of first importance. Finally, the sixth part provides a series of prayers to be prayed by those who minister to the dying person. Subsequent works within this genre did not always follow this order exactly, but they usually covered a similar agenda. The block book, *Ars Moriendi,* focuses on the temptations, rendering and illustrating them with a series of eleven prints, one for each of five temptations, one for each of five victories over temptation, and a final print depicting the

20. O'Connor, *Art of Dying Well,* pp. 1ff.

21. Its popularity is demonstrated in the striking fact that about 20 percent of the surviving block books (that is, books printed from engraved wood blocks) are copies of the *Ars Moriendi.* Dick Akerboom, "'Only the Image of Christ in Us': Continuity and Discontinuity between the Late Medieval *ars moriendi* and Luther's Sermon *von der Bereitung zum Sterben*," in *Spirituality Renewed: Studies on Significant Representatives of the Modern Devotion,* ed. Hein Blommestijn, Charles Caspters, and Rijcklof Hofman (Leuven: Peeters, 2003), pp. 209-72, 221.

22. See, for example, William Caxton's English version of 1490, *The Arte & Crafte to Know Well to Dye.*

moment of death itself. But even that short work contains the six items and begins with a commendation of death.

In search of an alternative to medicalized death, we turn back to an earlier episode in the history of dying, back to the fifteenth century and to the tradition that has come to be known as the *Ars Moriendi*. In the face of the anxiety and fear of the fifteenth century and in spite of the trouble in the church, the *Ars Moriendi* pointed the way toward dying well. Perhaps it can point the way for the twenty-first century as well. Perhaps, but perhaps not! Perhaps an examination of the *Ars Moriendi* of the fifteenth century will provide an alternative to a medicalized death that is equally problematic. At the very least, however, the *Ars Moriendi* might free our imagination a little. This episode in the history of dying may at least liberate us from the sense that we are simply fated to a medicalized death.

Can we retrieve the *Ars Moriendi?* We do not live in the fifteenth century, of course. We should not pretend to, and not many of us would want to. It was a time, as we have observed, of plague in Europe and of schism in the church. Nostalgia for the fifteenth century is not a temptation. Still, can we imagine a contemporary *Ars Moriendi* as an alternative to "medicalized" death? And if we can, what should a contemporary "art of dying" look like? What should we retrieve from the fifteenth century? And what should we reject? To address such questions, we turn back to the fifteenth century, back to the *Ars Moriendi,* examining it carefully, following the order of the earliest examples of the genre, describing each part as sympathetically as we can, trying to learn from it but sometimes quarreling with it as well. We begin, therefore, where *Ars Moriendi* began, with the "commendacion of death."

CHAPTER SEVEN

The "Commendacion of Death"

[D]ethe ys nothyng elles but agoyng owte off pryson and endyng off exyle, and dyschargyng off an hevy burden that ys the body, fynysshyng of all infyrmytees, escapyng off all perylles, destroy-ying off all euell thynges, brekyng of all bondys, payinge off all dette off naturall dewte, tornyng ayene in to hys contre and enteryng in to blysse and ioye.

Crafte and Knowledge For To Dye Well (1490)[1]

The first chapter of *Crafte and Knowledge For To Dye Well,* an anonymous manuscript from 1490, is "a commendacion of death" (p. 1). Such a begin-

---

1. *Crafte and Knowledge For To Dye Well* was an early English treatise of the *Ars Moriendi* tradition, a manuscript offering a translation of the French *Tractatis* into English (dated around 1490). The citations of this and other English *Ars Moriendi* texts are, unless otherwise noted, from the convenient anthology edited by David William Atkinson, *The English* Ars Moriendi, Renaissance and Baroque Studies and Texts, vol. 5 (New York: Peter Lang, 1992). This particular quotation is from p. 2. Hereafter it will be cited simply with page numbers from Atkinson in parentheses. I have usually preserved the antique English; where it may be difficult to understand I have provided contemporary language in brackets. Here: "Death is nothing other than the release from prison and the ending of exile, the discharging of the heavy burden that is the body, the end of all infirmities, the escape from all perils, the destruction of all evil things, the breaking of all bondage, the release from all obligations of natural duty, the journeying again to one's own homeland, and the entering into bliss and joy."

ning is typical of works in the *Ars Moriendi* genre. Indeed, such a beginning provides the context for the particular treatise called *Ars Moriendi* and for the whole genre. But do we really want to join them in commending death? The commendation of death may be not only the beginning of many of the treatises; it may also be the beginning of problems with them. Before we ask whether we should commend the "commendacion of death," however, we should let the tradition speak. The commendation in *Crafte* may be taken as illustrative.

The short preface to this work acknowledges that death is a dreadful and fearful thing, that even to "relygyous and deuoute persons" death "semeth wonderfull harde and ryght perlyous, and also ryght ferful and horryble." It is this dread and fear of death that prompt both *Crafte* and the rest of the *Ars Moriendi* literature. This is not so much Aries' "tame death" as death that needs taming. It is because death seems so dreadful and fearful that the author writes "for techying and comfortyng of hem that been in poynt off deathe." Already in the preface, however, that "techying and comfortyng" takes the form of a commendation of death; it is, *Crafte* says, our passage "owte off the wrechednesse of the exyle of thys worlde" (p. 1). If this world is our place of exile, a land of captivity, then death may be celebrated as "going home." And it was.

The first chapter of *Crafte*, like the preface, acknowledges that death is awful. The author cites Aristotle to make the point that death is "moste dredefull and all ferefull."[2] But immediately Aristotle's verdict on death is qualified and then rejected. *Crafte* insists that the "spirituall dethe of the sowle" is much more dreadful and fearful than the death of the body (p. 1). Indeed, for a Christian the death of the body ought to be considered neither dreadful nor fearful. Death is rather to be commended by the faithful.

In commending death *Crafte* draws upon various authorities, especially Scripture, of course, but also theologians and philosophers. One biblical text cited here, and regularly in the *Ars* literature, is Psalm 116:15:

---

2. Aristotle, *Nicomachean Ethics* 3.1115a: "the most fearful thing of all is death." Aristotle goes on to explain that death is the most fearful thing because "it is the end, and once a man is dead it seems that there is no longer anything good or evil for him." The remark comes in the context of Aristotle's discussion of courage. Few of the quotations offered by *Ars Moriendi* and *Crafte* are quite so easy to trace as this one. I have done my best to track the references down, but it has sometimes been impossible. The author seems frequently to be quoting from memory.

Precious in the sight of the LORD
  is the death of his faithful ones. (p. 1)

Crafte pauses to make the point that it is not just the deaths of saints and martyrs that are cherished by God, but also the deaths of repentant sinners who die in a state of true "repentance and contrycion" (p. 2). Next Revelation 14:13 is cited: "Blessed are the dead . . . who die in the Lord." And hard on the heels of that text, *Crafte* cites Wisdom of Solomon 4:7, "But the righteous, though they die early, will be at rest." They will go "to a place refreshynge." These texts of Scripture prompt the commendation that we set at the head of this chapter: "dethe ys nothyng elles but agoyng owte off pryson and endyng off exyle, and dyschargyng off an hevy burden that ys the body, fynysshyng of all infyrmytees, escapyng off all perylles, destroyying off all euell thynges, brekyng of all bondys, payinge off all dette off naturall dewte, tornyng ayene in to hys contre and enteryng in to blysse and ioye." Quite a commendation indeed. The argument from Scripture is clinched by a citation of Ecclesiastes 7:1: "the day of death [is better] than the day of birth." And the conclusion follows that Christians, including those who turn to God from sin on their deathbed, need not and should not be sorry at the prospect of death or troubled by it. On the contrary, if they would die well, they may and should die "gladely and wylfully." A Christian may and should suffer death patiently, "conformyng [his will] to Goddes wyll." In this way the "reason of hys mynde . . . rewleth hys sensualyte" (p. 2).

Crafte provides next a series of citations from the Roman Stoic Seneca. It cites him, for example, to underscore the point that "to dye wele ys to dye gladely and wylfully" (p. 2).[3] It cites him again to call attention to the importance of the reason of the mind ruling desires and to make the well-worn point that it is more important to live well than to live long (reinforcing the earlier citation of Wisdom of Solomon 4:7).[4] To live well is,

3. Cf. Lucius Annaeus Seneca, *Epistle* 61, "On Meeting Death Cheerfully," in *Seneca, Epistles 1–65,* trans. Richard M. Gummere, Loeb Classical Library 75 (Cambridge: Harvard University Press, 1917/2002), pp. 425-27: "[D]ying well means dying gladly. See to it that you never do anything unwillingly."

4. Seneca's epistle "On Meeting Death Cheerfully" continues, p. 427: "This is what I mean: he who takes his orders gladly, escapes the bitterest part of slavery, — doing what one does not want to do. The man who does something under orders is not unhappy; he is unhappy who does something against his will. Let us therefore so set our minds in order that we may desire whatever is demanded of us by circumstance, and above all that we may re-

for *Crafte,* to be conformed to God's will, and when and how one dies is determined by God's will. There is a certain Stoic fatalism in that claim. What the Stoic might have attributed to *Fortuna, Crafte* attributes to God's will. The Stoic fatalism is relieved somewhat by assurances from the fifth-century monastic theologian John Cassian that almighty God in wisdom and goodness providentially orders everything that happens, whether adversity or prosperity, to the good of God's children.[5] But whether death is attributed to fate or to providence, *Crafte* insists, echoing the Stoic Seneca, that since we cannot escape death, "we owghten to take oure deth when God wyll wylfully and gladely, withoute any grochying" (p. 3). "Grouching" may be natural enough in the midst of agony, but it is not the path of reason or virtue. That path is pointed out by another citation of Seneca to the effect that we should "suffre esely and blame natt that thow mayst natt chaunge ne voyde [endure easily and blame not what you can neither change nor avoid]" (p. 3).[6] *Crafte* adds another observation, again attrib-

---

flect upon our end without sadness. . . . To have lived long enough depends neither upon our years nor upon our days, but upon our minds." Cf. also Seneca, *Epistle* 93, "On the Quality, as Contrasted with the Length, of Life," in Seneca, *Epistles 93–124,* trans. Richard M. Gummere, Loeb Classical Library 77 (Cambridge: Harvard University Press, 1925/2006), pp. 2-5: "We should strive, not to live long, but to live rightly. . . . A life is really long if it is a full life, but fulness is not attained until the soul has rendered to itself its proper Good, that is, until it has assumed control over itself."

5. See John Cassian, "The Third Conference of Abba Chaeremon: On God's Protection," in John Cassian, *The Conferences,* trans. Boniface Ramsey, O.P., Ancient Christian Writers 57 (Mahwah, N.J.: Newman Press, 1997), pp. 465-91; see especially chapters 13–17. Seneca, too, could reflect on Providence. See, e.g., Seneca, *De providentia,* in Seneca, *Moral Essays,* vol. 1, trans. John Basore, Loeb Classical Library 253 (Cambridge: Harvard University Press, 1928/2003), pp. 2-47.

6. Mary Catherine O'Connor, *The Art of Dying Well: The Development of the* Ars Moriendi (New York: Columbia University Press, 1942), p. 26, identifies the quotation as from Publilius Syrus rather than from Seneca. I could not find the quotation in Seneca, but the thought is surely present. In his *De consolatione ad Polybium,* in Seneca, *Moral Essays,* vol. 2, trans. John Basore, Loeb Classical Library 254 (Cambridge: Harvard University Press, 1932/2001), pp. 356-415, Seneca says that fate *stant dura et inexorabilia* (p. 364). Then, of course, we can neither change nor avoid it. And he goes on to say that grief tortures us without accomplishing anything useful; "unless reason puts an end to our tears, fortune will not do so" (p. 367). *Crafte* may have outreached even Seneca on this point, however, for in the conclusion of this essay (p. 413) Seneca observes: "Reason will have accomplished enough if only she removes from grief whatever is excessive and superfluous; it is not for anyone to hope or to desire that she should suffer us to feel no sorrow at all. . . . Let your tears flow, but let them also cease, let the deepest sighs be drawn from your breast, but let them also find an end; so rule your mind that you may win approval both from wise men and from brothers." Cf. also

uted to Seneca, that the remedy for suffering is not "that thow be in another place, but that thow be another man,"[7] that is, a person whose reason governs desire. A certain "wyseman" is then cited in order to exhort the reader to become a new person, with a heart and soul always looking to God, always ready and eager to be with God.[8]

The conclusion of this commendation of death is that death should be welcomed, received as one would a "welbeloued and trusti frende" (p. 3). The reader is admonished to live his life "in pacience" and to die his death "in desyre" — specifically, in that longing of which Paul speaks in his letter to the Philippians (1:23), "my desire is to depart and be with Christ, for that is far better."

Should We Commend the "Commendacion" of Death?

One can and should acknowledge the author's motive here. As the preface states, the goal was to comfort the person facing death. And that comfort nurtured courage, too. It was *com-fortis,* a strengthening as well as a solace. Indeed, although *Crafte* does not later include courage among the virtues for dying well, perhaps the first virtue is courage, courage in the face of death and in spite of the fear of death.[9] The familiarity with death in the centuries of the plague had prompted both a preoccupation with death and a contempt for it. The *Ars Moriendi* tradition surely displays that preoccupation, but it may also ironically display the culture's contempt for death by its very effort to commend it. There is no irony in this commendation of death, but one gets the sense that the author protests too much. A charitable reading of this and other commendations of death would acknowledge, I think, that they are prompted by a deep love of life and a deeper love of God. These are intended to be words of comfort and of

---

Seneca, *De consolatione ad Marciam,* in *Moral Essays,* 2:21: "If sorrow will help, let us vent it. . . . But if no wailing can recall the dead . . . then let grief, which is futile, cease."

7. Again I could not find the precise quotation in Seneca. But the thought is surely present, echoing Seneca's remark in "On Meeting Death Cheerfully," *Epistle* 61, in *Epistles 1–65,* and the line from *De consolatione ad Polybium,* in *Moral Essays,* 2:367: "unless reason puts an end to our tears, fortune will not do so."

8. This "wyseman" is probably a reference to Ezekiel, and the passage is perhaps Ezek. 18:23-32 (so Atkinson, *The English* Ars Moriendi, suggests, p. 364 n. 13).

9. It is, perhaps, no accident that the opening citation from Aristotle came from his discussion of courage. See n. 2 above.

courage. The strategy was to render death less fearsome, less destructive, less threatening by commending it.

Even so, this is not a strategy Christians should adopt. And the fundamental reason is that it does not fit well with the Christian story. The very source that the *Ars Moriendi* tradition regarded as normative and most frequently cited, the Christian Scripture, resists that strategy and may be used to challenge and correct it. A fuller account of the biblical narrative as the context for thinking faithfully about dying well and about caring well for the dying will be given in the next part of the book. Here it is necessary only to consider the passages that *Crafte* cites in its commendation of death and to give enough of an account of the biblical narrative to challenge that commendation.

Consider, first, Psalm 116:15, the passage given pride of place in *Crafte* and a favorite of the *Ars Moriendi* literature:

> Precious in the sight of the LORD
>   is the death of his faithful ones.

The *Crafte* — and the *Ars Moriendi* literature generally — reads this psalm (and the Psalms generally) as though the psalmist was focused on life after death, as though he lived in perpetual hope of eternal and otherworldly bliss. But Psalm 116 is a psalm of thanksgiving for healing. Death is not commended in the psalm but regarded as an enemy and a threat. The psalmist reports that he had been very sick, near to death. "The snares of death encompassed me" (v. 3). But he did not practice hospitality to death, as if receiving a long-awaited friend. Rather, he says he had prayed to God, "O LORD, I pray, save my life!" (v. 4), and that the Lord had heard his prayer and answered it. The psalmist finds delight not in death but in life. The lesson he draws from this experience is that the Lord is gracious (v. 5), but the evidence of this grace is that the Lord preserved his life. God is to be praised, for God gives and preserves life. Finally, the psalmist vows to make a sacrifice of thanksgiving to God for preserving his life (v. 13). In this context, therefore, the psalmist's statement that death is "precious" in the sight of the Lord is not put forward to commend death, but to insist that God regards death as something costly, as the loss of someone or something dear. The Lord brings salvation not by bringing death, but by restoring life. God cherishes not the death of the saints but their life.

Many psalms evidently regarded death not as deliverance from exile, but as something like an endless exile. Death is not a passage into an eternal life spent in praise of God but a shadowy and joyless existence cut off from the praise of God. So, for example, in another song of thanksgiving for God's gracious gift of healing, the psalmist remonstrates with God,

> What profit is there in my death,
>   if I go down to the Pit?
> Will the dust praise you?
>   Will it tell of your faithfulness?
>
> (Ps. 30:9)

His premature death would have been loss to God, not profit, and a costly loss at that, a "precious" loss. Similarly in Psalm 88, the psalmist, after reporting that he had been sick from his youth onward and that he now faces the prospect of death, cries out to God:

> Do you work wonders for the dead?
>   Do the shades rise up to praise you?
> Is your steadfast love declared in the grave,
>   or your faithfulness in Abaddon?[10]
> Are your wonders known in the darkness,
>   or your saving help in the land of forgetfulness?
>
> (vv. 10-12)

In such lyrics the dead are regarded as dust, as shadows or shades *(rephaim)* of their former selves, unable to praise God. This is not, of course, the whole story of Scripture, or even of the Old Testament, but it is certainly enough to make us suspicious of reading Psalm 116:15 or other psalms to commend death.[11]

The second biblical citation in *Crafte* is Revelation 14:13, "Blessed are

---

10. "Abaddon" is the realm of the dead, roughly equivalent to "Sheol."

11. That the Psalms — indeed, the whole Old Testament (apart from the late apocalyptic passages like Dan. 12:2 and Isa. 26:19) — do not envision life after death is something of a consensus in contemporary biblical scholarship. It has not, it should be observed, gone altogether unchallenged. Mitchell Dahood, *Psalms III 101–150*, Anchor Bible 17A (Garden City, N.Y.: Doubleday, 1970), for example, reads many of the psalms as presupposing a life after death. I am not capable of judging the arguments invoking Ugaritic cognates, but he argues, for example, that "life" is "eternal life." (See the summary of his argument, pp. xli-lii.) His arguments, however, have not been accepted by most scholars, and the consensus remains a consensus. As I note later, a couple of psalms — notably Pss. 49 and 73 — may suggest an afterlife. See further the chapter "Death in the Psalms," in C. S. Lewis, *Reflections on the Psalms* (New York: Harcourt, Brace and World, 1958), pp. 34-43.

the dead who from now on die in the Lord." Revelation, however, does not here commend death itself. Rather it commends those who "keep the commandments of God and hold fast to the faith of Jesus" (Rev. 14:12). The beatitude John pronounces is an eschatological blessing, promising life and human flourishing in the good future of God, when "death will be no more" (21:4). In Revelation it is not death that is celebrated but God's victory over death. Death is an enemy, not a friend. Death rides "a pale green horse" and kills "with sword, famine, and pestilence" (6:8). It strikes fear in the hearts of all. To be sure, Revelation does call its readers to courage and endurance in the face of death, but its strategy is not to commend death, but to celebrate God's victory over death. God won that victory over death when he raised Jesus from the dead. Jesus is "the firstborn of the dead" (1:5). The final triumph over death will only come at the end. Then, according to John's vision, "Death and Hades gave up the dead that were in them"; then Death itself will be put to death (20:13). But that good future, God's final triumph over death, is not yet. God has "already" triumphed over death in the resurrection of Jesus, but our full participation in that triumph is still sadly not yet, even for the martyrs. The martyrs — no less than the living — have by God's grace already some share in it, but they too — no less than the living — must wait and watch and pray for God's final triumph over death. The martyrs cry out in lament, "How long?" They are given white robes and told to rest a little longer (6:10-11). The beatitude of Revelation 14:13 can hardly be read as a commendation of death.

The third text, Wisdom of Solomon 4:7, with its assurance of "rest" for the righteous who die young, may reasonably be interpreted as a commendation of death, but it is the exception that proves the rule. A premature death had been regarded by ancient Jews as a "bad death," and the premature death of the righteous was seen as a challenge to God's justice. This challenge to God's justice had evidently been taken up by "the ungodly." The Wisdom of Solomon was concerned to correct "the ungodly" argument that begins with the premise that "there is no return from our death" (2:5) and moves to a conclusion that justifies sensuality and oppression. The ungodly may conclude, "therefore, let us enjoy the good things that exist," taking our fill of pleasures and taking no thought for the oppression of the poor, and "let our might be our law of right" (2:6-11), but wisdom rejects such an argument. The Wisdom of Solomon meets that argument by calling attention to God's power and righteousness, and by denying the initial premise. The consolation here for those who die young is that they are spared the temptations of falling into evil. There are some things worse than death. Without mentioning Enoch by name, the passage goes on to use him as an example of those

> who pleased God and were loved by him,
> and while living among sinners were taken up.
>
> (4:10)[12]

They were taken up

> so that evil might not change their understanding
> or guile deceive their souls.
> For the fascination of wickedness obscures what is good,
> and roving desire perverts the innocent mind.
>
> (4:11-12)

God rescues the righteous youth from this world of wickedness and desire by death. There is a striking parallel in Seneca:

> Do you complain, Marcia, that your son did not live as long as he might have lived? For how do you know whether it was advisable for him to live longer? . . . Human affairs are unstable and fleeting, and no part of our life is so frail and perishable as that which gives most pleasure, and therefore at the height of good fortune we ought to pray for death. . . . [He then lists a series of possible afflictions of long life, from the loss of beauty and vigor to "the thousand taints of the soul," dissipation, and disgrace.] If you will consider all these possibilities, you will learn that those who are treated most kindly by Nature are those whom she removes early to a place of safety.[13]

The parallel is striking but not shocking, for this apocryphal book is itself a product of Hellenistic Judaism.[14] Like Seneca, it had assimilated Hellenistic patterns of thought.

---

12. Enoch's 365 years hardly seems like a short life, but he was younger by far than the other descendants of Adam listed in Gen. 5.

13. Seneca, *De consolatione ad Marciam*, in *Moral Essays*, 2:76, quoted in David Winston, *The Wisdom of Solomon*, Anchor Bible 43 (Garden City, N.Y.: Doubleday, 1979), pp. 140-41.

14. It was probably written in Alexandria in the first century before or the first century after Christ. Winston, *The Wisdom of Solomon*, argues for the first century after Christ, around the time of Philo, with whose Hellenistic Judaism, as Winston shows, the Wisdom of Solomon has great affinity.

The Wisdom of Solomon displays its indebtedness to Hellenistic patterns of thought also when it assumes the immortality of the soul.[15] That is an assumption shared, of course, by *Crafte*. "God created us for incorruption," Wisdom says,

and made us in the image of his own eternity,
but through the devil's envy death entered the world,
and those who belong to his company experience it.
But the souls of the righteous are in the hand of God,
and no torment will ever touch them.
In the eyes of the foolish they seemed to have died,
and their departure was thought to be a disaster,
and their going from us to be their destruction;
but they are at peace.

(2:23–3:3)

Even the Wisdom of Solomon, however, stops short of commending death finally.

God did not make death,
and he does not delight in the death of the living.

(1:13)

It is the ungodly who "invite death," who "summoned" it, and who consider death "a friend" (1:12, 16).

Crafte cites also Ecclesiastes 7:1, "the day of death [is better] than the day of birth." It surely sounds like a commendation of death, but to read it as such is to ignore the rest of Ecclesiastes. To be sure, Ecclesiastes is famous for its account of human life and effort as meaningless, "Vanity of vanities! . . . All is vanity!" (1:2; 12:8; and "vanity" passim). But the sage who wrote Ecclesiastes does not turn away from this world or this life toward a future bliss whose entry is death. He turns back to this world and this life and to their simple pleasures: "I know that there is nothing better for [people] than to be happy and enjoy themselves as long as they live" (3:12; see also 2:24; 3:22; 5:18-19; 8:15; 9:7-9; 11:7-12). It is this world and this life that are affirmed, even if human beings in their "wisdom" can make no sense of them. Thus it is enjoyment, not death, that Ecclesiastes "commends" (8:15).

15. It should be noted, however, that for the Wisdom of Solomon immortality is at its root a gift of God and due to the power of God; it is not simply a human possession or due simply to the nature of the soul (15:3).

In several places in Ecclesiastes death serves to underscore the "vanity" of things (e.g., 3:19-21; 12:1-8). It does not provide an entry to one's hope; it puts an end to it. "Whoever is joined with all the living has hope, for a living dog is better than a dead lion. The living know that they will die, but the dead know nothing" (9:4-5). The most hopeful thing Ecclesiastes says about life after death is that no one knows about it (3:22). But what sense can then be made of this verse cited by *Crafte*? It is part of a couplet,

> A good name is better than precious ointment,
>   and the day of death, than the day of birth.

(7:1)

The second line of the couplet is to be understood in poetic parallelism with the first line; one's good name, one's reputation, is not secure until the day of death. It may be hard to know exactly what point Ecclesiastes is trying to make here, but it is hard to believe that the author of "a live dog is better than a dead lion" is commending death.[16]

So far none of the texts cited by *Crafte* seem to commend death, but perhaps the crux of the matter, and surely the clinching citation for *Crafte*, is found in Philippians 1:23, "my desire is to depart and be with Christ, for that is far better." This is another of the favorite texts in the *Ars Moriendi* tradition, and appropriately so, for Paul is surely an example of faith and faithfulness in the face of death. Courage, patience, and hope are all on display in Paul and especially in his letter to the Philippians. Paul writes from prison (probably in Ephesus), where he evidently awaits condemnation and death (2:17). Despite his suffering and these threats, he rejoices (2:17). The cause of Paul's joy, however, is not death. It is not death that Paul commends but God and the cause of God. If death itself were to be commended, presumably Paul would have been less anxious about the recovery of Epaphroditus (2:25-30).[17] Death remains, for Paul, "the last enemy to be destroyed" (1 Cor. 15:26).

---

16. *Crafte* also cites, as we have observed, a certain "wyseman." If the wise man cited by *Crafte* is Ezekiel, and if the citation is from Ezek. 18:23-32 (so Atkinson, *The English* Ars Moriendi, p. 364 n. 13), then we need look no further than the end of the passage to become a little suspicious of citing this "wyseman" to commend death, for in Ezek. 18:32 the Lord declares, "I have no pleasure in the death of anyone."

17. Paul was hardly indifferent about whether Epaphroditus lived or died. Epaphroditus, who had been sent by the Philippians with gifts for Paul, had become "so ill that he nearly died," but "God had mercy" and he recovered (Phil. 2:27).

The cause of Paul's joy is the power of God that raised Jesus from the dead. He looks forward to "the day of Jesus Christ" (Phil. 1:6, 10), the day that will bring "the redemption of our bodies" (Rom. 8:23). In the meanwhile he shares boldly and patiently and happily in Christ's suffering for the sake of God's cause in the world. He wants "to know Christ and the power of his resurrection" (Phil. 3:10). He knows it already, of course, in a measure at least. He has known it since the day an appearance of the risen and exalted Christ knocked him from his horse on the road to Damascus. And since that day he had been ready to share in Christ's suffering and death "if somehow [he] may attain the resurrection from the dead" (3:11). The basis for Paul's courage and patience and hope in the face of suffering and death is not found in some commendation of death, but in the faith that one had been raised from the dead, the first fruits of God's triumph over death. He does not claim to "have already obtained" the resurrection, but he does claim that death does not have the last word, that not even death can separate us from the love of God in Christ Jesus.[18]

In Philippians 1:23 it seems clear that even the dead already mysteriously participate in the triumph of that love. The dead may rest from the struggle to serve God's cause in a world where the powers of sin and death continue to assert their doomed reign. Nevertheless, it is also clear that Paul's joy is not to be traced to the image of death as a "welbeloued and trusti frende" but to the triumph of God over death. That triumph colors even death with hope. Death has lost its power to terrify the one who shares in Christ's death and resurrection. It has surely lost its terror for Paul. There are worse things than death in Paul's view. He says as much. He is less concerned about his death than about his faithfulness in living and in dying. When he says, "this will turn out for my deliverance" (Phil. 1:19), he immediately defines that "eager expectation and hope" in this way: that he will not act shamefully but faithfully in service to the cause of God, "that by my speaking with all boldness, Christ will be exalted now as al-

---

18. Rom. 8:38-39. See also the consolation of 1 Thess. 4:13-18. Moreover, as Richard Hays argues, the pattern for Paul — and for reflection concerning the death of Jesus even before Paul — was provided by the royal psalms of lament. Those psalms give voice to real suffering and acknowledge the threat of death but trust that God will hear and answer. Paul and the early church understand Christ's death and resurrection in the light of the lament psalms, the lament psalms in the light of the story of Jesus, and their own suffering and death in the light of both. See Richard B. Hays, "Christ Prays the Psalms," in *The Conversion of the Imagination: Paul as Interpreter of Israel's Scripture* (Grand Rapids: Eerdmans, 2005), pp. 101-18.

ways in my body, whether by life or by death" (1:20). If we were to follow Paul and his example of courage and patience, our strategy in the face of death would not be to commend death but to remember and celebrate and anticipate the resurrection as God's victory over death.

As we have seen, in addition to these texts of Scripture, *Crafte* also cited Seneca to commend death. Indeed, it may be charged against this commendation of death that Seneca and Stoicism seem more in control of the argument than Scripture itself. This is, of course, hardly the first time Christian reflection about death had been influenced by Stoic thinkers. Already in the third century Cyprian's *Mortality* had made considerable use of Stoic consolation literature.[19] But the late medieval period saw a re-

19. Cyprian, bishop of Carthage, wrote (or preached) "on the mortality" to Christians threatened by both persecution and plague in the third century. The emperor Decius (249-251 C.E.) had ordered the death penalty for any who refused to sacrifice to the emperor, and a terrible plague had struck Carthage in 252 causing much death and great alarm. In the context of these two great threats of death, Cyprian reminded Christians that Jesus came into the world not to show people how to escape death but how to die. Cyprian's *Mortality* is fundamentally a call for patient endurance, attentive to both the cross and to God's faithfulness. In that context, however, Cyprian made considerable use of themes familiar to the consolation literature of the Stoics. He reminded the Christians of Carthage, for example, that death is a "rest" from the labors and sorrows of life (2), that death is common to all people (8), that they should not forget their responsibilities in the face of death (9; including the responsibility to care for the sick, 16), that they pass by death to immortality (22), and even that death is a return to one's "native land" (26). He even told them not to mourn (20, 24). These Stoic themes nearly overwhelmed the reminders of the gospel in *Mortality* (as they do in *Crafte*). Nevertheless, it remained clear that Cyprian's real consolation was the power of God. Christians are to hope in God, in spite of death. The devout Simeon was a "witness" by his peace in the face of death and by his confidence in God's promises (3). It is God's trustworthiness (6) that is finally to be celebrated, not death. And it is the resurrection of Jesus that is the final basis of hope (21). See Cyprian, *Mortality*, trans. R. J. Deferrari, in *Treatises*, Fathers of the Church, vol. 36 (New York: Fathers of the Church, 1958), pp. 195-221; the references in the parentheses above are to the chapters of *Mortality*.

Cyprian's *Mortality* was not the only option in the early church for dealing with death, however, nor was Stoicism the only philosophical resource utilized. Clement of Alexandria in *Stromateis* had earlier joined Middle Platonism to Christianity, affirming the immortality of the soul and praising death as the release of the soul from the body and from sin. Tatian, to the contrary, writing still earlier, had ridiculed the Greek view of "immortality of the soul" in his *Address to the Greeks*. Against every form of Greek dualism he insisted on the unity of body and soul. He insisted that the basis of Christian hope is the power of God to raise the dead. The Greeks, he said, pretend to be indifferent to the terrors of death, but if death is not a threat, then why, he asked, do they threaten Christians with it? Christians, on the other hand, he said, have contempt for death but even more contempt for sin. He called attention to Christ as paradigmatic for a Christian life and death, insisting that Christians

newed interest in the Stoics — in large part due to the efforts of Renaissance humanists. Stoic thought, however, does not make a good fit with the Christian story.

The Stoics placed death in the category of "indifferent things." To be sure, one could distinguish within that category things to be preferred (e.g., wealth and health) and things not to be preferred (e.g., poverty and sickness), but these preferences were not regarded as moral preferences or as morally relevant to the moral life. The moral life was a life in harmony with nature, that is, a life of consenting to whatever happens.[20] So Stoics recommended "contentment" (Greek *autarkeia*), lest the desire for the things preferred disrupt one's consent to whatever happens. Such "contentment" is the evidence of the "true Stoic" and the way to happiness. As Epictetus said, the true Stoic was one who "though sick is happy, though in danger is happy, though dying is happy, though condemned to exile is happy, though in disrepute is happy."[21] For the Stoic the world was fundamentally rational, governed by a divine *logos*. It was Nature with a capital *N*, fate with the face of a divine reason.[22] Because the Stoic regarded whatever happened, including death, as "natural," as governed by a divine reason, he should submit to it as a rational agent as to a natural law and accept it with equanimity. By using his own reason to live in harmony with na-

---

must be willing to die for the faith but never ready to sin in order to stay alive. See Tatian, *Oratio ad Graecos and Fragments*, ed. and trans. Molly Whitaker (Oxford: Clarendon, 1982). Tatian and his teacher Justin Martyr seem to me to provide an account of death that fits the biblical story better than the Stoicism of Cyprian or the Platonism of Clement. See further the little book by Jaroslav Pelikan, *The Shape of Death: Life, Death, and Immortality in the Early Fathers* (Nashvillle: Abingdon, 1961), which provides an account of the views of death in Tatian, Clement of Alexandria, Origen, and Irenaeus.

20. Epictetus, *The Encheiridion* 8: "Do not seek to have everything that happens happen as you wish, but wish for everything to happen as it actually does happen, and your life will be serene." Epictetus, *The Discourses*, vol. 2, trans. W. A. Oldfather, Loeb Classical Library (Cambridge: Harvard University Press, 1959), p. 491.

21. Epictetus, *The Discourses* 2.19.24; in Epictetus, *The Discourses as Reported by Arrian, the Manual, and Fragments*, vol. 1, trans. W. A. Oldfather, Loeb Classical Library (Cambridge: Harvard University Press, 1956), p. 367.

22. Stoic thinkers did not adhere to a rigid orthodoxy; they disagreed about many things, including the account to be given of death. There was, however, a core conviction that the good life was a life in agreement with "Nature." Nature was regarded as a divine rationality that permeates the universe and rules the world, so that everything that exists or happens must be regarded as determined by "Nature." This divine rationality that permeates the universe could be called "reason" (or *logos*), "Zeus," "fate," "providence," "god," or "nature," but a good life was life that conformed to it.

ture, by willing whatever happened, the true Stoic would be freed from the passions of grief (or joy). Attachments make such equanimity difficult, of course, and the Stoics recommended that people be ready to surrender such attachments, that they regard possessions, family members, and, indeed, life itself as matters of indifference. Then it would be easy to bid them farewell when it came time to die.[23] It is finally only the passions that can interfere with such contentment (which was often named *apatheia* in Greek). So, for the Stoic, as for *Crafte*, one can achieve contentment when his reason rules his passions, when one lets the "reason of his mind rule his sensuality" (*Crafte*, p. 2). Stoics achieve contentment by quitting the passions; they avoid fear and grief by ceasing to hope. To quote Seneca, "'Cease to hope and you will cease to fear.' Just as the same chain fastens the prisoner and the soldier who guards him, so hope and fear, dissimilar as they are, keep step together; fear follows hope. . . . The present alone can make no man wretched."[24] That is Stoic contentment.

Paul's contentment is quite different. It is true that Paul can use the same Greek word for "contentment" *(autarkeia)*. When he advises the Philippians to "rejoice in the Lord always" (Phil. 4:4), and he reports that he has learned "to be content" *(autarkes)* whatever happens (Phil. 4:11), it may sound a little like the lines from Epictetus quoted above. But Paul's "contentment" must not be confused with Stoic "contentment," or his "joy" with the "happiness" of the Stoic. Paul does not invite people to become passionless (and he never uses the Greek word *apatheia*); he invites people to share the passion of Christ. He does not urge people to surrender hope; he urges them to hope in God. It is not fear that follows such hope but courage. He does not propose conformity to Nature, participation in the cosmic Reason, or the subjection of the passions to the rule of reason; he proposes instead participation in the cross and resurrection of Christ and submission of the whole person to the reign of God. "Rejoice in the Lord always; again I will say, Rejoice. Let your gentleness be known to everyone. The Lord is near. Do not worry about anything, but in everything

---

23. See, e.g., Epictetus, *The Discourses* 4.110-112; *Enchiridion* 3, 7.

24. Seneca, *Epistle* 5, "The Philosopher's Mean," in *Epistles 1–65*, p. 23. The internal quotation is from Hecaton, a Stoic philosopher from around 100 B.C.E. Cited in Peter G. Bolt, "Life, Death, and the Afterlife in the Greco-Roman World," in *Life in the Face of Death: The Resurrection Message of the New Testament*, ed. Richard N. Longenecker (Grand Rapids: Eerdmans, 1998), p. 65. On Seneca's concern to exterminate the passions, see further Martha Nussbaum, *The Therapy of Desire* (Princeton: Princeton University Press, 1994), chapters 9–12.

by prayer and supplication with thanksgiving let your requests be made known to God. And the peace of God, which surpasses all understanding, will guard your hearts and your minds in Christ Jesus" (Phil. 4:4-7). That is hardly Stoic contentment.

It is also true that the doctrine of providence can sometimes sound suspiciously like Stoic fatalism, and it surely does in *Crafte*. When the place that cosmic reason has in Stoicism is simply given to God, then the doctrine of providence comes too close to Stoic fatalism. The Christian doctrine of providence, however, rejects the Stoic notion that all things happen by fate or by *Fortuna*. It affirms that nothing that happens puts us beyond the constant care of God; it affirms that God provides, that God will not allow sin and evil to have the last word in the world God made good, that God's care and power can be trusted even in the worst of times. It does not make sin or suffering or death "good" or commend the evil as the work of God.[25] Christian talk of providence will frequently have an "in spite of" attached. *In spite of* the agony of Christ's death, providence affirms that God's love was at work. *In spite of* oppression and hunger and poverty and violence, providence insists that God is still at work and that God has not abandoned God's cause of love and justice. *In spite of* sickness and death, providence affirms that God is present with God's care and saving purpose. The doctrine of providence should not prompt us to talk as though oppression or sickness or death are themselves God's intentions. It does not call us to be indifferent or apathetic about the evils that infect our lives and our common life. On the contrary, it calls us to hope in God and faithfully to stand firm in that hope *in spite of* death and every evil.[26]

The problem, however, is not just that the Stoic notion of "contentment" does not quite fit Pauline "contentment" or that Stoic fatalism is not

25. That was the error of those whom Calvin accuses of misunderstanding the doctrine of providence in his treatise against the Libertines. See John Calvin, *Treatises against the Anabaptists and against the Libertines*, ed. and trans. Benjamin Wirt Farley (Grand Rapids: Baker, 1982). Calvin, who himself is sometimes accused of fatalism, is quite explicit about rejecting those he calls "the new Stoics, who count it depraved not only to groan and weep but also to be sad and care ridden. . . . [W]e have nothing to do with this iron philosophy which our Lord and Master has condemned not only by his word, but also by his example. For he groaned and wept both over his own and others' misfortunes" (*Institutes* 3.8.9).

26. See further the profound and touching wrestle with the notion of providence in Ellen T. Charry, "May We Trust God and (Still) Lament? Can We Lament and (Still) Trust God?" in *Lament: Reclaiming Practices in Pulpit, Pew, and Public Square*, ed. Sally A. Brown and Patrick D. Miller (Louisville: Westminster John Knox, 2005), pp. 95-108. Her reflections respond to the death of her husband, Dana, at age fifty-six.

to be confused with the Christian doctrine of providence. The problem is also that Stoic accounts of death hardly fit with the New Testament's proclamation of the resurrection of the body. There were, to be sure, diverse accounts of death among the Stoics. Early Stoics typically agreed with the Epicureans that death was "nothing," that there was no life after death, even if they lived quite different lives in the face of that nothingness. Later Stoics, including Seneca, sometimes displayed the influence of Platonic and Neoplatonic conceptions of an immortal soul. And it is that conception of an immortal soul that is finally in control of the commendation of death in *Crafte* and in the *Ars Moriendi*.

The commendation of death in *Ars Moriendi* is indebted finally more to Platonism and to the Renaissance revival of Platonism than to the Stoics, even if Plato is not explicitly cited. The Renaissance had retrieved Platonic and Neoplatonic thought against the influence of Aristotle. It is not, of course, as though Platonic notions were first utilized by Christian theology in the fifteenth century.[27] Nevertheless, there was a revival of Platonic

27. As we have noted (n. 19 above), already in the third century Clement of Alexandria joined Middle Platonism to the Christian gospel. His student Origen was in some ways even more influenced by Middle Platonism. (He seems to have held, for example, that immortal souls exist prior to their entrance into bodies and that through death will be restored to their original condition in unity with God. Origen himself was never declared a heretic, but those ideas were condemned at the Council of Constantinople in 553.)

In the fourth century, after the conversion of Constantine, when the church moved from the status of persecuted minority to a position of privilege in the Roman Empire, the influence of Jewish patterns of thought diminished and the influence of Platonic thought increased. It was also at this time that asceticism and virginity began to replace martyrdom as the marks of exemplary Christians. Thankfully, the Old Testament was never displaced as authoritative Scripture, but it was sometimes read in ways that accommodated it to Platonism. (Philo had shown the way to do this in his first-century fusion of Judaism and Platonism, and Clement of Alexandria and Origen had learned from him in their efforts to join Platonic thought to Christianity.) And thankfully, the quotidian life of the body in this world was not displaced as an arena for discipleship.

Ambrose was consul of the region of the empire that included Milan and was a student of philosophy before being pressed into service as bishop of Milan in the fourth century. He was deeply impressed by the philosophical work of Plato and the later Platonists. His indebtedness to Plato is on display when he treats death as liberation of the soul from its union with the body in his treatise *De bono mortis* ("Death as a Good," trans. M. P. McHugh, in *Saint Ambrose: Seven Exegetical Works*, ed. P. M. Peeples et al., Fathers of the Church: A New Translation, vol. 65 [Washington, D.C.: Catholic University of America Press, 1972]).

Ambrose would play a part in Augustine's conversion. Augustine reports that he first went to hear Ambrose preach because he was interested in his rhetoric rather than in his gospel. Nevertheless, as he says in his *Confessions*, "Though I did not realize it, I was led to

thought in the late Middle Ages. The center of that revival, certainly, was Florence, where Marsilius Ficinus (1433-99) worked to translate not only Plato and Plotinus but also Pythagoras. His *Platonic Theology* provided a summary of Platonic philosophy, emphasizing the immortality of the soul, a dualism of matter and spirit, and contemplation of the divine. Ficinus argues that contemplation of the divine requires a detachment from the material world, that it requires knowledge of and desire for God, and that it culminates in the vision and enjoyment of God.[28] The revival of Platonic thought in the Renaissance, however, was hardly initiated by Ficinus or limited to Florence. In movements like the *Devotio Moderna* among the Brethren of the Common Life and in the mystical theology of people like Jean Charlier Gerson, Plato had been retrieved. And in the *Ars Moriendi* tradition the influence of Plato (and Pythagoras) may be discerned in the construal of death as the relocation of the soul, in the construal of the body as a tomb and prison for the soul, and in the construal of salvation as salvation *from* the world rather than *for* the world.[29] Then life may be construed as an exile and death as a liberation and as the end of exile. Then death could be celebrated and commended.

The Christian Scripture, however, provides a different context for thinking about death. It starts with a celebration of the creation. The world God made is not God, but it is good. God made the world and loves it. The human creature is embodied, and as a psychophysical unity is part of that world made good and loved by God. Salvation is not a matter of finding some crack in the material world through which to slip into some other

---

him by you so that, with full realization, I might be led to you by him" (*The Confessions of St. Augustine* 5.13, trans. Rex Warner [New York: New American Library, 1963], p. 108). Augustine also reports that reading the Platonists (7.9) and conversations with Christian Platonists (especially Simplicianus, 8.1-2) had also been used by God in his conversion. Ambrose and the Platonists were deeply formative of Augustine's early work. It is fair to say, with David Albert Jones, that his exegetical and pastoral work and his controversies with the Manicheans and the Donatists would lead to "a shift in his thought to a position distinct from, and in some important ways antithetical to, the sort of Platonist Christianity that he had once shared with Ambrose" (David Albert Jones, *Approaching the End: A Theological Exploration of Death and Dying* [Oxford: Oxford University Press, 2007], p. 39). Even so, it is also fair to say that the great Augustine bequeathed to Western Christianity a theological tradition with an acknowledged indebtedness to Platonic thought. (See, e.g., not only the citations of the *Confessions* above but also *City of God* 8.5, 9ff.; 9.1; 10.1.)

28. See Paul Oskar Kristeller, *The Philosophy of Marsilio Ficino* (New York, 1953).

29. Only at the Lateran Council of 1513 was the immortality of the soul promulgated as an official dogma of the church.

world, some spiritual world. Salvation comes not when souls leave this world but when God comes to this world. God comes to save, not by rescuing God's people from the world but by being with them in it. And he comes to save the world, not just souls. Israel's hope for the future is finally that God will break the power of sin and death, and that hope is vindicated when Jesus is raised, "the first fruits of those that have died" (1 Cor. 15:20). That resurrection is the basis for Christian hope in the face of death, but the scope of that hope remains cosmic. Heaven and earth do not become paradise and hell; they remain the world God created and that God will renew in a "new heaven and a new earth." Jesus' body is not a tomb; after an interval of Holy Saturday it leaves the tomb behind. And so, finally, Scripture says, will we all. To be sure, there is a contrast between "the flesh" and "the spirit," but that contrast bears no resemblance to the dualism of body and soul. It is the contrast of submission, body and soul, to the power of sin and submission, body and soul, to the power of the Spirit.

In that context the commendation of death as a "welbeloued and trusti frende" (*Crafte*, p. 3) hardly fits. The image of death as a "friend" surely does stand in stark and obvious contrast to the image of death as the "enemy" in a medicalized dying. Nevertheless, Paul's image, that death is "the last enemy" (1 Cor. 15:26), is the image that should govern a Christian imagination. The contrast to be made is the contrast between death as "the enemy to be defeated by the greater powers of medicine" and death as "the enemy to be defeated by the greater power of God." The image of death as "the enemy to be defeated by the greater powers of medicine" is nurtured and sponsored by the Baconian project. The hold it has on our imagination is displayed in the martial images we use for physicians and medical research, when we regard, for example, physicians as "fighters" and we engage in a "war on cancer."[30] The image of death as an "enemy to be defeated by the greater power of God" is nurtured and sponsored, as in Paul, by the resurrection of Jesus from the dead. It is important to be careful about the ways we understand and use the image of death as "enemy."

It is important to acknowledge also that the image of death as "friend" can be understood and used in more than one way. The image I refuse to commend is the image of death as a "friend that liberates our souls from their regrettable union with bodies." That image is nurtured and sponsored by Platonic (and Gnostic) dualism, and it is on display, I

---

30. See William F. May, *The Physician's Covenant: Images of the Healer in Medical Ethics* (Philadelphia: Westminster, 1983), pp. 64-66.

think, in the commendation of death in *Crafte*. When Cardinal Bernardin, however, talked of "befriending death" and said his cancer had taught him to regard death "as a friend," he evidently used a different image, death as a "friend who teaches us to depend upon God and provides an opportunity for witness to Christ."[31] His *Gift of Peace* is a wonderful book, and Cardinal Bernardin can hardly be accused of Platonic dualism. The earlier caution holds, of course; it is important to be cautious about the ways we understand and use also the image of death as "friend." And when our imagination is captured by the resurrection of Jesus from the dead, we will, I think, prefer the image of death as "enemy to be defeated by the greater power of God."

We should be suspicious of the strategy of commending death in Platonic fashion. We may celebrate the victory of God over death, but we should not ignore the sadness and pain of a Friday we call good and the long wait of that Saturday before Easter. We should not condemn and forsake the world God made and loves, the world that we receive with our bodies and that we love, for the sake of some spiritual otherworld. This commendation comes too close to a facile escape from the pain of loss. It comes too close to a denial of death. We would do better to acknowledge the tragedy, even while we delight in the hilariously good news that God has won the victory over the powers of sin and death. We would do well to look not for an escape from the world but for a blessing upon the world.

When we attempt in the next part of this book to imagine a contemporary *ars moriendi*, we will begin not with a commendation of death, but with a celebration of life and of God's power over death. Even so — or especially so — the victory over death has robbed death of its sting, of its terrors. The strategy cannot be to commend death, but the objective of *Ars Moriendi* to provide comfort and courage in the face of death need not be surrendered. There can be a saintly serenity in the face of death.

31. See Joseph Cardinal Bernardin, *The Gift of Peace* (Chicago: Loyola University Press, 1997); the last chapter is entitled "Befriending Death." See also Henri J. M. Nouwen, *Our Greatest Gift: A Meditation on Dying and Caring* (New York: HarperCollins, 1995). And see also M. Therese Lysaught, "Love Your Enemies: Toward a Christoform Bioethics," in *Gathered for the Journey: Moral Theology in Catholic Perspective*, ed. David Matzko McCarthy and M. Therese Lysaught (Grand Rapids: Eerdmans, 2007), pp. 307-28. I have great regard for these works, and none of them can be accused of Platonic dualism. I wish that in Nouwen's work the resurrection would have been more than an afterthought. In Lysaught's essay, much to her credit, I think, the image of death as "enemy" is preserved; "loving one's enemy" suggests in this context a response other than violent resistance.

There can be deliverance from the anxiety and dread of death. There can surely be a readiness to acknowledge that at the end of life and at the limits of human powers God can still be trusted. While we will resist the commendation of death, we must not make of life a second god. Precisely because death will not have the last word, we need not always resist it. And because the triumph over death is finally not a technological victory but a divine victory, we will resist not only the commendation of death but also its medicalization.

CHAPTER EIGHT

The "Temptacions" and the Virtues

He shall give his angels charge over thee, to keep thee in all thy
ways.

Psalm 91:11 KJV

Lord, let at last thine angels come,
To Abraham's bosom bear me home,
That I may die unfearing.

J. S. Bach, *Passion according to St. John*

"The secunde chapitre ys of temptacions of men that dyen."[1] The *Ars
Moriendi* tradition assumes that the dying will encounter temptation. And
no small part of this self-help literature is intended to help the dying to
overcome these temptations. Indeed, that is the main focus of the block
book *Ars Moriendi,* and it is on that work with its artful figures that we will
concentrate in this chapter.

---

1. *Crafte and Knowledge For To Dye Well* (hereafter *Crafte*), in *The English* Ars Moriendi, ed. David William Atkinson, Renaissance and Baroque Studies and Texts, vol. 5 (New
York: Peter Lang, 1992), p. 3. Hereafter citations from this work will be placed in the text.

The Temptation to Lose Faith

In the first figure (fig. 1, p. 112) we meet Moriens, the dying Everyman. He lies on his bed, emaciated. At the bedside stand three doctors, evidently discussing the case, but this is hardly a medicalized death. We need not be privy to their conversation to know that the man is dying. The medical prognosis seems clear enough, but given the other characters in this death-bed scene, it is the spiritual prognosis that concerns us. There at the head of the bed are the Virgin Mary, Jesus, and God the Father. It's promising. Mary is praying. Jesus is robed in glory. The Father has the book of life. If they keep company with Moriens and he with them, there is every reason for confidence.

There are, however, also those demons, those beastly, grotesque little creatures, and they are working hard on Moriens. One, floating above the bed, is pointing downward, and the little scroll next to him leaves no doubt about the significance of his gesture. "Hell is prepared for you," it says. A second demon seems intent upon seizing Moriens, bedsheet and all. A third hideous little monster joins her voice — or scroll — to the horror, urging Moriens to deny the faith, "Do as the pagans do." It is tempting; the pagan king and queen toward whom he gestures look pretty comfortable while they pray before their idol. A fourth nudges the shoulder of Moriens, but his message is hardly one of consolation; his scroll invites Moriens to kill himself, while at the lower right a man with a knife at his throat displays one technique.[2] Moriens is tempted to lose faith, to deny the faith. It is the first and fundamental temptation of dying in *Ars Moriendi*.

The temptations are not simply stages. The temptation to lose faith is

2. The female figure standing beside the man with a knife to his throat is a puzzling image. She carries a scourge and palms, the very equipment of Christ in figure 6. Palms, moreover, were frequently used in iconographic depictions of martyrs and saints. And the scourge suggests participation in the suffering of Christ. In that case, and in stark contrast to the figure of the suicide that she stands beside, she is a saint. Perhaps these two figures stand in the foreground as representative of the choice Moriens confronts, the two ways open to him, standing firm in the faith in the face of death or surrendering to the demons. That is my best guess. But what if she stands not as a contrast but as a companion to the figure that accompanies her? That was my first impression, and it is hard to dismiss. If she is to be regarded as companion, then her scourge may suggest the flagellant movement, regarded as a superstitious heresy. Indeed, *Crafte* (p. 40) does warn that if the devil cannot cause Moriens to lose faith, he works "to dysceyue him with some maner off supersticiones and false errors and heresyes." Perhaps, then, this female figure represents such superstition. I want to thank Peggy Palmer of Virginia Theological Seminary for her help with the consideration of this figure.

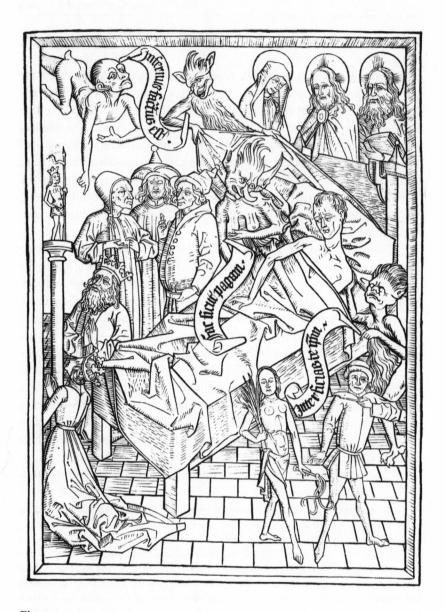

Figure 1

set first because it is of such fundamental importance. On the facing page of text, Augustine is quoted to make the point that faith is the foundation of all virtue and the source of a person's well-being.[3] Besides citing Augustine, *Crafte* (p. 3) includes a number of biblical citations to underscore the significance of faith. It cites Paul to insist that "no one can lay any foundation other than the one that has been laid" (1 Cor. 3:11). It cites the book of Hebrews to make the point that "without faith it is impossible to please God" (Heb. 11:6). And it cites John to warn that "those who do not believe are condemned already" (John 3:18). Little wonder, then, as the figure displays and as both the facing page and *Crafte* assert, when Moriens is dying, the devil works "with all his might" to tempt him to turn from the faith.

The Virtue of Faith

Mercifully, in the second illustration (fig. 2, p. 114) a good angel visits Moriens. At his bedside stand again the Virgin Mary, Jesus, and God the Father. Moses and a host of saints, most invisible except for their haloes, have also joined them.[4] A dove, representing the Holy Spirit, rests on the headboard of the bed. Moriens is not abandoned. He is accompanied by God and by the saints of God. The angel encourages Moriens, "Stand firm in faith." On the facing page that message is given more fully. The angel reminds Moriens of the importance of faith, quoting Scripture (Heb. 11:6; John 3:18; see above) and Saint Bernard's teaching that "faith is the primogenitor of all virtues."[5] The angel invites Moriens to consider the great "cloud of witnesses" (Heb. 12:1) who by their faith "received approval" (Heb. 11:2). It mentions Old Testament exemplars of faith, Abraham, Isaac, Jacob, Job, and others, but it also calls attention to the faith of the apostles and of the martyrs.[6] It reminds Moriens, for example, that it was by faith

3. *Crafte*, p. 3: "ffythe ys foundment off all goodnesse and begynning of mannes healthe." I have been unable to identify the source of this quotation. Atkinson, *The English Ars Moriendi*, p. 364 n. 16, suggests Augustine, *De utilitate credendi*, as a possible source. There are some corresponding ideas there, but no corresponding phrase.

4. The depiction of Moses with horns reflects an ancient mistranslation of Exod. 34:29. Where it says that Moses' face "shone," some translators had read "horns."

5. I could not identify any passage from Bernard of Clairvaux identical to the one quoted.

6. In *Crafte* the dying person is also invited to consider the exemplars of faith. A few do not survive the abridgment of *Ars Moriendi*. One such is "the woman off Achor." It is a curi-

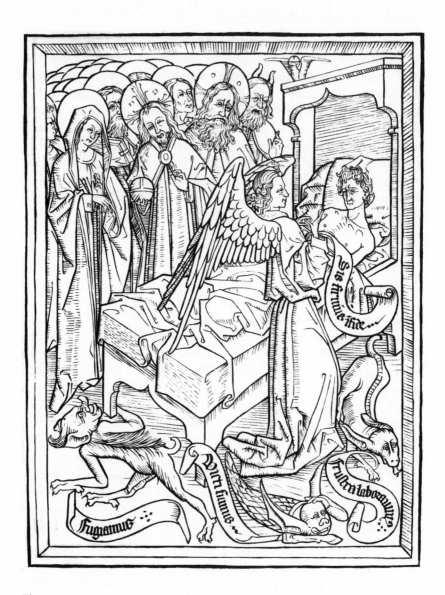

Figure 2

that Peter walked on water. And it reiterates the promises of Christ that all things are possible to the one who believes (Mark 9:23); whatever one prays for in faith will be done (Mark 11:24). Finally, the angel encourages Moriens to resist the devil and to remain steadfast in his faith (1 Pet. 5:9).

In an aside to those who might attend the dying person, both the facing page in *Ars Moriendi* and *Crafte* urge them "when a man ys in hys agonie of dying, with a hygh voyce oftyn tymes to sey the crede before hym that he that ys seke may be fortyfied in stablenesse off the feythe" — and that the demons may be driven away, for they cannot bear to hear it (*Crafte*, p. 4).

With the help of this good angel and its encouragement, Moriens evidently does not abandon the faith. The demons scatter across the bottom of the page, looking more ludicrous than ominous now. They slither away bearing scrolls announcing their defeat and frustration. The prognosis for the soul of Moriens is good, even if there is no change in the prognosis for his body, but even his body looks a little less anxious. The matter is not yet settled, however. The question mark after *frustra laboravim* ("have I labored in vain?") indicates that the frustrated demons have not yet given up. Nevertheless, after victory in this first temptation, as *Crafte* assures the dying man, the devil's might need not cause alarm. Though the devil is "the father of lies" (John 8:44), no lie is as powerful as God's truth (*Crafte*, p. 4).

The Temptation to Despair

The demons return in the third figure (see fig. 3, p. 116), in greater numbers and even more hideous in appearance, to tempt Moriens to despair. This is the second temptation, the temptation to lose hope. When a man suffers the agonies of the body in dying, then the devil is busy in the effort to induce spiritual agony as well, reminding him of his sins in order to tempt him to surrender hope.[7] The demons in the illustration accuse Moriens of

---

ous reference, presumably a reference to Hosea's vision in Hos. 2:14-15 of God's faithfulness that restores the covenant. God promises to "allure" Israel, to "bring her into the wilderness, and speak tenderly to her." Then "the Valley of Achor will be a door of hope" rather than a place of unfaithfulness as it was when the people entered the promised land initially (Josh. 7:20-26). "There she shall respond as in the days of her youth, as at the time when she came out of the land of Egypt." If this is right, then it is a quite stunning example of faith after a history of unfaithfulness and an encouragement to one who would repent on the deathbed.

7. The facing page makes this point. Cf. also *Crafte*, p. 5: "ffor whan a seeke man is

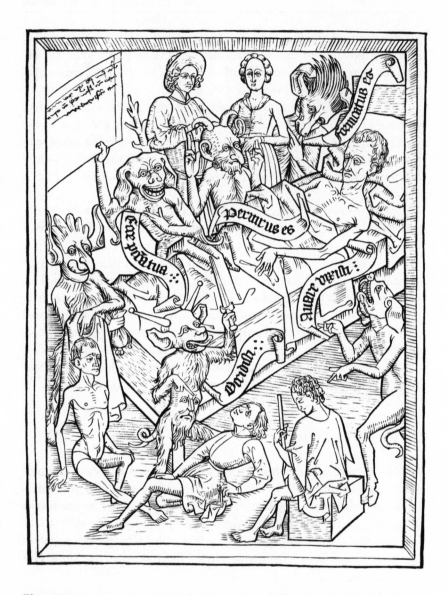

Figure 3

various sins. At the top of the figure one demon accuses him of being an adulterer *(Fornicatus es)* and points to a woman as evidence. On the right another accuses him of avarice *(Avare vixisti)* and points to a man presumably left in need because of his greed. A third, at the foot of the bed on the left side of the illustration, provides further evidence of the avarice of Moriens. He bears no scroll of accusation, but he holds a full sack of coins and a man's shirt as he points to a naked man ruined by Moriens's failure to be generous. Another at the foot of the bed has drawn a dagger and points to a man while he accuses Moriens of murder *(Occidisti)*. A fifth accuses him of perjury *(Perjurus es)* while he points toward a man injured by his lie. And a sixth holds up a list of the sins of Moriens and instructs him to behold his sins *(Ecce peccata tua)*. Moriens is a sinner. What hope can there be for his soul?

As the facing page makes clear, the demons can use Scripture and the just requirements of Scripture to their own advantage in tempting the sick sinner to give up hope. The second temptation is related, of course, to the first, for it is the loss of faith that brings despair, prompting the sinner to give up the trust and confidence he ought to have in God.[8] But if God is a righteous judge who condemns sin, as Scripture and these demons remind us, then what hope can Moriens have for his soul? Perhaps the demons will be victorious after all.

The Virtue of Hope

Lest the demons have cause to rejoice, another angel visits Moriens in the fourth engraving (see fig. 4, p. 118), encouraging him, "You need not despair." Hope is possible, after all. And the evidence surrounds the bedside. There they are, sinners all, brought through the judgment by the grace of God. Is the accusation fornication? But there is Mary Magdalene, with her reputation as a sinner, and ready again with her costly ointment.[9] Is the ac-

---

sore tormented and vexed with sorowe and seekeness of hys body, than the deuyll ys most besy to supreadde sorowe to sorowe with all the weyes that he may."

8. *Ars Moriendi* is obviously concerned with Moriens's despair concerning his soul; it is not despair over his body or the loss of worldly goods like health or family or friends. That despair will be called avarice, and avarice will be the final temptation.

9. The medieval church largely accepted the judgment of Gregory the Great that Mary Magdalene, Mary of Bethany (the sister of Lazarus), and the unnamed sinner of Luke 7 were the same person.

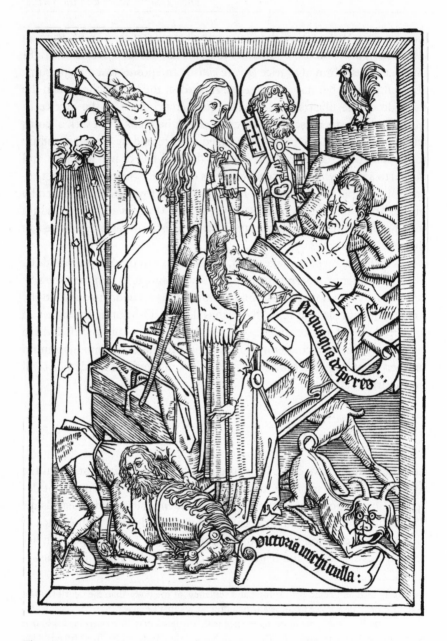

Figure 4

cusation avarice? But there is the thief on the cross. Is the accusation murder? But there is Paul, or Saul of Tarsus, struck down from his horse on the way to Damascus to persecute and kill. And is the accusation perjury? But there is Peter, holding the keys of the kingdom, and on the headboard the cock whose three crows marked his own perjury. And there in the background are the heavens opening, with a path for sinners. There is evidence enough of the great grace of God upon repentant sinners, evidence enough to put a stop to despair, evidence enough to send the demons once more slithering away. One hurries off, bearing a scroll announcing his defeat, while another takes cover under the bed. Moriens may trust in God for forgiveness, may hope for life, even as he lies dying.

Once again the facing page reports more fully the angel's message of consolation and hope. The angel reminds Moriens of Psalm 51:17 and of its promise that God will not despise "a broken and contrite heart." It repeats Ezekiel's promise that the wicked who turn from their ways will be saved (Ezek. 18:27). It quotes Bernard to announce that the mercy and pity of God is greater than any wickedness of man,[10] and Augustine to insist that God is more powerful to save than any sin is to condemn.[11] But it also warns Moriens that to despair is a great offense against God; to abandon hope is to act as if God were not to be trusted. The angel reminds Moriens of the cross of Christ and of the many examples of sinners who learned to hope in God in spite of their sin. Those depicted in the engraving are included, of course — Mary Magdalene, the repentant thief on the cross, Paul, and Peter — but for good measure the angel mentions also Matthew and Zacchaeus, the publicans, the woman caught in adultery (John 8), and Mary of Egypt.[12] With such assurances and examples Moriens should not and need not relinquish hope (Heb. 10:35).

The message of the angel in *Ars Moriendi*, abridged from the longer

[margin note: despair]

---

10. Cf. St. Bernard de Clairvaux, *On the Song of Songs*, translated by a religious of C.S.M.V. (London: A. R. Mowbray, 1952), pp. 55-60.

11. Cf. Augustine, "Tractate 49," in *Tractates on the Gospel of John 28-54*, trans. John W. Retting, Fathers of the Church, vol. 88 (Washington, D.C.: Catholic University of America Press, 1993), pp. 238-59. Augustine comments here on the raising of Lazarus (John 11). If this is in fact the source cited by *Ars Moriendi*, it is striking that Augustine's attention to the power of God to raise the dead has been eclipsed by the power of God to forgive sins. *Ars Moriendi* is again characteristically silent about resurrection of the body.

12. Written records of Mary of Egypt date to the sixth century. Briefly, the story is that she had been an actress and a harlot who experienced a conversion on a pilgrimage to Jerusalem when she was seventeen. Upon repentance, Mary lived as a hermitess in the Jordanian desert for the next forty-seven years.

text, leaves out a little, of course. One item of significance, left out because of the limits of a single page of text, invited further attention to the cross. When *Crafte* nurtures hope and confidence by pointing to the cross, it cites Bernard's invitation to meditate on the cross. "Take hede and see hys hede ys inclyned to saue the, and hys mouth to kysse the, hys armes spredde to cylppe the, hys handes thrilled to yeue the, his side openyd to loue the, hys body alonge strygth to gyfe all hym selfe to the. Therefore ther shulde no man dyspayre off foryenes, but fully haue hope & confidence in God."[13]

With the help of this good angel Moriens evidently does not abandon hope. But the issue is not yet settled, and that demon hiding under the bed awaits a new opportunity.

The Temptation to Impatience

And that opportunity comes with the next engraving (fig. 5, p. 121). It is the temptation to impatience. Only one demon is shown, but perhaps that one under the bed from the previous illustration is still there making it uncomfortable. At any rate, the single demon seems to be doing a good job. Moriens has already overturned the table to which his daughter was bringing food. Now he kicks at a man, presumably his doctor, who is evidently himself a little impatient with such rude treatment. Meanwhile his wife makes excuses for him: "See what suffering he endures." Yes, but see as well what suffering those who care for Moriens endure when he is impatient. The single demon claims a victory: "How well I have deceived him!"

The facing page acknowledges that great pain and suffering can accompany dying and that such make patience difficult. But it also identifies the temptation to impatience as a temptation "against charity," which demands that we love God above all things. The devil would destroy our love of God and corrupt our other loves. So the first three temptations are temptations to violate faith, hope, and love, and the greatest of these is the temptation against love. The pain and suffering of the deathbed are especially dreadful to those who are not ready to die, or who die against their

13. *Crafte*, pp. 5-6: "Take heed and see his head is inclined to save you, and his mouth to kiss you, his arms spread to embrace you, his hands pierced to bless you, his side opened to love you, his stretched body striving to give all himself to you. Therefore, no one should despair of forgiveness, but have hope and confidence in God." O'Connor identifies the quotation as from St. Bernard, "In Feria IV Hebdomadae Sanctae sermo," in *Patrologia Latina*, ed. J.-P. Migne, 217 vols. (Paris, 1844-64), 183:270.

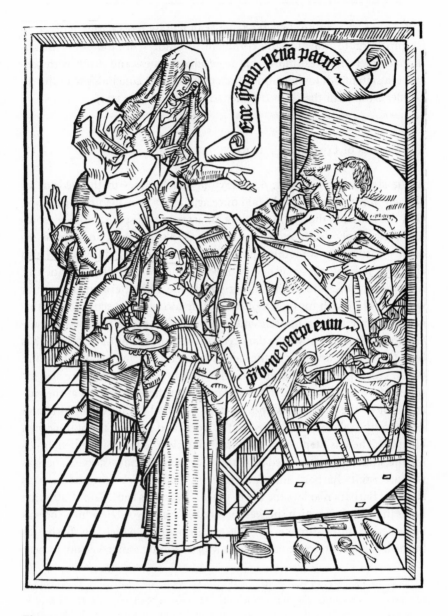

Figure 5

will. Those who do not love God above all will be most easily tempted to be impatient, to murmur and complain. To underscore the point the author cites Jerome's testimony that to receive sickness and death with sorrow is a sign of not loving God sufficiently.[14] And it concludes with the reminder from Paul that love is patient and kind (1 Cor. 13:4).

The Virtues of Love and Patience

In the sixth engraving (fig. 6, p. 123) an angel comes to the bedside of Moriens once again and to his aid once again, this time inspiring patience. God the Father is there, too, holding an arrow and a scourge. They represent presumably death and suffering, but God's face does not express sadistic pleasure, but something like love. Those whom God loves God also chastens. To know that may help Moriens to endure the suffering patiently. Moreover, at the side of the Father stands the Christ, crowned now not with glory but with his crown of thorns. He too carries a scourge, but this is the scourge that he himself endured before his cross. He, too, has suffered and died. He knows the dark recesses of our caverns of gloom. He has been there. And now he is at the side of Moriens, sharing his suffering and death, keeping company, keeping faith with Moriens. His presence also inspires Moriens to patience in his suffering. But there are others at the side and foot of the bed, saints and martyrs who had endured suffering and death for the sake of God's cause in the world and for the sake of their own integrity. There is Stephen in the foreground, at the foot of the bed, holding the stones that had killed him as if they were precious stones. There as well are Saints Barbara and Catherine and Laurence, celebrated martyrs all. Saint Barbara displays the tower in which she was kept. Saint Catherine holds the wheel on which she was tortured and the sword by which she was beheaded. Saint Laurence has the gridiron upon which his flesh was burned.[15] Their presence encourages Moriens to be a martyr, too, to bear

14. I have not been able to identify the source. Atkinson, *The English* Ars Moriendi, p. 365 n. 31, suggests that the source is Jerome, "Homily on Mark 9:1-7," in *Homilies of St. Jerome*, vol. 2, trans. Marie Liquori Ewald, Fathers of the Church, vol. 57 (Washington, D.C.: Catholic University of America Press, 1965), pp. 159-68, but I did not see the precise phrase there (or elsewhere in Jerome).

15. These three martyrs were among the most venerated and popular of saints in the Middle Ages. The accounts of the life and death of Saint Barbara are largely legendary. The story is that she was the daughter of a wealthy heathen man who carefully guarded her by

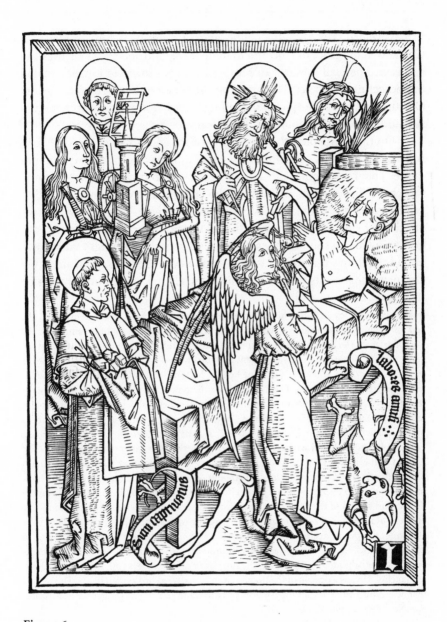

Figure 6

witness *(martus)* by his patient endurance of suffering to his confidence in God and in the grace of God and to his love for God above all else, even life and ease. These all minister to Moriens, who is shown no longer agitated but peacefully at prayer. The malicious little demons are frustrated again. One tumbles out of the picture, scrolling his frustration, and another scurries under the bed announcing his defeat.

On the facing page the inspiration of the angel is given words. "Turn from impatience," it says, and it proceeds to make the case against impatience. That case begins with a warning, a citation from Gregory, "No one shall have the kingdom of heaven who complains and is impatient."[16] It promises that the suffering before death is a purgatory for the dying, provided it be suffered as it ought, that is to say, "patiently and freely with gratitude," for we should be grateful to God in both the things that console us and the things that afflict us. It is the mercy of God, it says, again citing Gregory,[17] that sends temporal punishments here lest the punishments be

---

shutting her in a tower. When his father ordered a bathhouse built near her dwelling, she had three windows put in it as a symbol of the Trinity. Finally, she told her father that she was a Christian. Her father then brought her before the prefect of the province, who first ordered that she be tortured until she recant and finally condemned her to death. Her father carried out the death sentence, beheading her. On his way home from beheading his daughter he was struck by lightning. The dying would call upon her as an intercessor to assure the reception of the sacraments of penance and Eucharist in their dying hour. On that last point see further Mathilde van Dijk, "Traveling-Companion in the Journey of Life: Saint Barbara of Nicomedia in a *Devotio Moderna* Context," in *Death and Dying in the Middle Ages*, ed. Edelgard E. DuBruck and Barbara I. Gusick (New York: Peter Lang, 1999), pp. 221-37. The story of Catherine is that she confronted the emperor Maximinus for his cruel persecution of the Christians and provided a learned account of the Christian faith. The emperor summoned scholars to dispute with her in an effort to get her to apostatize. Catherine won the debate, and several of the scholars summoned to dispute with her became Christians. The empress, too, impressed by the learning of this young woman, became Christian. They were all summarily put to death. Catherine herself was condemned to be tortured and put to death on the wheel. The wheel was, however, miraculously destroyed. Then the angry emperor had her beheaded by the sword. The story of Saint Laurence is both better attested and less fanciful. He was a deacon of the Roman church, martyred by Valerian in 258. The story is that he was burned to death on a gridiron. See further the entries in *The Catholic Encyclopedia* (New York: Appleton Co., 1908).

16. Atkinson, *The English* Ars Moriendi, attributes the quotation to Gregory, *Dialogues* 4, but I could not identify it there. See *Saint Gregory the Great: Dialogues,* trans. Odo John Zimmerman, Fathers of the Church, vol. 39 (Washington, D.C.: Catholic University of America Press, 2002), pp. 189-275.

17. Again, although Atkinson suggests that the line comes from Gregory's *Dialogues* 4 (*Saint Gregory the Great: Dialogues,* pp. 172-74), I have not found it there.

eternal. Moreover, the sufferings of the deathbed, the angel assures Moriens, are nothing compared to the happiness of eternal salvation. Then the angel again reminds him of the cross, of the patience of Christ displayed there, and of the saints who followed him to death, having learned from Jesus a quiet and humble heart (Matt. 11:29), and who were given rest for their souls.

The Temptation to Pride

Having endured the temptations to lose faith, hope, and charity, Moriens is not quite done — nor are the demons quite done with Moriens. There is another — and terrible — temptation waiting. It is depicted in the seventh engraving (fig. 7, p. 126). It is a horrible picture, and a great temptation. It is the temptation to "vainglory," to pride. The demons look confident, and well they might. It is a clever strategy they have adopted for this temptation. If they lost the previous battles for the soul of Moriens, perhaps they can turn those defeats to their advantage and tempt him to pride. They failed when they tempted him to give up the faith, so now they praise him as commendably firm in the faith and offer him a crown. One of the hideous demons, the one lurking at the head of the bed, carries out this strategy, putting a crown in the hand of Moriens while saying, "You are firm in faith." They failed when they tempted him to despair, but perhaps they can use that very defeat to tempt him now to pride. Putting aside the accusations that he had been a terrible sinner, a murderer and a fornicator and a liar and an avaricious old miser, perhaps they can finally prevail if they praise him as a great human being, worthy of a crown. Another of the demons, the one in the center by the side of the bed, evidently has that assignment, offering a crown while announcing that he deserves it. They failed in the temptation to impatience, but perhaps they can get him to boast about his great patience if they praise him for it. And the two diabolical little creatures on the right do exactly that. The scroll they share reads, "You have persevered in patience." A fifth demon also delivers a crown — and the temptation. "Exalt yourself," he says.

The facing page warns against this temptation, against complacency and spiritual pride. Especially if Moriens can claim to be firm in faith and strong in hope and patience, he must work to avoid pride. It sounds like a catch-22. If the devil doesn't get you on despair, he will get you on pride. If you manage to resist him in his efforts to bring you low, he will get you for

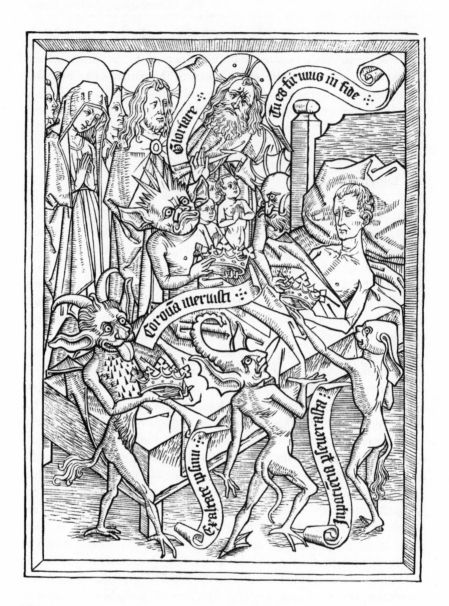

Figure 7

being exalted. If the dying manage faith, hope, and charity, they are liable to boast. And if they manage humility, they are liable again to despair. Nevertheless, the facing page makes it clear that it is a blasphemous presumption to think one could stand justified before God on the basis of the little faith one has held onto steadfastly or the little hope one has not relinquished or the little patience one has charitably displayed. Pride is the way of the devil, the way to hell.

The horrific picture in figure 7, however, is not unrelieved. There in the background stand the Virgin Mary, praying, the risen Christ, and God the Father, who carries a flag with a scroll of its own, *"Gloriare,"* "to boast." The message, I think, is Paul's: "Let the one who boasts, boast in the Lord" (1 Cor. 1:31). There is again, moreover, a company of others, humble saints in the background. Among that company, notably, are three small children, also praying. They are reminders, of course, of Jesus' word, "Whoever becomes humble like this child is the greatest in the kingdom of heaven" (Matt. 18:4). But the crowns are enticing. The flattery feels good. Moriens is in trouble.

The Virtue of Humility

He is in trouble, that is, until angels visit again in the eighth engraving (fig. 8, p. 128). This time three angels are pictured. Perhaps that is a sign of just how strong the temptation to pride can be. One angel, a consoling angel, bends over Moriens and encourages him to humble himself. The message of the scroll is simply that, "Humble yourself." A second angel, hardly consoling, warns Moriens just how fateful and deadly a sin pride is. The warning is in the scroll, "The proud are punished," and in the lower right corner of the image, to which he points. There the punishment for pride is displayed: the fanged mouth of a hound of hell devours the proud, including a friar.[18] The flames of hell escape its mouth, but none of the proud. The third angel prays at the foot of the bed. Once again the Virgin Mary, Jesus, and the Father are present, looking on solicitously, and the Spirit in the form of a dove has joined them. The other figure, with a bell and a crosier, is Saint Anthony. Anthony was remembered and revered not only as the founder of monasticism but also as an exemplar of holiness and humility. He was, moreover, celebrated for his care of the sick, regarded as endowed

18. *Crafte*, p. 12, also refers to "helle houndes" in a prayer to be delivered from them.

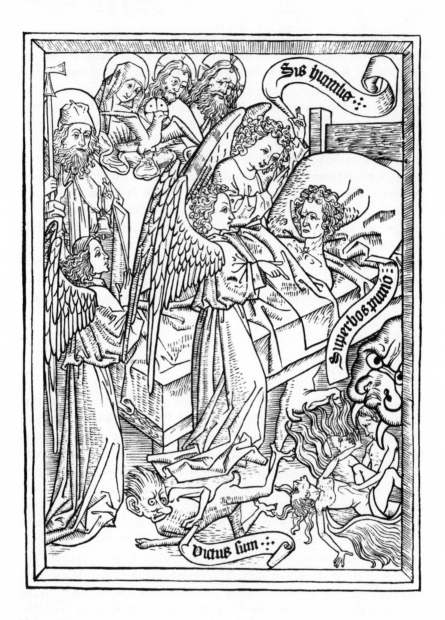

Figure 8

with miraculous powers, but also remembered as attentive to herbal reme-dies. The monastic order dedicated to his patronage, the Antonites, ran hospitals in association with its monasteries, and had distinguished itself by its care of the sick.[19]

The facing page gives a fuller account of the message of the first an-gel. The angel tells Moriens to ascribe his continuing in faith, hope, and patience "solely to God," reminding him of the word of Christ, "apart from me you can do nothing" (John 15:5). Moriens is called to think not so much about himself, whether in pride of his good works or in despair of his sin; he is called to attend to God. Looking to God, not to himself, he can escape the catch-22 that seems to have him caught between despair and pride. He can resist this temptation to pride if he rests confidently finally in God's grace, not in his own virtue. Trust in God, the angel says in effect. It is, I think, the best answer both to anxiety and presumption in the face of God's judgment. The angel warns him that the one who exalts himself will be humbled, and promises him that the one who humbles himself will be exalted (Matt. 23:12; etc.). The facing page also expands upon the warning of the second angel, reporting that the devil himself was cast from heaven for his pride and that he and all the proud with him are doomed to hell. The third angel, the angel at prayer, is itself a model of humble attention to God. The facing page, however, calls attention to that other model of hu-mility pictured in the wood-block print, Saint Anthony. "Take for your model Saint Anthony," the angel says. "To him the devil said, 'Anthony, you have conquered me, for when I wished to tempt you to pride, you were humble, and when I wished to bring you to despair, you were steadfast in hope.'"[20] It is evidently enough for Moriens to humble himself, for the de-

19. Anthony's story had been told by Athanasius in his *Life of Anthony*. See Athanasius, *"The Life of Antony" and "The Letter to Marcellinus,"* trans. Robert C. Gregg (New York: Paulist, 1980). The tau-shaped cross on the top of a long staff is characteristic of representations of Anthony and of the Antonite order. The monastery and hospital at Isenheim were associated with the Antonite order, and Grunewald's famous Isenheim Altar-piece also includes depictions of Anthony. See Andre Hayum, *The Isenheim Altarpiece: God's Medicine and the Painter's Vision* (Princeton: Princeton University Press, 1989).

20. This particular story, however, is not found in *The Life of Anthony*. Mary Catherine O'Connor, *The Art of Dying Well: The Development of the* Ars Moriendi (New York: Columbia University Press, 1942), p. 31 n. 125, suggests that it was attributed to An-thony "in the *exemplum*," because, that is, the life of Anthony was regarded as the example of just such humility. A very similar story was told of Macarius the Great, another "desert fa-ther," a little later than Anthony: "The devil said, 'Macarius, I suffer a lot of violence from you, for I can't overcome you. For whatever you do, I do also. If you fast, I eat nothing; if you

mons slither away again, one to that familiar hiding place under the bed, and the other admitting defeat with his scroll. The prognosis for the soul of Moriens takes another turn for the better.

The Temptation to Avarice

But the final temptation awaits; it is avarice, as the facing page of text announces. In the engraving (fig. 9, p. 131) the temptation is undertaken by three demons. The temptation is subtler than the avarice of the miser. There is no depiction of tidy stacks of gold coins. Instead one demon points toward a fine house, a fine horse with its fine groom, and a fine little wine cellar inside the fine house, where a thief can be seen helping himself to a little wine. How can Moriens let this go? "Consider your treasures," the demon says. A second demon points toward a man and a woman who have evidently come to visit. How can Moriens let such good friends go? He should consider his friends, the demon says. And a third demon, almost solicitously, gestures toward a woman and two children, one still an infant. They are evidently the family of Moriens. How can he abandon them? How can he leave them? What will become of them? Such anxious thoughts may set Moriens's mind on "things of earth" and drive out thoughts of God. So the demons hope, at any rate.

Avarice, the facing page warns, tempts the "secular and carnal." It is to be "preoccupied with temporal and outward things." The devil tempts those who are dying with an inordinate love of the things of this earth, things like a wife and children, friends, and possessions. Moriens should put these things out of his mind and attend to God, considering the greater riches of heaven. But the attachments are real and hard to surrender.

The Virtue of "Letting Go"

Once again, however, an angel attends him, supporting and consoling him (fig. 10, p. 132). He exhorts Moriens to let go, not to hold on too tightly to

---

keep watch, I get no sleep. There is only one quality in which you surpass me.' Macarius said to him, 'What is that?' The Devil answered, 'Your humility; that is why I cannot prevail against you.'" *The Desert Fathers: Sayings of the Early Christian Monks*, trans. Benedicta Ward (New York: Penguin Books, 2003), p. 156. My thanks to Brett McCarty for identifying this passage.

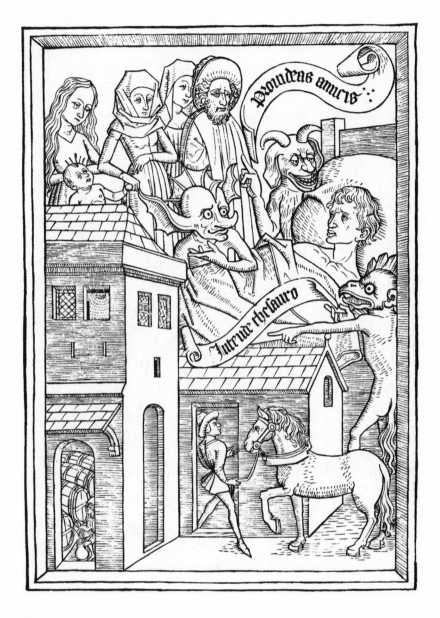

Figure 9

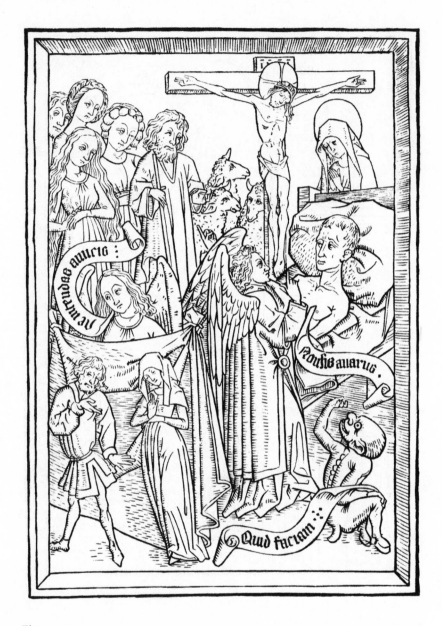

Figure 10

earthly goods, to resist the temptation to avarice. There is Mary again, who let go her own son. And there he is, hanging on the cross. He did not count even equality with God as a thing to be grasped (Phil. 2:6-8). He let go his heavenly glory and then surrendered his life for his sheep. They are there, too, or three of them at least, with the Good Shepherd standing at their side. To the left of the Good Shepherd are three women and the head of a man. Perhaps these are family and friends who can be (and must be) entrusted to the care of that Shepherd. (One of the women is identical to the young woman fairly presumed to be Moriens's daughter in figure 9.) The other little scene in this engraving is, I judge, perhaps his widow put on display by some matchmaker. Whatever this scene is exactly, an angel hides it from the view of Moriens by holding a curtain up. The angel also bears a scroll, "Do not concern yourself about those you love." If Moriens were to see this scene, he might reject the advice of the angel. The single demon is not clever enough to rip the curtain from the hands of the angel, exposing the vulnerability of his wife; instead he looks as if he is trying to snatch the scroll that bears the warning against avarice.

The facing page again expands on the message of the angel, warning Moriens against avarice and reminding him that none of these earthly goods and treasures are able to confer upon him his eternal salvation. Moriens is invited to hold tight to God, not to earthly things. Indeed, they are now impediments on his way to God. He is instructed to renounce them. The angel quotes Luke 14:33, "None of you can become my disciple if you do not give up all your possessions," and Luke 14:26, "Whoever comes to me and does not hate father and mother, wife and children, brothers and sisters, yes, and even life itself, cannot be my disciple." It is a hard word from the angel, but he comforts Moriens with the assurance that those who let go of these things "will receive a hundredfold, and will inherit eternal life" (Matt. 19:29). So Moriens may renounce the things he has loved in this world and die willingly. Finally the angel blesses him with the blessing of Christ: "Blessed are the poor in spirit, for theirs is the kingdom of heaven" (Matt. 5:3). Having let go of earthly things, Moriens is free to go to God happily. The demons have been defeated once again and finally. At the bottom of the figure, the scroll of the little devil, frustrated because he is unable to snatch away the message of the angel, admits defeat.

The Death of Moriens

After the demons have been defeated and the temptations resisted, the final engraving depicts the death of Moriens (fig. 11, p. 135). He holds a candle, still lit, supported by a monk, but he breathes his last breath, and his soul, depicted as a miniature replica of Moriens, escapes from his body to be greeted by a quartet of angels in the upper left-hand corner. The Christ on the cross, probably at the moment he commended his own spirit to God, dominates the rest of the upper half of the engraving. But there at the cross is also the Virgin Mary, Mary Magdalene, and an assembly of disciples and saints. (This is the second appearance of Mary Magdalene, now not so much as the penitent sinner who anointed Jesus, but rather as the faithful follower ready to anoint his body for burial. Mary Magdalene is also, of course, the first witness of the resurrection in John's Gospel, but there is no reference to resurrection in *Ars Moriendi*.)

While the upper half of the engraving is peaceful, if sorrowful, in the face of death, the lower half of the picture is filled with rage, rage at the passing of the light. Six ludicrous little demons rant across the bottom of the scene, raging not because they love life more than Moriens did, but because they have lost the struggle for his soul, their scrolls expressing their frustration.

The facing page contains directions concerning the prayers that the dying should utter while awaiting death. These are the prayers recommended in the later sections of the longer versions, and we need not consider them here. But we should at least note that near the end *Ars Moriendi* advises the dying person to have a faithful friend available to read the prayers if he should become unable to say them. And at the very end it laments the fact that "there are few who will assist those who are near death with interrogations, admonitions, and prayers for them. Because of that, and because the dying often do not wish to die quite yet, their souls are seriously imperiled."

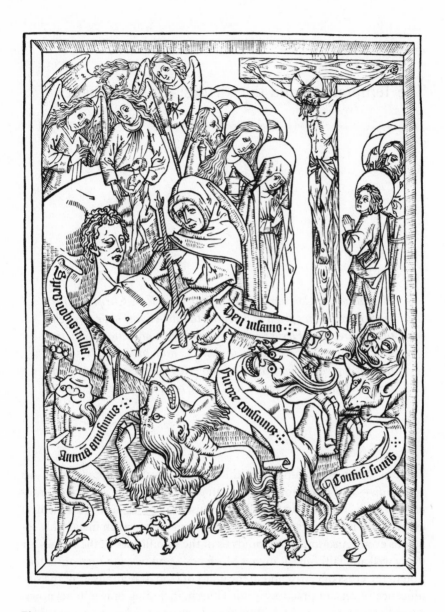

Figure 11

CHAPTER NINE

The Temptations and the Virtues: An Assessment

Blessed be the God and Father of our Lord Jesus Christ! By his great mercy he has given us a new birth into a living hope through the resurrection of Jesus Christ from the dead, and into an inheritance that is imperishable, undefiled, and unfading, kept in heaven for you, who are being protected by the power of God through faith for a salvation ready to be revealed in the last time.

1 Peter 1:3-5

There is much to commend in the account of the temptations in *Ars Moriendi* — and much to retrieve in an effort to imagine a contemporary *ars moriendi*. There is, first of all, the refusal to reduce death to a medical event; death is here regarded as a human event — and as an inalienably religious event. *Ars Moriendi* reminds us of the significance of the virtues for dying well and faithfully. It invites Moriens — and us — to turn our attention to the cross of Christ and to the grace of God. It reminds us of the significance of certain practices of the church, including prayer. It acknowledges the importance of a faithful friend or friends who can care well for the dying. All this and more should inform the effort to imagine a contemporary *ars moriendi*.

It is obvious from the very first illustration that *Ars Moriendi* provides an alternative to a medicalized death. The physicians are there, but they are bit players in the drama of Moriens. As we have noted, the primary complaint of the bioethics literature against the medicalization of death has been that medicalized death renders patients passive while it makes doctors the primary actors, the agents, the people who make decisions. The Baconian refusal to acknowledge that anyone is "overmastered" by disease effectively eliminates the "dying role" and assigns the patient to the "sick role," and one distinguishing feature of "the sick role" is that the sick are relieved of their responsibilities (except for getting to a physician and doing what the doctor says). In *Ars Moriendi*, however, it is acknowledged that Moriens is dying and recognized that he has decisions to make. In contrast to the medicalized dying to which we are heirs, here there is a "dying role" and candid reminders that the dying are moral agents, that they have responsibilities, that they have decisions to make. Moreover, these are not just medical decisions. These are fundamental choices, choices about one's identity and fidelity in the face of death. These choices are not just about some present moment cut off from past and future; these are choices about how to meet the future and about how to own the past as one's own past. These are choices about one's self, one's character, one's virtues. Shall Moriens meet the future, including death and the judgment of God, with faith and hope and patience? Shall he own his past as his own with repentance? It is repentance that allows Moriens not to be fated by that past, neither now as he lies dying nor in his future. And it is faith, hope, and patience, with repentance, that allow Moriens not to cling desperately to life but to be carefree and to die well and gracefully.

To be sure, the dying are not always able to make these decisions. Weakness and weariness and pain and other things can incapacitate them. That is reason enough to have given thought to such matters — and to have formed the requisite virtues — before one reaches the deathbed. And that is reason enough to reject any conspiracy of silence concerning death. As we have also noted, the silence and denial that surround medicalized death have been a primary complaint of the death awareness movement. But here, too, *Ars Moriendi* presents an alternative to medicalized death. Here there is no conspiracy of silence, no denial of the reality of death (even if, as we have complained, the "commendacion of death" denies the real evil of death). All this is to be commended.

Still, this account of the temptations of Moriens and of the virtues necessary to overcome them is not without its problem. It does provide an alternative to medicalized dying but not an alternative that we should attempt to retrieve without qualification. Consider first the scene itself, the deathbed drama of Moriens's temptations.

The Deathbed Drama

For *Ars Moriendi* the deathbed is the scene of great drama and of the greatest temptations, for it is the scene of the final battle for the soul of Moriens. It is the cosmic conflict played out in miniature, the last judgment brought within the microcosm of the bedroom. But the deathbed scene and the drama of Moriens may well seem to us a little *too* dramatic. At least it should prompt some misgivings and questions.

One might complain, for example, that the drama leaves Moriens too much a mere spectator of the war between the demons and angels for his soul. But that complaint seems mistaken. Moriens is, after all, the one who must make decisions, who must resist the demons and follow the advice of the angels. This little self-help manual is not simply a program for people to use to identify the players at an event at which they are spectators.

Alternatively, I suppose, one might complain that it looks a little too much like a trial by ordeal, like a final inquisition to see whether Moriens can pass. Then the spiritual beings that surround him might be inquisitors, tormentors, witnesses, or judges, but they would all remain finally mere spectators of Moriens's ordeal. This complaint too, however, seems mistaken. These spiritual beings are not merely spectators; they are indeed actors in this drama, and the drama is not finally simply a judicial ordeal. If it were, it could only inspire fear, not the comfort and courage *Ars Moriendi* evidently intends to inspire by reminding Moriens of the greater power of God in this contest.

Still, there may be reasons for some misgivings here. One might well complain that, whatever the intention of *Ars Moriendi*, the dramatic attention to the judgment of God at the deathbed and to its significance for the destiny of the soul of Moriens can only serve to heighten the anxiety of dying.

That may be so for many contemporary readers, but in defense of *Ars Moriendi*, the people for whom this little self-help manual was intended started with both the fear of death and the fear of God's judgment. The fifteenth century was a fearful time. The fear of death is understandable enough, given the recurrent plagues. But it was also a time, according to Jean Delumeau at least, of unprecedented attention to one's own guilt and shame and to the threat of God's judgment.[1] The fear of God's judgment,

---

1. We have already cited Jean Delumeau, *La peur en Occident: XIVe-XVIIIe siècles, une cité assiégée* (Paris: Fayard, 1978), for the argument that the centuries following the Black

nurtured by celebrated preachers like Franciscan Bernardino of Siena (1380-1444), was intended to be salutary, leading to repentance and salvation. But it could be argued that the role of dread and terror in pastoral practice created a culture of fear and guilt in the fifteenth century, an image of God as vengeful, and an imagination in which a robust confidence in God was undercut by the presence and power of demons.[2]

Before we turn this complaint against *Ars Moriendi* into a complaint against the whole of the fifteenth century and reject both, we should be a little careful. In the first place, *Ars Moriendi* is an attempt to help Moriens recover a robust confidence in God and in the grace of God. And in the second place, perhaps we should make an effort to appreciate the connection between the fear of death and the fear of God's judgment. Perhaps that connection seems a little off-putting to us simply because we live in a culture accustomed to a "no-fault" morality. Consider the second point first.

The emphasis on God's judgment and the fear of God's judgment is surely unmistakable in *Ars Moriendi*. The deathbed scene is, after all, the scene of the final judgment transferred to the bedroom of Moriens. But we should give it credit, I think, for its acknowledgment that God is, in the phrase of Rudolf Otto, *tremendum et fascinans*,[3] both terrifying and fasci-

---

Death were a particularly fearful period. In his *Sin and Fear: The Emergence of a Western Guilt Culture, Thirteenth-Eighteenth Centuries* (New York: St. Martin's Press, 1990) he argued that the fear of death in those centuries was accompanied by an excessive fear of God's judgment. He traces that fear of judgment to the practices of the "examination of conscience" that had been nurtured by the decision of the Fourth Lateran Council to require annual confession. He called attention not only to the Penitentials, the manuals for the confessors, but also and especially to the sermons of Dominicans and Franciscans who invited people to repentance by warning them of the fierce wrath of God. Jonathan Edwards's "Sinners in the Hands of an Angry God" had plenty of fifteenth-century precedents. Delumeau noted, for example, that the celebrated Franciscan Bernardino of Siena (1380-1444) distinguished at least eighteen types of suffering in hell. In his *Rassurer et protéger: Le sentiment de securité dans l'Occident d'autrefois* (Paris: Fayard, 1989), a study of the efforts to reassure people of the grace of God, he counts the *Ars Moriendi* literature among those efforts to prompt repentance by attention to the wrath of God. A thoughtful survey of the work of Delumeau is provided by Thomas Worcester, "In the Face of Death: Jean Delumeau on Late-Medieval Fears and Hopes," in *Death and Dying in the Middle Ages*, ed. Edelgard E. DuBruck and Barbara I. Gusick (New York: Peter Lang, 1999), pp. 157-74.

2. So, for example, Franco Mormondo, "What Happens to Us When We Die? Bernardino of Siena on 'The Four Last Things,'" in *Death and Dying in the Middle Ages*, pp. 109-42.

3. Rudolf Otto, *The Idea of the Holy*, trans. John W. Harvey (London: Oxford University Press, 1936).

nating. This is a piety that both desires God and fears God. It is a spiritual-ity that regards God as the only final satisfaction for the eros of the soul but also as the one before whom we cannot stand without a shudder. It de-sires finally a relationship with God, but it fears that it is unworthy of a re-lationship of blessing. If we find this unappealing, we should at least ac-knowledge that we rather than the fifteenth century are the outliers here. This ambivalence is not only more typical but also more authentic than the modern supposition that God is simply "nice." A long line of theologi-cal worthies would take the side of *Ars Moriendi* concerning that point. John Calvin comes to mind.[4] And there is Augustine's line from the *Con-fessions* praising God for God's revelation, "You beat back the weakness of my sight, blazing upon me with your rays, and I trembled in love and in dread."[5] And more recently Thomas Merton declared, "The Word of God which is [the believer's] comfort is also his distress. The liturgy, which is his joy and which reveals to him the glory of God, cannot fill a heart that has not previously been humbled and emptied by dread."[6] Faith in God al-ways involves, as Schleiermacher would say, "a feeling of ultimate depen-dence," but it also always typically — and rightly — involves something more, a feeling of inadequacy, of remorse, of shame.[7]

God is God. And we are not! It is not simply a matter of power. It is not simply that God possesses the might, the absolute might, to make claims upon Moriens — and upon all of us — and to compel their fulfill-ment. It is rather that God has the right, the absolute right, to claim our service and praise, for God is absolutely worthy to be served and praised.[8] And it is not simply that Moriens is objectively guilty, that he — or any of us — could be found guilty in the judgment and be liable to punishment. That is true enough, I suppose, in a confrontation with the holiness of God. But although Moriens might quite reasonably worry that he will be found guilty and might reasonably fear punishment, there is something else, something more, in the experience. There is also what Martin Buber

4. His account of "piety," for example, joins the reverent fear of God to the love of God and confidence in his benevolence; *Institutes* 1.2.1.

5. Augustine, *Confessions* 7.10, trans. Rex Warner, p. 149.

6. Thomas Merton, *Contemplative Prayer* (New York: Doubleday, Image Books, 1996), p. 27.

7. On Schleiermacher see Otto, *Idea of the Holy*, pp. 9-11, and "How Schleiermacher Rediscovered the *Sensus Numinis*," in Otto, *Religious Essays*, trans. Brian Lunn (London: Ox-ford University Press, 1931), p. 76.

8. See Otto, *Idea of the Holy*, chapter 8, pp. 50-59.

observed, that "the bearer of guilt is visited by the shudder of identity with himself."[9] The experience of guilt cannot be reduced to the fear of punishment. Even without the judgment and the threat of punishment, the experience of guilt is found in the sense that I *deserve* to be caught and punished. While I proceed unhindered in the ordinary pursuit of pleasure, it is possible to avoid the question of my guilt.[10] But a verdict or an impending verdict can force the question. Then guilt acknowledges the rightness of a guilty verdict; it "approves the other's disapproval of me."[11] And for Moriens the impending encounter with God and with the judgment of God gives new focus and intensity to the ordinary human experience of guilt. It is not just that he is unable to stand in God's presence, but also that he is not worthy to do so. He knows that he is not worthy of the happiness the presence of God promises. So, while he is drawn into the presence of God as his own highest blessing, in the presence of God his life and his very self are offensive to him. To be called into the presence of God is at once a blessing and a threat to the all-too-human self that Moriens — and each of us — is.

Moreover, and crucially, for Moriens this experience of God as threat, as *tremendum,* this fear, this dread, this shuddering, is not the last word. *Ars Moriendi* helps him by helping him to rely on the grace that allows him to avoid the punishment he would otherwise deserve, by assuring him that he need not fear the punishment, and by healing the wounded self-awareness that could only approve God's disapproval. *Ars Moriendi* reminds him not only how vastly his desire for happiness exceeds his worthiness but also how vastly the grace of God exceeds his unworthiness. The drama of the deathbed temptations should not heighten Moriens's anxiety but should nurture in him a robust confidence in God and in the grace of God. True, the devil works "with all his might" to get the dying to lose faith

9. Martin Buber, "Guilt and Guilt Feelings," reprinted in *Guilt: Man and Society,* ed. Roger W. Smith (Garden City, N.Y.: Anchor Books, 1971), cited by Merold Westphal, *God, Guilt, and Death* (Bloomington: Indiana University Press, 1984), p. 75.

10. Westphal, *God, Guilt, and Death,* p. 79, identifies five techniques by which we avoid the question of our guilt: (1) denial of responsibility (e.g., "I was only following orders"), (2) denial of injury (e.g., "Nobody got hurt" or "It was acceptable collateral damage"), (3) denial of the victim's innocence (e.g., "They had it coming" or "They belong to the evil empire"), (4) appeal to higher loyalties (e.g., "How could I abandon my friends?" or "How could I abandon my country?"), and (5) condemnation of condemners (e.g., "Who are you to condemn?").

11. Westphal, *God, Guilt, and Death,* p. 78.

and hope and charity, to be proud and avaricious. True, grotesque demons invade his room and trouble his thoughts. Nevertheless, there is every reason to have confidence in God. From the beginning God is present. From the beginning Christ keeps company with Moriens. From the beginning the Virgin prays for him. And visits from angels always follow the invasions of the horrific little demons, who are consistently driven off the page frustrated. The devil and the demons are doomed to be defeated again and again. Moriens is assured that the might of the devil need not cause alarm. The devil is not as strong as the love of God, and the lies of this "father of lies" are not as powerful as the truth of God. Again and again the angels — and the text — encourage and console. Again and again they remind Moriens of the pity and the mercy of God, which are greater than both his wickedness and the little faith and hope and love that he can manage.[12] This little self-help manual is no more intended to frighten and depress its user than any other late medieval conduct book, whether on hunting or etiquette.[13] It reminds Moriens that God is gracious and invites him to the experience of God as *fascinans,* as attractive, as the exalted source of ecstasy, rapture, beatitude, bliss, and blessing.

Too many contemporary believers — not to mention the cultured despisers of religion — tend to reduce the religious life to its attractive dimension, eliminating the experience of God as *mysterium tremendum.* I think the dying frequently know better, and I think any contemporary *ars moriendi* had better be prepared to deal with guilt and fear honestly and graciously.

That said, however, a complaint can be registered about this death-

---

12. *Crafte and Knowledge For To Dye Well* (hereafter *Crafte*) makes the same point. At the end of its chapter on "the temptacions," *Crafte* assures the dying person again (as it had in the first temptation) that the devil is finally powerless against the grace and power of God. The text cites Paul's word of promise that "God is faithful, and he will not let you be tested beyond your strength, but with the testing he will also provide the way out so that you may be able to endure it" (1 Cor. 10:13). It is the grace of God that enables Moriens to withstand the temptations of the deathbed and to overcome the devil. It is the grace of God that enables Moriens to increase in virtue: in faith, in hope, in charity, in humility, and in devotion to God. The victory is sure. If he submits himself fully into the hands of God, then with God's help, "he shall sewrely opteyne and haue the victory in all maner of tempacions, seekness & tribulaciones, euellyes & sorowes, & dethe ther to" (p. 9). *Crafte and Knowledge For To Dye Well,* in *The English* Ars Moriendi, ed. David William Atkinson, Renaissance and Baroque Studies and Texts, vol. 5 (New York: Peter Lang, 1992).

13. Mary Catherine O'Connor, *The Art of Dying Well: The Development of the* Ars Moriendi (New York: Columbia University Press, 1942), p. 5.

bed drama. By transposing the judgment scene from the end of history to the bedroom of Moriens, *Ars Moriendi* distorts the judgment. To be sure, the last judgment is played out in miniature on the deathbed. But the displacement means a narrowing of vision from the cosmic horizon of Christian hope to the fate of an individual soul. Moreover, in that cosmic horizon the judgment of God is a good thing. In Scripture when God comes to judge the world, God puts it right, God straightens it out. God's judgment will prompt sighs of relief among the oppressed and afflicted and shouts of joy among the trees and the hills (Pss. 96:12-13; 98:7-9). Moreover, the one to whom all judgment has been given (John 5:22) is the very one who was sent because God so loved the world (John 3:16), the very one who came that we might have life (John 10:10). The narrowing of vision from a cosmic horizon of the world set right to a focus on the passage of an individual soul to bliss runs the risk of reducing hope to something egocentric. It is, of course, personal. But brought safely through the judgment by the mercy of God, we are privileged to have a share in the good future of God for the world God has made and will set straight. To use Peter's phrases, "by [God's] great mercy" we have "an inheritance" that surpasses our imagination but that nothing can destroy or wither, "a salvation ready to be revealed in the last time" (1 Pet. 1:3-5).

Moreover, the last judgment follows the resurrection. The resurrection of Jesus (the basis of hope in Scripture and in 1 Pet. 1:3) and our solidarity with Christ in a resurrection like his at the end of time go unmentioned in *Ars Moriendi*. In the cosmic conflict settled by resurrection and the judgment of God, death is a power aligned with sin. It is not commended as a friend to be welcomed.

A different charge has sometimes been brought against the deathbed drama of Moriens. The complaint is that Moriens is represented too much as a solitary individual, isolated and alone in this confrontation with God. *Ars Moriendi*, according to this complaint, is insufficiently attentive to the community.[14] The charge, however, is quite unfair as it stands. Moriens is hardly represented as a solitary individual. True, death itself cuts him off from family and friends, but already in the first engraving he is accompanied by God the Father, Christ the Son, and the blessed Mary. And in the

---

14. So, for example, Brian Patrick McGuire, *Jean Gerson and the Last Medieval Reformation* (University Park: Penn State University Press, 2005), p. 347: "Gerson's message can be interpreted as one of an isolated individual who abandons all hope and bonds with other people and turns to God alone."

second engraving a host of saints have joined both them and him. There are moments, to be sure, when he must feel quite alone, as in the third engraving, that cavern of hopelessness, accompanied only by the demons and accusing memories. Still, it is clear even there that the solitary death is an unhappy death, a bad dying, a dying that jeopardizes the soul of Moriens. Indeed, *Ars Moriendi* reminds him that he is not alone, that he is surrounded by a great cloud of witnesses (Heb. 12:1), who keep showing up along with the angels. The love of God surrounds him; angels and the saints in heaven accompany him, and if the advice of *Ars Moriendi* is followed, so does a faithful friend. The faithful friend or friends who care for him ask the questions of faith, read the prayers, and echo the warnings and comfort of the angels — including the admonition not to think too much of "worldly attachments" like family and friends and possessions. Without such faithful friends the soul of Moriens is placed in jeopardy.[15] If he is reclusive in his sickness, his solitude only provides greater opportunities for Satan to conjure up the temptations to unbelief, despair, impatience, pride, and avarice. It is not good to die alone. To die well is a death in communion with the catholic church, with the saints in heaven and on the earth.

Still, there is reason to be sympathetic with this complaint, especially as a complaint against the advice that Moriens turn away from family and friends, surrendering those relationships as "worldly attachments." *Ars Moriendi* does disparage "worldly" and "carnal" relationships. We will return to this complaint when we consider the virtues commended by the angels. Here we observe that *Ars Moriendi* does not recommend turning from the ties that bind us to family and friends because it regards Moriens as a solitary individual. We have seen that this is not the case. Rather, it recommends turning from these relationships because they are "worldly" and "carnal" rather than "spiritual." Its disparaging of these relationships can be traced to the same dualism of body and soul that prompted the commendation of death. That dualism prompts not only the disparaging of embodied human life and the commendation of death, not only the disparaging of the material world God made and gives and the embrace of some "other" world, but also the disparaging of "carnal" relationships and the preference for "spiritual" relationships.

With this disparaging of the body, this disparaging of "carnal" relationships, *Ars Moriendi* risks allowing death a premature triumph. The risk is not that Moriens will die sooner but that death makes good on its

15. See the facing page of figure 11. See also *Crafte*, p. 17.

threats earlier. As we noted when we discussed the ironies of a medicalized death, death threatens to alienate us from our own flesh, from our communities, and from God. The dualism assumed in *Ars Moriendi* risks its own ironies; in the face of death dualism can sponsor the alienation from our flesh, and by this disparaging of "carnal" relationships it can support the alienation from our communities. If the irony in medicalized death was that the threats of death were allowed a premature triumph for the sake of our biological survival, the irony here is that they are allowed a premature triumph for the sake of the love of God. *Ars Moriendi* insists that we should love God above all, and properly so, but in its dualism (as in some mystical and aesthetic traditions) that is taken to call us from our "carnal" love of family and friends. On the contrary, in my view, the God we are to love above all is the God who gives the good gifts of this world and our bodies and husbands and wives and children and parents. And if that is so, then the duty to love God above all calls us also to be grateful for God's gifts, to delight in them, to mourn their loss. When we suggest in the next part of this book a contemporary *ars moriendi*, we must leave behind not only the commendation of death but also the disparagement of carnal relationships in *Ars Moriendi*.

The Virtues

Consider also the account of the virtues in *Ars Moriendi*. All that deathbed drama, after all, simply stands in the service of nurturing resistance to the temptations of Moriens and sustaining the virtues for dying well and faithfully. Five temptations were listed. The first was the temptation to lose faith. The second was the temptation to despair, to lose hope. The third was the temptation to impatience, the temptation to lose charity. The fourth was the temptation to pride. And the fifth was the temptation to avarice. The remedies for these temptations were the virtues of faith, hope, love that is patient, humility, and serenity.

The temptations are not to be regarded as stages of dying. Although Moriens proceeds from one to the other, the little self-help manual is alert to the problem that the one who is dying may encounter any one of them at any time and any one of them more than once while dying. Old wounds can open up again, and despair can threaten again. Or, one can go limping between pride and despair, with humility and hope seemingly at odds. But the virtues are finally a unity. The temptation to lose faith is set first because faith in God is fundamental for all the others, not because it is a different thing than all the others. It is faith that exists as hope and works as charity. It is faith that evokes humility and the freedom from anxiety about "worldly" things.

Although we will retrieve both this emphasis on the significance of the virtues for dying well and these particular virtues in their rich diversity and their unity, we must also question and qualify certain features of the account of the virtues in *Ars Moriendi*.

Faith

As the angel said, citing Bernard, "Faith is the primogenitor of all virtues." But what is faith? It is worth observing once again that the Spirit rests on the bedpost of figure 2. Perhaps Bernard is remembered here, too, without being cited, for Bernard, commenting on Psalm 90:9, "You, O Lord, are my hope," had called attention to faith as a gift of the Spirit: "Brothers, to savor this [Psalm 90:9] is to live by faith. No one can pronounce the sentence, 'because you, O Lord, are my hope,' except the person who is inwardly persuaded by the Spirit that, as a prophet admonishes, he casts his burden upon the Lord, knowing that he will be cared for by him, as in keeping with what the apostle Peter said, 'Cast all your anxieties on him, for he cares about you.'"[16] Faith in Bernard is not some last desperate work. It is a gift of the Spirit that persuades us of the truth of what the prophets and the apostles say. It is a kind of knowledge, then, but it is not simply an intellectual knowledge, for the truth is that God cares and can be trusted. It is an experiential knowledge that takes root in our heart and passes into our daily life — and into our dying. It is a lively confidence not only that God is, but that God cares. It is loyalty to God and to the cause of God. It gives birth, as Bernard says, to hope and to all the virtues.

So to live by faith — and to die in faith — is to "savor" that care with confidence and hope. It allows Moriens to cast his anxieties upon the Lord. By faith he can find both comfort and courage for his dying. By faith he can "look to" and follow "Jesus the pioneer and perfecter of our faith, who for the sake of the joy that was set before him endured the cross" (Heb.

---

16. Bernard of Clairvaux, Sermon 9.6 on Psalm 90, in his *Sermons on Conversion*, trans. Marie-Bernard Said, O.S.B., Cistercian Fathers Series, no. 25 (Kalamazoo, Mich.: Cistercian Publications, 1981), 22.7. The internal citation of Peter is 1 Pet. 5:7.

12:2). By faith he can join that great cloud of witnesses in Hebrews 11 who endured suffering and death in loyalty to God's cause. Confident of God's care, he can overcome anxiety (1 Pet. 5:7); loyal to God, "steadfast in faith," he can overcome even the devil (1 Pet. 5:9). By faith he may be assured that suffering and death are not the last word, that "the God of all grace, who has called [him] to his eternal glory in Christ, will himself restore, support, strengthen, and establish [him]" (1 Pet. 5:10).

All this is commendable, I think, and a contemporary *ars moriendi* will retrieve it. Even so, a question or two must also be registered. First, did the *Ars Moriendi* tradition always preserve this emphasis of Bernard on experiential knowledge in its account of faith? In *Crafte,* for example, faith is defined in ways that seem to privilege intellectual assent and obedience to the church's laws. There faith is to give full credence to "the pryncypall articles of the feyth, but also to all holy wrytte in all maner of thynges and fully to obeye the statutes off the Churche off Rome" (p. 4). There is in *Crafte*'s account of the first temptation no mention of faith as trust, as a lively confidence in the grace and care of God. The stress in *Crafte* risks reducing the significance of faith and faithfulness in the face of death to the intellectual acceptance of a deposit of tradition and to obedience to canon law.[17]

This complaint is not to deny that faith exists as a kind of knowledge; it does, also in Bernard. This knowledge, moreover, is not simply the knowledge that God exists; it is the knowledge of God's character and cause. It is that knowledge, the knowledge of God's character and cause, that shapes both faith and faithfulness. The more fundamental question that must be raised, then, concerns the account of the character and cause of God presupposed in *Ars Moriendi*. *Ars Moriendi* clearly affirms that the virtue of faith is not simply to trust any old god; it is not faith in some god invented by the philosophers or imagined in the conceit of someone's "ultimate concern."[18] Faith in such gods is folly, and is frequently broken in dying. This is faith in the God of Israel and of Jesus, the God whose char-

---

17. There is also reason to worry a little that the creed is treated like a charm, like magic, when both the angel of *Ars Moriendi* and *Crafte* (p. 4) commend to those who might attend Moriens the practice of repeating the creed in a loud voice as a way to drive the demons away.

18. I suppose everyone has "faith" of some sort, some person or thing in which one places trust and whose cause one serves. As H. R. Niebuhr said, "to be a self is to have a god." H. R. Niebuhr, *The Meaning of Revelation* (New York: Macmillan, 1952), p. 80. In a sense everyone lives by faith. And dying sometimes breaks such faith, such trust and confidence. That is one of the reasons people suffer in their dying.

acter and cause are made known in the story Scripture tells. So far, there is no quarrel. But how we tell that story makes a considerable difference to how it passes into our daily living and into our dying. How we plot that story makes a considerable difference to the way we understand the character and cause of God — and so also to the way we enact our trust and perform our faithfulness. And the question is whether *Ars Moriendi* gets that story quite right.

It is a story that begins with creation, that continues with God's covenant and care in spite of human sin, that centers in the crucified and risen Jesus of Nazareth, and that ends in resurrection and the renewal of this world. It is not a story in which God's world or our bodies are damned (even if they are currently damaged). It is not a story in which God's cause is to save individual souls from the world (or from their bodies), but a story in which God's cause is to save the world (and to redeem our bodies — Rom. 8:23). The passage that stands at the head of this chapter, 1 Peter 1:3-5, and the whole of the New Testament may be called as witness to two points about the story. First, the resurrection of the Lord Jesus Christ stands at the center of the story and as the source of our hope, our faith that God cares and can be trusted. And second, the cause of God, the salvation that is already at work in the world, will finally be "revealed in the last time."[19] By its neglect of Christ's resurrection (and our own) and by the shrinking of cosmic hope to the salvation of souls, *Ars Moriendi* risks distorting the shape of faith and faithfulness. Faith is not faithfully displayed in an asceticism that is born of dualism and takes flight from this world to some "other world." It is displayed in delight in God and in the gifts of God, which include this world and this embodied life, and in confidence that at the limits of that life God can still be trusted to care and to save. The story is that God saves the world, a world and a salvation in which we have by grace already a share.

19. This is an "inheritance" that surpasses our imagination but that nothing can destroy or wither. That it is "kept in heaven" does not mean that you have to go to heaven to get it, and it surely does not mean that "salvation" is simply a matter of going to heaven when you die. "Heaven," as biblical scholar N. T. Wright says, is simply a reverent way to talk of God. He illustrates his point in this way: "If I say to a friend, 'I've kept some beer in the fridge for you,' that doesn't mean that he has to climb into the fridge in order to drink the beer." God's good future, our inheritance, a new heaven and a new earth, are kept safe with God. And by the same power that raised Jesus from the dead, God will reveal that good future here in this world "in the last time." See N. T. Wright, *Surprised by Hope: Rethinking Heaven, the Resurrection, and the Mission of the Church* (New York: HarperOne, 2008), pp. 151-52.

Hope

Faith exists as hope, to be sure. *Ars Moriendi* and Bernard have that right. Dying is a great threat to hope, and despair is a great threat to dying well. Dying can break the faith, the confidence, we have in some things and some people. Something like that happens in a medicalized dying. When we, catechized in the Baconian project, trust technology to relieve the human condition of its misery and its mortality, when we suppose that no one, and especially not we ourselves, will be "overmastered by their diseases," then that faith is fragile when we are dying. And when that faith is broken, despair can take its place. It works the other way, too. In the absence of any hope or confidence in God that death will not have the last word in God's creation, the medical resistance to death can grow desperate, and dying can become increasingly medicalized. Then we have the ironic consequences of a premature alienation from our flesh, from our communities, and from God that we described in the first part of this book.

Ars Moriendi, of course, is not particularly interested in the despair that can follow the unmasking of technology and the mastery of nature as false "gods" as we lie dying. It is interested, rather, in the despair that can follow the unmasking of our confidence in our own righteousness. That confidence, too, is confidence in a false "god," and it will almost certainly be broken with the little review of one's life that usually accompanies the acknowledgment that one is dying. When that confidence is broken, it can indeed bring despair. And the antidote for such despair is not one more desperate attempt to achieve one's own righteousness while we are dying; the antidote is hope, hope in God rather than in the little good we did well, hope in God in spite of the sins that have marked and marred our lives.

As we noted, *Ars Moriendi* cites Bernard to announce that the mercy and pity of God are greater than any wickedness of man. With hope Moriens can look to Jesus on the cross and see there the mercy of God. Bernard's invitation to meditate on the cross was given in *Crafte,*[20] and it assured Moriens that no one need despair of God's forgiveness. With hope he can join those sinners who learned to hope in God: Peter and Paul, Mary Magdalene and the thief on the cross. With hope he can see the heavens open to sinners like him, as in figure 4.

20. See above, chapter 8, note 13.

This is not hope in our own righteousness but hope in God. For all its attention to the sins of Moriens, *Ars Moriendi* knows that the contemplation of God's goodness and mercy must take precedence over the contemplation of our sins. Perhaps Bernard is remembered again without being cited, for he had said quite plainly, "Sorrow for sin is indeed necessary, but it should not be an endless preoccupation. You must also dwell on the glad remembrance of God's loving kindness, otherwise sadness will harden the heart and lead it more deeply into despair."[21]

Again there is much here to commend. It may be asked, however, whether *Ars Moriendi* has too restricted a vision of the temptation to despair. The temptation to despair in the face of death is not just prompted by the poverty of our own little righteousness in confrontation with the worthiness of God. It is also prompted by the fact of death itself, by the fact that my life will soon be over, by the fact that I will soon be no more. The antidote to such despair is still hope in God, to be sure. But the basis of that hope is not just the cross of Christ, in which we may see the disposition of God to forgive, but also and especially the resurrection of Christ, in which we may see the power of God to give life to the dust, to make all things new, even us. But *Ars Moriendi* is silent about the resurrection. Perhaps that silence is not so curious, given the assumption of the immortality of the soul and the commendation of death, but it is a silence that distorts hope. The basis of our hope is not the immortality of the soul. The basis of our hope is the power of God to raise the dead. And the scope of our hope is not limited to the salvation of an individual soul, transported to heaven. The scope of our hope is the cosmic sovereignty of God, in which we by God's grace may share. A hope that reduces God's cause to the salvation of souls suggests an egocentric faith and a shrunken hope.

Patience

Impatience can surely make dying more difficult. And as figure 5 displays, the impatience of Moriens makes his dying difficult not only for him but also for those who would care for him.[22] Impatience finds its remedy in the

21. Bernard of Clairvaux, *Sermons on Conversion* 11.2.
22. It works the other way, too, of course, that the impatience of caregivers can make dying difficult, but *Ars Moriendi* is not a self-help manual for caregivers (even if it does address them in a few asides) but for the dying.

virtue of patience, and patience, as *Ars Moriendi* insists, is the work of love. It cites 1 Corinthians 13:4 to make the point. "Love is patient; love is kind."

Ars Moriendi evidently understands the "love" of 1 Corinthians 13 to have God as its object rather than other members of the Christian community, and that may prompt a question or two. First, Paul seldom uses "love" to talk of a Christian's disposition toward God, and it is unlikely he did so in 1 Corinthians 13. Hard on the heels of the twelfth chapter, 1 Corinthians 13 is part of a polemic against the spiritual elitists in Corinth, against those who boasted about their spiritual gifts but did not love the less gifted. The first three verses are enough to make that plain, but we might remember the claims of chapter 12 that each Christian is gifted and that each is gifted "for the common good" (12:7). To boast about one's gift, to use it in an elitist fashion, is not to use it as the Spirit intended. As faith is active in love of the neighbor (Gal. 5:6), so love of the neighbor is active in patience and kindness (1 Cor. 13:4).[23] These are the routine works of love in community, in the "one body" (12:13), the body in which "if one member suffers, all suffer together with it" (12:26).

It may seem a mere quibble. After all, the commandment to love God is the first and great commandment. But when the love of the neighbor is left out of consideration, we get a shrunken image not only of love, but also of love's patience. Indeed, we get a shrunken image of the cross. When Moriens is invited to look to the cross of Christ and to the patient love displayed on that cross, he is invited to see, of course, Christ's devotion to God the Father and to God's cause. He loved God more than his own ease, more than life itself. For the sake of God's cause he walked a path that led to suffering and death quite willingly. But when Moriens attends to that cross, one may hope that he also sees Christ's love for the neighbor and for the enemy. That is the pattern of the cross, the willingness to suffer with and for others. So, at least, 1 Corinthians 13 suggests. The elitists who claimed that they were already fully spiritual did not get it. They denied the solidarity with any who suffer that is the pattern of the cross, the solidarity with any who suffer in the "one body." In their preoccupation with themselves and their spiritual status, they neglected the responsibility to love the neighbor, to be patient with a neighbor, to have compassion. But that love for the neighbor, that patience, that compassion is, Paul says, the

---

23. "Patient" and "kind" are verbs in the Greek, not predicate adjectives; "love patiences" and "love kindnesses" would be odd but accurate translations, capturing the emphasis on the works of love.

best index of their spiritual status, for it is the mark of God's good future and the evidence that members of this one body participate in that future already. "Love never ends" (1 Cor. 13:8). That love is relevant both to those who would die faithfully and to those who would care for them. And any effort to imagine a contemporary *ars moriendi* will have to include that love, with its patience and compassion.

There is, however, another problem here. *Ars Moriendi* invited Moriens to look to Christ and also to the martyrs to learn compassion. The martyrs had learned from Jesus a humble and quiet heart in the face of suffering and death, and they witnessed by their patient endurance of suffering that some things were more valuable than ease, some duties more compelling than survival. That is surely right, and it is an emphasis that must be preserved, retrieved, in any contemporary *ars moriendi*. But it does not make suffering itself a good or death itself commendable. They are evils to be endured for the sake of other and greater goods, other and greater duties. *Ars Moriendi* goes badly wrong when it (citing Jerome) insists that to receive sickness and death with sorrow is a sign of not loving God sufficiently. The cross does not make masochists of us. And the love of God is not inconsistent with loving the world God loves or the bodies God gives or the "carnal" relations in which bodies inevitably involve us. And if they are worth loving, then their loss is worth grieving. It was the Stoics, not Christ, who had no place for sorrow in the face of suffering and death. And as we have noted, Stoic "contentment" and Christian patience are not the same. It is Stoicism, not Scripture, that condemns lament. Christ's patience was not incapable of lament, and a contemporary *ars moriendi* will make a place for lament. Attention to Christ as the paradigm for a Christian's faithful dying itself allows — and requires — it.[24]

24. I leave aside another legitimate complaint. The construal of patient suffering as a satisfaction of time in purgatory risks giving an egocentric justification for suffering. To be sure, in *On Loving God* Bernard of Clairvaux identified four stages of love: to love self for one's own sake, then to love God for one's own sake, then to love God for God's sake, and finally, to love even one's self for God's sake. And he says, moreover, that in the third stage to love the neighbor is no longer difficult. Still, one might prefer Calvin's complaint about preoccupation with one's own salvation: "It is not very sound theology to confine a man's thoughts so much to himself, and not to set before him as the prime motive of his existence zeal to show forth the glory of God" ("Reply to Sadolet," in *Calvin: Theological Treatises*, ed. and trans. J. K. S. Reid, Library of Christian Classics, vol. 22 [Philadelphia: Westminster, 1954], p. 208).

Humility

Surely *Ars Moriendi* is right: pride gets in the way of dying well. Pride pretends to self-sufficiency, whether the self-sufficiency of our own righteousness or the self-sufficiency of our own resources to keep suffering and sickness and death at bay. Pride pretends to have no need of either the grace of God or the grace of another human being. It refuses to acknowledge neediness, and it is therefore no good at gratitude.

As my mother used to tell me, and as the sage once said, "Pride goes before a fall" (cf. Prov. 16:18). Life frequently has a way of bringing down those who exalt themselves, but if life does not do it, dying will. Death is the great leveler, after all. And dying almost inevitably reminds us of our neediness. The refusal to acknowledge neediness makes difficult not only gratitude but also receiving the gift of care from another.

The temptation to pride may be especially strong in our culture, which places such emphasis on autonomy and control. We pity those we see as "needy," and, while we may exercise a condescending helpfulness, we want it clear even in our helpfulness that we are not needy ourselves. We will have to return to "the conceit of philanthropy," which can poison the work of caregivers. But pride can also poison the task of receiving care, making those in need of care resentful about "being a burden" and unable to receive care graciously.

Such pride is finally folly. We are simply not as independent and autonomous as we like to pretend. We all start, after all, as babies, and we remain dependent upon others all through our lives. To acknowledge gratefully our dependence upon God and upon other human beings is a mark of wisdom and a key to living well and dying well.[25]

Ars Moriendi may restrict its account of pride too much to the self-

---

25. Alasdair MacIntyre, *Dependent Rational Animals: Why Human Beings Need the Virtues* (Chicago: Open Court, 1999), observes that we are all always somewhere on a continuum of disability. "[T]here is a scale of disability on which we all find ourselves. Disability is a matter of more or less, both in respect of degree of disability and in respect of the time periods in which we are disabled" (p. 73). He rejects the dichotomy between disabled and nondisabled. Identifying ourselves with the disabled is an important part of acknowledging our dependence, and acknowledged dependence is, as MacIntyre argues, a key to human flourishing. He also observes that people with current disabilities are dependent upon the imaginative and creative involvement of the surrounding community. His position is not opposed to technological interventions, but it rejects as a "failure of imagination" communal support for the disabled (or for the dying) that is restricted to technological intervention.

righteousness that pretends to have no need of God's grace, but it is surely right to identify pride as a temptation and a measure of humility as the antidote. And it is surely also right to insist that attention to God and to the grace of God can nurture humility. Attentive to God, we can acknowledge our neediness and no longer fear it. Attentive to the grace of God, we need not pretend that it is our little righteousness that makes us worthy of God's care (or anyone else's) and we need not anxiously hoard the little resources we think we have against vulnerability.

"Letting Go"

Thus pride is related to avarice, to the anxious tightfistedness that is unwilling to let go of the possessions by which we think to establish our independence and our security against need. That temptation, of course, is the final temptation of Moriens, the anxious refusal to "let go." And there is something profoundly right in this. The anxious refusal ever to let go, whether of our possessions or of our family members or of our friends or of life itself, is something closer to idolatry than to affection.

Let go of them, of course, we finally must. Death will take them from us. That is the threat of death. To die is to be dispossessed, to be sundered from the things and the people we love. And let go of them we finally may, for at the limit of our lives God may still be trusted. With faith in God we can let even ourselves go, confident in God's power and grace. That confidence, with its attendant freedom from anxiety, is the antidote for avarice.

Still, there is something deeply flawed about the way *Ars Moriendi* understands this temptation and its antidote. We have complained previously about the disparagement of "worldly attachments," and so we can be brief here. Granted that my parents and wife and children are not gods; they are nevertheless the good gifts of God. To treat these relationships as trivial, to disparage these "carnal" relationships, is not a mark of great spiritual maturity but of ingratitude. If they are worthy of my love while I live (and they are), then they are worthy of my grief at being sundered from them. Dying well requires that I do not cling to them anxiously as if I could expect them to save me from my mortality (or as if they have no hope without me), but it also requires that I do not discard them as distractions or prematurely alienate myself from them. That is to give death a premature triumph. Dying well requires attention to these relationships, not neglect of them. Words of gratitude and praise, requests for forgiveness and the granting of forgiveness, provision for their future well-being, and words of love and affection — all of that and more belong to "letting go."

The angel cited the hard words of Jesus against possessions and about "hating" those to whom we are tied with natural bonds of affection (Luke 14:33, 26). I take these hard words to be warnings against idolatry, and I acknowledge that the good gifts of God can be rendered idols, but I insist that they remain nevertheless good gifts of God. And I simply confess that I have never found the consolation of Matthew 19:29 about receiving "a hundredfold" what we have left very consoling. I do not want a hundred wives. I love the one I have. I do not want a hundred children. I love the ones I have. One other or a hundred others are not a substitute for the ones I love.[26] With C. S. Lewis I "hope that the resurrection of the body means also the resurrection of what may be called 'our greater body'; the general fabric of our earthly life with its affection and friendships."[27]

The strength of this temptation to Moriens suggests that he loves life and loves the material world. But the problem is not that he loves what God made good. The problem is not that he loves what God also loves. The problem is to let go of that anxious grasping. And the antidote for that anxiety, for this avarice, is not to be found by substituting for this world some disembodied and "spiritual" otherworld, to which our souls will be transported. The answer is to be found in the good future of God, the kingdom of God, the renewal and redemption of this world and of these bodies. The answer is to be found in God's power and promise to give life to the dust, to raise the dead. God's good future is sure to be. God's grace and power secure our identity and our hope. Then we can be carefree, serene, even in the face of death. Then we can hear the command "Be not anxious" as a blessing.

All these virtues — faith, hope, a love that is patient, humility, and

---

26. These "hard sayings" were prompted by the urgency of the announcement of the coming kingdom of God and by the social context. They remain appropriate challenges to our culture when "family values" are given an ultimacy that they do not warrant. They seem to render Jesus dismissive of family relationships and obligations, but Matt. 15:4-6 demonstrates that he was not. It was, moreover, in discipleship, not in death, that they "left" possessions and friends. To those whose relationships with their families were severed because they had become followers of Jesus, the promise of compensating relationships in the kingdom (and already in the relations of "brother" and "sister" within the church) may indeed have been consolation. But such sayings should not be read or used as consolation for the dying (or the grieving).

27. C. S. Lewis, *The Four Loves* (New York: Harcourt, Brace and World, 1960), p. 187.

serenity — support another virtue, namely, courage in the face of death and in spite of the fear of death. In the preface of *Crafte* it was clear that the motive for this self-help literature was to comfort the person facing death, but that comfort, as we noted, was not just solace but *com-fortis,* a strengthening, courage. Their comfort was their courage, and all these virtues nurture it and sustain it.

CHAPTER TEN

"Interrogaciones," "Instruccions," and Prayers

Q. *What is your only comfort in life and in death?*

A. *That I am not my own, but belong — body and soul, in life and in death — to my faithful Savior Jesus Christ. He has fully paid for all my sins with his precious blood, and has set me free from the tyranny of the devil. He also watches over me in such a way that not a hair can fall from my head without the will of my Father in heaven: in fact, all things must work together for my salvation. Because I belong to him, Christ, by his Holy Spirit, assures me of eternal life and makes me wholeheartedly willing and ready from now on to live for him.*

The Heidelberg Catechism, Lord's Day 1[1]

The "Interrogaciones"

The third chapter of *Crafte and Knowledge For To Dye Well* "contyneth the interrogaciones that schulde be askyd of thym that been in deth bedde whyle they may speke and vnderstand."[2] Its provision of a little catechism

---

1. "The Heidelberg Catechism," in *Psalter Hymnal* (Grand Rapids: CRC Publications, 1987), p. 861.

2. *Crafte and Knowledge For To Dye Well* (hereafter *Crafte*), in *The English Ars Moriendi*, ed. David William Atkinson, Renaissance and Baroque Studies and Texts, vol. 5 (New York: Peter Lang, 1992), p. 9. Page references to this work will be placed in the text.

with questions and answers concerning faith, repentance, and the assurance of God's pardon is typical of works in the *Ars Moriendi* genre.

Crafte, of course, did not invent this device of questions and answers as a way to profess the faith. Nor was it an innovation to use such a device in ministry to the sick. O'Connor believes that such "interrogaciones" of the sick belonged originally with penance and were joined to the anointing of the sick (or extreme unction) very early.[3] Even the particular questions and answers used in *Crafte* were not new. *Crafte* provides in fact two separate little catechisms, the first attributed to Anselm (1033-1109),[4] and the second to Jean de Gerson.

The questions would ordinarily be put by a priest, of course, but priests were in short supply in the centuries of plague; so it is good that they find a place in these self-help handbooks. If there is no priest at hand, or no friend to read them to the dying person, then Moriens should consider these questions "in hys sowle" (p. 11). And in preparation for death, these questions and answers could be memorized so that they could be remembered and recited in the hour of death, whether in response to the "interrogaciones" of a priest or a friend or "in hys sowle." The proper answers could provide assurance that Moriens need fear neither death nor the judgment of God.

The seven questions attributed to Anselm are these: (1) Are you glad that you die in the faith of Christ? (2) Do you acknowledge that you have not done what you should and that you have done what you should not? (3) Do you repent of these sins? (4) Would you amend your life, should you survive? (5) Do you believe that our Lord Jesus Christ, God's Son, died for you? (6) Do you thank him with all your heart? (7) Do you believe that you can be saved only by Christ's passion and death? The catechism instructs Moriens simply to say yes in answer to each of these questions.

Following these questions and their answers there is an instruction to give thanks to God "whyle thy soule ys in thy body" (*Crafte,* p. 9) and to trust completely and only in the passion and death of Christ while one is dying. "To thys dethe comytte fully." Then should any anxiety about God's judgment and damnation arise (as in figure 3), if "thyne enemy putte in to

3. See Mary Catherine O'Connor, *The Art of Dying Well: The Development of the* Ars Moriendi (New York: Columbia University Press, 1942), p. 34.

4. O'Connor, *Art of Dying Well,* pp. 34-35. See Anselm, *Admonitio morienti et de peccatis nimium formidant,* in *Patrologia Latina,* ed. J.-P. Migne (Paris: 1844-55), 158:685-88. The "Anselm catechism" may in fact be older still; the questions were widely used in medieval liturgies. For a brief history of the "Anselm questions," see O'Connor, pp. 33-35.

thy mynde that God well deme the," Moriens is told to say, "Lord, I putte the dethe off oure Lord Ihu Cryste betwene me & mine euyll dedys, betwene me and thy iugement, otherwyse I well nat stryve with the." Finally, the dying person is instructed to say three times, "into thy handes I comytte my sowle." It is, of course, the prayer of Jesus on the cross (Luke 23:46). If Moriens is unable to say these words, then those caring for him or standing by should say, "in thy handes Lorde, we commende hys sowle" (p. 9). Thus Moriens may die confidently and "nat dye euerlastyngly" (p. 10).

The Anselm "interrogaciones" are "sufficient," *Crafte* says, but following Gerson it recommends that people receive a fuller inquiry and instruction concerning "the state and the hele of hyr sowles" (p. 10). The alternative set of questions, also seven, expands upon the questions of Anselm. So, for example, the first question is no longer simply whether one is glad to die in the faith of Christ. It asks whether one accepts the creed and what is taught in Scripture (as interpreted by "the holy and trewe doctours off holy chyrche"), whether one rejects all the heresies rejected by the church, and then finally whether one is glad to die in the faith of Christ. And, for good measure, it adds, "& in the vnity and obedience off holy churche."

The expansions upon the second, third, and fourth questions reflect the mystical theology of Gerson. The second question, concerning the acknowledgment of sins, cites Bernard of Clairvaux, one of Gerson's favorites, to commend humility and to assert that the fear of God is both the beginning of wisdom and the beginning of a soul's health. The third question, whether the dying person repents of these sins, is expanded to inquire whether repentance is prompted not only by the fear of God's judgment "but rather more for loue of God & ryghtwysnes" (p. 10). It contains the invitation to repent for any disordered love, that is, any failure to love God above all things. And the fourth question expands the question concerning the commitment to amend one's life with attention to the temptation of worldly attachments. It includes an inquiry whether that commitment to amend one's life includes a readiness to forsake all earthly things, including life itself, "thy lyfe off thy body," for the sake of loving God.

Two questions are inserted that bring repentance and the commitment to amend one's life to bear on the dying person's responsibilities in dying. The fifth question here reminds Moriens that the love of Christ, from whom he has the hope of forgiveness, requires forgiveness and reconciliation with others. It asks whether he has forgiven those who have wronged him and sought the forgiveness of those whom he has wronged. The sixth question here asks whether restitution has been made for any "mysgoten" goods. The final three questions of Anselm's "interrogaciones" are combined into one final question in this second set: "beleuest thou fully that Cryste dyed for the and that thow mayst neuer be saued, but be the meryte of Crystes passyon, and thankest theroff God withall thyn herte as moche as thow mayst?" (p. 11).

Crafte then assures Moriens that, if he can answer yes to all these questions, he may be assured of the health of his soul and its salvation. The chapter ends with another reminder that Moriens should commit himself fully to the passion of Christ: "Late hym remembre hym and thynke on the passion off Cryste, for therby all the deuylles temptacions and gyles be moste ouercome and voyded" (p. 11). It is the crucial piece of advice to Moriens.

The "Interrogaciones": An Assessment

I admit that I am a fan of catechisms, having been nurtured on the Heidelberg Catechism. I memorized it as a growing boy at the insistence of both the pastor who taught the "catechism class" and my parents. I remember struggling to recall the words without fully understanding them, usually failing my father's initial oral examination, but always receiving his praise when I finally got it right. Those sessions seemed tedious then, but I look back on them with a certain fondness. I can remember my father admonishing me at the end of some of his examinations, "And now remember, son, it's not enough just to memorize these words. You must take them to heart and try to live by them." It sounded like strange advice to me then, but although I do not remember the whole catechism by any means, some of the questions and answers have come back to me again and again. The first question and answer has provided comfort and courage in the face of reminders of my own mortality.

Q. What is your only comfort in life and in death?

A. That I am not my own, but belong — body and soul, in life and in death — to my faithful Savior Jesus Christ. He has fully paid for all my sins with his precious blood, and has set me free from the tyranny of the devil. He also watches over me in such a way that not a hair can fall from my head without the will of my Father in heaven: in fact, all things must work together for my salvation. Because I belong to him, Christ, by his Holy Spirit, assures me of eternal life and makes me wholeheartedly willing and ready from now on to live for him.

When my hair fell out as a result of chemotherapy, the catechism reminded me that God's care was still my constant companion. This comfort was indeed a *com-fortis* to me. The same question and answer had found its way onto the lips and into the hearts of my parents — and many others who knew "the Heidelberg" — as they lay dying.

Anselm's little catechism would no doubt have served similarly to comfort and encourage those who had memorized it. One might quibble a little with the lengthier catechism. The emphasis shifts a little from faith as a robust confidence in the grace of God to faith as an intellectual acceptance of certain propositions and to obedience to the statutes of the church. Moreover, the love of God above all things seems to be taken to require a depreciation of "carnal" goods. But we have registered these complaints before and need not revisit them. On the other hand, there is considerable wisdom in the inclusion of the duties of forgiveness and restitution at the end of life, included by the lengthier catechism in questions five and six. Indeed, to some extent at least, such duties honor rather than diminish the significance of "worldly attachments." They should not be forgotten when we attempt to imagine a contemporary *ars moriendi*.

The "Instruccion": Christ as Paradigm

The third chapter of *Crafte* ended with the crucial piece of advice to "remember Jesus" and his passion, to "thynke on" it. In the fourth chapter, simply entitled "an instruccion" (p. 11), that advice is repeated and developed. That "instruccion," to remember Jesus and to imitate him in his dying, is central to the effort of *Crafte* and many other works in the *Ars Moriendi* genre to help Moriens to die well and faithfully. It is essential to both the comfort and the courage they intend to nurture. Jesus' death is paradigmatic for a Christian's faithful dying.

The "instruccion" begins by citing Gregory the Great, "Euery doyng off Cryste ys oure instruccion & techyng."[5] It is, however, especially the story of Christ's passion to which *Crafte* — and the whole *Ars Moriendi*

5. Gregory frequently called for the imitation of Christ, but I could not locate this precise phrase.

tradition — invites attention. Jesus' death is the great paradigm for a Christian's dying; "suche thynges as Cryst dyd dyinge on the crosse the same shulde euery man do att hys last ende." *Crafte* then lists five things that Christ did on the cross: he prayed, he cried out to God, he wept, he commended his soul to God, and he gave up his spirit ("wylfully he gaff up the gost on the cross"; p. 11). *Crafte* observes, moreover, that in his prayers Jesus made use of the Psalms, and as evidence it mentions Psalm 22:1, "My God, my God, why have you forsaken me?" and Psalm 31:5, "Into your hands I commit my spirit."

These five things Moriens should also do. He should pray. He should cry out to God; *Crafte* insists that his cry, unlike Jesus' cry, should be and must be for the forgiveness of his sins. He should weep; Crafte insists that his tears should be tears of repentance. He should commit his soul to God, saying, "Lord God, in to thy handes I commende my spyryte, for trewly thow thy selfe bought hit dere" (p. 12). And he should "wylfully" give up his spirit; he should die willingly, conforming his own will to the will of God.

Next *Crafte* provides, in accord with its instruction to pray, a collection of prayers for the dying person to use (for as long as he can).[6] The first pleads for the mercy of God: "O thow hygh Godhed and endeles goodnes, most mercyable & gloryous trynite, thow art hygest loue and charyte. Haue mercy on me, wreched and synfull man, for to the I commend fully my sowle." The next is a longer prayer addressed first to God the Father and then to God the Son, pleading once more for mercy, commending the soul to God, and now petitioning by Christ's merit for entry into "paradyse and blys" (p. 12). Then Moriens is invited to repeat often the prayer of Psalm 116:15-17: "Lord, . . . You have loosed my bonds. / I will offer to you a thanksgiving sacrifice." This invitation is given with the assurance (citing Cassiodorus) that to say this verse three times in good faith at the end of life assures the forgiveness of sins.

These prayers are followed by still others. Moriens is invited to pray to the Virgin Mary that she would intercede for him with her Son. He is instructed to pray to the angels (and especially to his guardian angel) that they would accompany and protect him in his dying. He is told to pray to the apostles, saints, martyrs, confessors, and virgins, and especially to any saint who has been most loved by the dying person during his life, that they too would protect him and welcome him to heaven.

6. The prayers seem to be taken from the work of Jean de Gerson (O'Connor, *Art of Dying Well*, p. 37).

There is then this prayer that *Crafte* recommends to Moriens (and attributes to Augustine): "The peese off oure Lorde Ihu Cryste, and the vertew off his passyon, and the sygne of the holy crosse and the maydenhed off oure blessyd lady, Seynt Mary, and the blyssyng of all seyntes, and the kepying off all aungelles, and the suffrages off all the chosen peple off God be betwene me and all my enemyes, visible & ynvisible, in thys oure off my dethe" (p. 13). And a final prayer is offered, with the instruction that Moriens say it three times: "graunte me Lord a clere ende that my soule shall neuer downwarde, but yeve me euerlasting blysse that ys the reward off holy dying" (p. 13). These prayers are to be said by Moriens, but if he is unable to say them all, then *Crafte* instructs that they be read aloud in his presence by a person who is with him.

The "Instruccion": An Assessment

The instruction is surely right to command our attention to Jesus as the paradigm for faithful dying. Whatever the differences among Christian communities, they would seem to agree about this, that all the stories of our life and of our common life ought to be tested somehow by the story of Jesus. And surely the stories of our dying ought to conform somehow to the story of Jesus' death and passion. Our effort to imagine a contemporary *ars moriendi* in the next part of this book will take this as the fundamental clue from the fifteenth century, that the story of Jesus' dying is somehow normative for a Christian's dying and caring for the dying. Following the tradition of the *Ars Moriendi* on this crucial point, we will find reasons, I think, to depart from it on several other points. But following it on this point, we may also find the resources to imagine a contemporary *ars moriendi* and to resist the medicalization of death. That, however, is the task for the next section of this book.

Even so, we may already note that *Crafte* seems not to notice the inconsistency of its earlier adoption of a Stoic attitude toward death, which made no place for lament, and its own account here of "suche thynges as Cryst dyd dyinge on the crosse." In its account of Jesus' prayers, it noted that he prayed using the Psalms, but the psalms Jesus prayed and that *Crafte* noted (Pss. 22 and 31) were psalms of lament. If we follow *Crafte* in commending the death of Jesus as paradigmatic for a Christian's dying, then we will have to correct it when it gives no place for lament.

We should, moreover, also note one other problem here. *Crafte* focuses so much on Jesus' death as atonement, as a death for the forgiveness of our sins, that it risks losing sight of the human tragedy of death. It puts at risk the very paradigmatic significance of Jesus' death that it is at pains to underscore. The focus falls so much on the atoning death, on the death of Jesus *for* our sins, that the solidarity of Jesus *with* the dying and suffering (and the solidarity of the dying with him) is put at risk. The paradigm breaks. So, while, like Christ, we should cry out to God, our cries, unlike Christ's, should be cries of repentance, cries for the forgiveness of our sins. And while, like Christ, we should weep, our tears, unlike Christ's, should be tears of repentance. The point is not to deny that Christ's suffering and death have atoning significance; the point is rather to suggest that the atoning significance is precisely the point at which the paradigmatic significance of the story of the cross breaks down. We need not — and we should not — pretend that our suffering and dying are somehow redemptive, surely not in the sense that our suffering now may ease our suffering in purgatory. Nevertheless, the crucial point remains that the death of Jesus is paradigmatic for a Christian's faithful dying in ways I hope to display in the next section.

Some of those ways are already noted in this "instruccion," and we cannot leave this section of *Crafte* without commending its invitation to Moriens to pray. Prayer was among the practices that helped Moriens to die well, and it surely must be included among those practices that will help contemporary Christians to die well and faithfully. Further attention to prayer, too, however, must await the next section. Here let it be enough to worry a little that prayer can be corrupted into magic, into a technology to get what we want. That risk is real, it seems to me, when *Crafte* suggests that reciting the prayer of Psalm 116:15-17 guarantees that one's sins will be forgiven.[7]

An "Instruccion" to Friends and Caregivers

The fifth chapter of *Crafte* is entitled "an instruccion vnto hem that shullen dyen" (p. 13), but it is actually an instruction to the friends and caregivers of Moriens. This may be a self-help manual, but it is aware that a good dying requires good friends. The chapter begins with the observation

7. An additional complaint might be registered about the misreading of Ps. 116 as a commendation of death. It is not. It is a psalm of thanksgiving for the recovery of health, for being restored to life. But we have registered that complaint before.

that many people are in what we would call denial. Even the "relygyous & devoute" tend to assume they will not die any time soon. It may be self-deception, but *Crafte* says it is a self-deception wrought by the devil. That observation prompts *Crafte* to instruct friends and all who would care for the sick to warn them and to invite them to care for their souls' well-being when their bodies seem in perilous condition. It is a matter of first importance, then, that friends and caregivers instruct the sick to seek "spyrytuell medycyne and remedy off hys soule."

Crafte reminds its readers of a "certain decretall" of Gregory IX that had insisted upon the priority of spiritual care, observing that "bodyly sekenes cometh of sekenes off soule" and requiring that doctors refrain from treatment until the dying person had sent for the priest, or in the quaint language of *Crafte,* that "euery bodyly leche . . . yeue ne sekeman no bodyly medycyne vnto the tyme that he hath warned & enduced huym to seche hys spiritual leche [every physician for the body . . . give no medicine for the body unless he has warned and induced the sick man to call for his spiritual physician]."[8]

8. The Fourth Lateran Council (1215) had decreed that:

Since bodily infirmity is sometimes caused by sin, the Lord saying to the sick man whom he had healed: "Go and sin no more, lest some worse thing happen to thee" (John 5:14), we declare in the present decree and strictly command that when physicians of the body are called to the bedside of the sick, before all else they admonish them to call for the physician of souls, so that after spiritual health has been restored to them, the application of bodily medicine may be of greater benefit, for the cause being removed the effect will pass away. We publish this decree for the reason that some, when they are sick and are advised by the physician in the course of the sickness to attend to the salvation of their soul, give up all hope and yield more easily to the danger of death. If any physician shall transgress this decree after it has been published by the bishops, let him be cut off from the church till he has made suitable satisfaction for his transgression. And since the soul is far more precious than the body, we forbid under penalty of anathema that a physician advise a patient to have recourse to sinful means for the recovery of bodily health. (Lateran IV, 22)

The translation is from R. J. Schroeder, *Disciplinary Decrees of the General Councils* (St. Louis: Herder, 1957), p. 236; cited by Darrel W. Amundsen, *Medicine, Society, and Faith in the Ancient and Modern Worlds* (Baltimore: Johns Hopkins University Press, 1996), p. 201. This canon was included in the *Decretals* of Gregory IX (5.38.13) and so made its way into canon law.

Several things are worthy of note in the decree. The first is obvious: it asserts the precedence of spiritual care over medical care. The decree insists on the priority of the spiritual medicine of confession and sacrament in part, at least, because "bodily infirmity is sometimes caused by sin." There is an assumption here of a connection between sin and sickness,

Death was not yet "medicalized," and it was not likely to become "medicalized" as long as Gregory had his way. Care for the sick and dying

---

an assumption that presumably was widely held. It implies an intimate relation of body and soul in the living human person, signaled by what we might today call psychosomatic disorders. To be sure, many medieval thinkers had learned from Job or from Jesus to hesitate before accusing the sick of some particular sin. Still, it was generally understood that sickness should prompt repentance, and this assumption of a connection between sin and sickness could burden the ill with a sense of guilt. Confession, as the decree says, may be curative. The spiritual medicine could restore spiritual health, and then the medicine for the body would be rendered either superfluous or more effective in healing.

The point of the decree is evidently not to assure that confession is made before the death of the patient but rather to assist the patient's recovery. Physical life and health were regarded as great goods. And physicians were regarded as the servants of God and of those goods. Only let them not be presumptuous. Let them not forget that their skills and knowledge, their medicines and their successes, come from God. Let them not forget that their patients are not just bodies, but religious persons.

However commonplace the *contemptus mundi* (contempt for this world) was in the literature of the late Middle Ages, and it was commonplace, the church did not forget that life and health are good gifts of God. One treatise, influential throughout the late Middle Ages, *De miseria humane conditionis* (On the wretchedness of the human condition), had been written by Innocent III, the pope who convened the Fourth Lateran Council, when he was still a cardinal. But however wretched the human condition (and especially old age) in the view of Innocent III, life was still a good gift from God. It may be broken and spoiled by sin, but it remained the work of the Creator.

Moreover, the church was hostile neither to science nor to medicine. Neither was regarded as the enemy. Indeed, the church had founded most of the universities and hospitals, and even when some of these institutions passed into the control of municipal governments in the thirteenth and fourteenth century, they continued to have the support of the church. To confirm this judgment one need only consider the penitential literature of the time. That literature, designed to aid confessors in their work, had been stimulated by the requirement of annual confession to one's own priest — another canon of the Fourth Lateran Council that was included in the *Decretals* of Gregory. Together with the inquiries of the confessors, penitential writings required of physicians that they be competent, that they keep abreast of developments in medicine, that they consult colleagues when in doubt about a case, and that they not harm a patient by negligence or ignorance (Amundsen, p. 203).

Still, it is not finally the health or life of the body that is the primary concern of the Fourth Lateran Council. While the decree makes it plain that physical life and health are to be regarded as great goods, it also makes plain that they are never to be regarded as the greatest goods. Some things were more important than health, more important even than physical life itself. The final stipulation of the decretal pronounces an anathema on the physician who would recommend illicit means to recover health or to preserve life. It does not stipulate what those illicit means are. The penitential literature, however, did sometimes identify the illicit means. Among the sinful means were fornication, masturbation, and magical incantations. The authors of the penitential literature did not always agree about the list, but

was not to be reduced to medical care, and medical care was surely not to be reduced to an effort to cure. The patient was not to be reduced to body, and surely an embodied person not to his or her pathology. Gregory's decretal had insisted on the priority of spiritual care, and it had not been forgotten in the fifteenth century. There were reminders of it not only in the *Ars Moriendi* literature but also in medical writings of the day.[9]

Crafte complains, however, that the counsel of this decretal is usually ignored, that people "seken sonner & besylyer [sooner and more actively] after medycynes for the body than for the sowle" (p. 13). So *Crafte* repeats the advice, as if repetition could remedy the neglect. To be a good friend or a good physician one must exhort Moriens above all to make peace with God, to receive the sacraments, and to order his affairs, making a will and testament.

Then *Crafte* complains again that too many will not even hear of the likelihood of their death. And to that complaint *Crafte* adds another, even more interesting to modern ears. It complains about a practice of giving too much hope for recovery to the sick, about "a veyn and a false cheryng and comfortyng and feyned behotyng of bodyly hele" (p. 14). *Crafte* worries (citing Gerson)[10] that, trusting such false assurances of their recovery, some will die unprepared for God's judgment and risk damnation. *Crafte* counsels a different course. Friends and caregivers should tell the sick honestly of the peril they are in, even if it frightens them. They are to tell the truth, not offer deceptive assurances of recovery.

Crafte instructs friends one more time to exhort their sick friend to confession. Even if he is in great peril spiritually, they should not despair but encourage him to make confession, to turn from his life of sin, and to be assured of God's mercy. The friends are to be no less honest about his spiritual health than about his physical health, even if this too frightens him. Isaiah's warning to King Hezekiah is provided as a model. "Hit ys better and ryghtfuller that he be compuncte and repentaunte with holso

---

they all agreed that the effort to preserve life did not license anything and everything (Amundsen, pp. 267-68).

9. So, for instance, one anonymous physician, writing a tractate in 1411 concerning the plague, advises his colleagues to tell the patient "to set himself right with God . . . as is set forth according to the Decretals"; then he continues by giving advice about the examination of the patient's urine and feces and pulse. Cited in Amundsen, *Medicine, Society, and Faith*, p. 300.

10. Jean de Gerson, *Opusculu Tripertitum*, in *Opera Omnia*, ed. Louis Ellier Du Pin (Hildesheim: George Olms Verlag, 1987 [a reprint of Antwerp 1706]), 1:449.

feare and drede, and so be saued, than that he be dampned with flatteryng and false dissimulacion" (p. 15). In this context *Crafte* assures them of the legitimacy of deathbed repentance, citing Gregory and Augustine as accepting the authenticity of repentance on the deathbed. The friends are then urged to help the sick sinner to resist the temptation to despair, and *Crafte* suggests that for that task they might make use of some of the material in its second chapter. Indeed, friends should help the sick resist all the temptations, utilizing the other admonitions and comforts provided in the second chapter of *Crafte*. They are told to inquire whether the sick sinner is under any censure of the church, and if so, to exhort him to make it right that he may be absolved.

Many other acts of care for the soul of Moriens are suggested. Friends are urged to recite for him "deuoute historyes and deuoute prayers," especially those in which he delighted while he was healthy. They are told to help him in his self-examination by rehearsing the commandments of God. They are instructed to use the interrogations and the prayers given in the manual, even if he can only answer "with consente of his herte." They are told to present him with the crucifix and to sprinkle holy water on him, for the demons cannot tolerate these things. And if it is not possible to do all these things, then the friends should at least do what they can. But they should not, *Crafte* urges, neglect to pray.

There is one more instruction for the friends of Moriens. They are told not to call to his mind his "carnal friendys" or his wife, or his children. The friends prove themselves to be spiritual friends by helping Moriens to focus solely on his "spirituell helthe" (p. 15).

The chapter closes with a warning to all. When death comes, devotion flees; "whan dethe or grete sekenes falleth vpon the, deuocion passeth oute ffro the" (p. 16). Because it is not easy to die well and faithfully, *Crafte* admonishes its readers, including the friends of the dying person, to learn the craft of dying while they are still "in hele [in good health — not in hell]" (p. 16). This is as close as *Crafte* gets to what will become a commonplace in the subsequent tradition, that to learn to die well we must first learn to live well.[11] And because it is not easy to die well and faithfully, it is important that Moriens be accompanied. Many — indeed, "all a cyte" — should come together to the aid of a sick man near death.

11. Perhaps first and most notably in Erasmus, *Preparing for Death* (1534), trans. John N. Grant, in *Collected Works of Erasmus*, vol. 20, *Spiritualia and Pastoralia*, ed. John W. O'Malley (Toronto: University of Toronto Press, 1998), pp. 392-450.

An "Instruccion" to Friends and Caregivers: An Assessment

There is much here to commend. If earlier we noted that some worried that Moriens was represented as a solitary individual in his contest with the demons, this part should put that worry finally to rest. Dying well takes a community.

The community must be relied upon, first of all, to tell Moriens honestly that he may be approaching death. That honesty stands in obvious contrast not only to the self-deception to which the sick, as *Crafte* acknowledged, were tempted also in the fifteenth century, but also to the silence and denial of the medicalized death of the twentieth century. In the medicalized death of the twentieth century, as we have noted, one could hardly count on physicians or friends to tell you that you were dying. There would be a conspiracy of silence and deception to keep such a prognosis unknown. It might be observed, I guess, that even if dying well is taken to mean dying without knowing that one is dying, it takes a community. The silence and denial surrounding medicalized death require something of a conspiracy and social sanction for the deception. But community cannot be built upon lies; deception finally alienates. And a medicalized death, as we have observed, gives the alienation from community that death threatens a premature triumph.

The community can be and must be relied upon also to accompany Moriens in his dying. It may not abandon him to the physicians or to his solitude. To die well is acknowledged to be hard, and it requires help from one's friends. This attention to the help caregivers can and must offer to the dying is also commendable. The attempt of the next chapter to imagine a contemporary *ars moriendi* may not ignore consideration of the responsibilities to care well for the dying. And no small part of that care for the dying, both in *Crafte* and in any retrieval of the *Ars Moriendi* tradition, is found in simply being present, keeping company, and then doing what one can to help and comfort Moriens.

We may, in this context, commend one other point hinted at by *Crafte*. To tend to the dying, to care for them, contributes to one's learning to die well oneself. To witness another dying well or badly is instructive for those who would die well themselves.[12]

---

12. The point is made more explicit in subsequent works within the genre. See, e.g., Erasmus, *Preparing for Death*, pp. 447-48: "[W]e shall profit greatly by being frequently at the bed of the dying. We will then avoid what we have seen to be detestable in them and will imitate what is righteous and holy."

Still, we must register once again the complaint that has become something of a refrain. There is again a depreciation of "worldly" and "carnal" attachments. And it threatens to give a premature triumph to the alienation from our bodies and from our "carnal" community associated with death.

One other little aside in this chapter deserves our praise and will help to form a contemporary *ars moriendi*. It is the simple instruction to the friends, do not neglect to pray.

Prayers

What was a "little aside" in the fifth chapter becomes the focus of the final chapter of *Crafte*. In its sixth chapter it provides a collection of prayers and blessings for friends and caregivers to use as Moriens lies dying.

The chapter begins with the rueful complaint that only a few know the craft of dying well and "wyll be nygh and assiste" the dying (p. 17). To help both those who are at hand accompanying Moriens and Moriens himself, the prayers are provided. They were not the creation of *Crafte;* they had, as O'Connor observes, liturgical origins.[13] There are prayers addressed to God the Father, to Christ the Son, to Saint Michael, and to the Virgin Mary. The prayers to God and to Christ attend to the love of God and the cross of Christ and plead for mercy and pardon for all the sins of Moriens. The prayer to Michael asks for protection from evil spirits and "the dragon off hell" (p. 18). The prayer to Mary asks her to help with the anguish and against the enemies of Moriens. The prayers are followed by two commendations, or blessings, that commend the soul of Moriens to God and bless him as he goes. The second of these is an ancient one:

> Go Crysten soule owte of thys worlds, in the name of the almyghty Fader that made thee of naught, in the name of Ihu Cryste, hys Son, that suffred his passion for the. And in the name of the Holy Gost . . . cherubyn & seraphyn mete with the, patriarches and profytes, apostiles and euangylistes, martyres, confessoures, monkes, heremytes, mayden and wydowes, chyldren & innocentes help the. The prayers of all prystes and dekens . . . helpe the that in pease be thy place, and thy

13. O'Connor, *Art of Dying Well,* p. 40.

dwellynge in heuynly Ierusalem euerlastyngly, bi the mediacion of oure Lord Ihu Cryste that ys medyatoure betwen God and man, Amen. (*Crafte,* pp. 19-20)

And that blessing is *Crafte's* last word.

Prayers: An Assessment

The prayers are quite beautiful. But perhaps most notable is what is absent. There is no mention in any of these prayers of the resurrection. There is no mention of the resurrection of Christ as the basis of the Christian hope, and no mention of the resurrection of the Christian, the redemption of our bodies, or the renewal of God's creation as the object of our hope.

But that is the place an effort to imagine a contemporary *ars moriendi* should begin, and to that task we finally turn.

PART THREE

Faith and Faithfulness in the Face of Death: Toward a Contemporary *Ars Moriendi*

Love is strong as death.

Song of Solomon 8:6

In the first part of this book we attended to the medicalization of death in the mid–twentieth century. While we celebrated the advances in science and medicine that provided new powers to preserve life, we also noted that the rejection of that old wisdom that some are simply "overmastered by disease" had led not only to great accomplishments but also to the medicalization of dying. We complained that the medicalization of dying prematurely alienated people from their own bodies, from their communities, and from God. Ironically, the threats of death were allowed a premature triumph in the name of preserving life.

In that first part we attended also to the chorus of voices that had challenged the reduction of death to a medical event. And while we joined our voice to that chorus, we also complained a little about the complaints of standard bioethics and the death awareness movement. We questioned the wisdom of the single-minded emphasis on patient autonomy in standard bioethics. And we challenged the mantra of the death awareness movement that "death is natural." But we acknowledged that communities of faith bear the responsibility for teaching people how to die well and faithfully, and we admitted that the churches have been too often silent about death and too ready to surrender dying to medicine.

In the second part, looking for an alternative to medicalized dying, we turned to the fifteenth century and to the *Ars Moriendi*. In that self-help handbook for dying well the church was not silent, and it refused to surrender dying to medicine. It surely did present an alternative to medicalized death — but not an altogether satisfactory alternative. Indeed, when it began by commending death as liberation from the body, it sounded more Platonic than Christian. It may have made dying easier, but the cost was high. In its otherworldly orientation, it risked in its own way a premature alienation of people from their bodies, from their "worldly" communities of family and friends, and from God's good creation (if not from God). Ironically, death made its power felt in the very commendation of it.

Still, by its invitation to faith and faithfulness in the face of death, the *Ars Moriendi* can prompt twenty-first-century Christians to consider again what it might mean to die well and faithfully. And for that consideration it provided some important clues, the most important being the paradigmatic significance of the death of Jesus. But there are other clues as well: its attention to the significance of the virtues for dying well, its recognition of the importance of the community of faith (and that in a self-help handbook), and its commendation of the practice of prayer. The tradition of *Ars Moriendi* can be retrieved — but it must also be criticized — in the light of Scripture. Since Scripture is regarded as normative by the *Ars Moriendi* tradition itself, such a selective retrieval is surely warranted.

This part of the book will suggest some important features of a contemporary *ars moriendi*. It will take the invitation of *Ars Moriendi* to think about faith and faithfulness in the face of death by following the clues left by that little self-help handbook, by remembering the story that Scripture tells, and especially by considering the paradigmatic significance of the story of Jesus. This is not a self-help manual on the art of dying, but I hope it will be instructive for whoever would undertake the task of writing something like *Dying Well for (Christian) Dummies* (and I hope someone will).[1]

It starts not with a commendation of death but with a commendation of life, attending especially to the story of the resurrection. It moves

---

1. Perhaps that hope has already been fulfilled. In the final days of the preparation of this manuscript, InterVarsity Press was kind enough to send me a galley copy of Rob Moll, *The Art of Dying: Living Fully into the Life to Come* (Downers Grove, Ill.: IVP, 2010). It is a fine book, and I am happy to recommend it.

then not directly to the temptations and to a consideration of the virtues but rather to the "instruccion" of *Ars Moriendi* to remember and follow Jesus, attending to the stories of Jesus' passion and death. Then the way will be clear, I hope, to attend again to the temptations and to the virtues for dying well, virtues formed by the story of Jesus.

In the fourth section, recalling the little catechism of *Ars Moriendi,* we will attend to contemporary catechesis, to the task of the church to form faith and to nurture faithfulness and virtue in the face of death by its instruction and its practices. We will follow *Ars Moriendi* by emphasizing one of those practices, prayer. And we will retrieve the wisdom of *Ars Moriendi* that dying well and faithfully is made easier by the presence of others who care well and faithfully for the dying.

CHAPTER ELEVEN

A "Commendacion" of Life

Thine be the glory, risen, conquering Son;
endless is the victory thou o'er death hath won.

Endom Budry, "Thine Be the Glory"[1]

The Resurrection

On a Sunday morning some women went to the tomb where Jesus had been buried.[2] What they found there, or didn't find, changed the world. Life would never again be quite the same — nor death.

---

1. Endom Budry, "A toi la glorie," trans. R. Birch Hoyle, in *Rejoice in the Lord*, ed. Erik Routley (Grand Rapids: Eerdmans, 1985), #327.

2. The story of the discovery of the empty tomb is found in all four Gospels: Mark 16:1-8; Matt. 28:1-8; Luke 24:1-12; and John 20:1-13. The story has been subject to considerable scholarly debate. Because the empty tomb is not mentioned in the summaries of the proclamation of the early church (e.g., Acts 2:14-39; 1 Cor. 15:1-7) or anywhere else in the New Testament, some have suggested that the story is a late invention, a pious fiction. (So, for example, Willi Marxsen, *The Resurrection of Jesus of Nazareth* [Philadelphia: Fortress, 1968], p. 161.) Many have called attention to the discrepancies in the details: Were there several women (as in the Synoptic Gospels and in my retelling here), or one? Was there a young man (as in Mark and in my retelling here), or an angel, or two men, or two angels? Was Galilee the place for the promised appearance of the risen Christ or a place of memory? Each Gospel tells the story in its own way, and I hold no brief for the historical accuracy of each of the details in each of the stories, but the substantial reliability of the story of the empty tomb

It was an ordinary day, a day when the mundane patterns of life in and around Jerusalem resumed after the Sabbath. But on this ordinary day, an extraordinary thing had happened. The women were still grieving, thinking perhaps that the hole in their lives left by his death might shrink a little if they could just be close to his dead body. Perhaps they could at least show his body a little care, a little respect. But the body was not there. There was just a young man in a white robe. It was not Jesus, but he knew they were looking for Jesus. "He has been raised," he said. There was no doubt that he had been dead. These women had seen the crucifixion, had seen the body taken from the cross. He was dead. "He has been raised," the young man said. "But it cannot be," the women must have thought. "Dead is dead, and he *was* dead. It cannot be that he was raised, unless God . . ."

It cannot be, unless God is faithful to his promises. It cannot be, unless God is at work to end the rule of sin and death in God's own world. It cannot be, unless God had now won the great victory that was promised. The passive voice of the messenger was the hint of it. It was God who was active here, God who had raised Jesus from the dead.

The empty tomb, of course, proves nothing really. The women were not quick to the inference that it was God at work. Maybe it was not God; maybe the body was moved or stolen. The empty tomb proves nothing, but it does raise some questions. Whose work is this? What is going on?

Later on that same day, the disciples saw Jesus, or at least someone or

---

has much to be said for it. The first point to be made is simply that it has multiple attestation; it is told not only by Mark (and Matthew and Luke, following him) but also independently by John. Moreover, if the story were a late invention, it would be more than a little strange that in the narrative it was women (or a woman) who discovered the empty tomb. Women were not regarded as reliable witnesses in the first century. That prejudice would have prompted inventors of such a story to have Peter or John (cf. John 20:3-10) or some other male discover the empty tomb. And to make just one other point, the early announcement in Jerusalem that Jesus had been raised would not have lasted a day if someone could have produced his body. The belief in the resurrection of Jesus was not the conclusion of a historical argument, but in the Jewish world of the first century the claim that he had been raised would have been easily falsified by producing his corpse. Those who did not believe the announcement that Jesus had been raised acknowledged that the tomb was empty even as they provided some other explanation for that strange fact. They might claim that the disciples stole the body (Matt. 28:11-15), or at least that someone took him (cf. John 20:2, 13), but they evidently agreed that the tomb was empty. The stories, surely, are not the sort of history that an Enlightenment historian would like, but we may be confident about their substantial reliability. The Evangelists were not attempting to provide an archivist's report; they were proclaiming the gospel, but they were proclaiming the gospel *because* they were convinced that Jesus had been raised and the tomb was empty.

something that sure looked like Jesus.[3] They, too, were not quick to believe that Jesus had been raised from the dead. The Gospels are quite clear that the initial response was disbelief. Luke reported that when the women told the disciples about the empty tomb, they dismissed it as "an idle tale" (Luke 24:11). The disciples on the way to Emmaus did not even recognize Jesus as Jesus until he had interpreted Scripture for them and broken bread with them (Luke 24:13-32). And even after the report of the women and the disciples from Emmaus, even after they had heard of an appearance to Simon Peter, when Jesus appeared to all of them at once, they were "startled and terrified, and thought that they were seeing a ghost" (24:37). "In their joy they were disbelieving," Luke says (24:41). This was a story too good to be true. It could not be, unless God . . .

The other Gospels make the same point in their own ways. Matthew reports that when Jesus appeared to them in Galilee, "some doubted" (Matt.

---

3. The stories of the appearances of Jesus have also been the subject of considerable controversy. That Jesus appeared to the disciples (and to many others) was surely part of the earliest proclamation of the gospel (e.g., 1 Cor. 15:1-7; Acts 10:36-45; 13:17-41). But again there are discrepancies in the details that elude any easy harmonization. Mark gives no account of an appearance, only the promise of one to the disciples in Galilee (Mark 16:7; Marxsen reads "there you shall see him" in that verse as a reference not to an appearance of the risen Jesus but to the appearance of Christ at the parousia at the end of time [Marxsen, *Resurrection of Jesus*, p. 164]. That reading seems implausible, however, both because of other references to the resurrection in Mark [e.g., Mark 9:10] and because of the reference to Peter [cf. 1 Cor. 15:5]). Two of the other Gospels tell a story of an appearance to the women (in Matt. 28:9-10) or to Mary Magdalene alone (in John 20:14-18). Matthew, Luke, and John all tell a story of an appearance of Jesus to the disciples. Matthew sets it in Galilee (Matt. 28:15-20), while Luke and John set it in Jerusalem (Luke 24:36-43; John 20:19-23). In addition, Luke tells the story of an appearance of the risen Jesus to two disciples on their way to Emmaus (Luke 24:13-32) and reports an appearance to Peter (Luke 24:33-35). John tells the story of a second appearance to the disciples when Thomas was present (John 20:24-29). And John 21 tells the story of an appearance of Jesus to the disciples by the Sea of Tiberias (or Galilee, John 21:1-14). Again I hold no brief for the historical reliability of all the details in these stories, but the substantial reliability of the tradition that Jesus appeared to members of his community — or at least that there were people who claimed to have seen Jesus — is undeniable. Again, the claim to have seen Jesus does not "prove" the resurrection. There are plenty of other explanations, no less familiar to them than to us: hallucination, ghosts, dreams, etc. The belief that Jesus had been raised is not the conclusion of a historical argument, whether the premise is an empty tomb or the report of an appearance. Still, when these two are put together, it is not historically unreasonable to believe that Jesus was raised from the dead. Of course, one may still insist that it's impossible, but that is a metaphysical argument (and probably a fundamental choice about how to construe the world we live in), not a historical argument. And the reply is still, "It *is* impossible, unless God . . ."

28:17). And John tells the story of "doubting Thomas" (John 20:23-29). These were not some gullible primitives who did not understand (as we modern people do) that dead is dead. They knew that. And judging from the stories of those disciples on the Emmaus road and of Thomas, they were ready also to acknowledge that the hope they had harbored that Jesus was the Messiah, "the one to redeem Israel" (Luke 24:21), was also dead. These were not enthusiasts who refused to acknowledge the facts. Dead is dead, and he *was* dead. It cannot be that he was raised, unless God . . .

However reticent they may have been to believe that Jesus had been raised, these Jewish women and men had resources to understand the significance of that event that the Gentiles did not have — and that we have largely lost. We need, therefore, first to try to understand those Jewish resources, the Jewish context for this astonishing claim that Jesus had been raised, if we hope to understand its significance.

Israel's Hope and Consolation

As we noted previously when we complained about the way that *Ars Moriendi* read several Old Testament passages as commendations of death, the Old Testament had a fairly consistent view of death and of "the dead." As the wise woman of Tekoa put it to David, "We must all die; we are like water spilled on the ground, which cannot be gathered up" (2 Sam. 14:14). That was the rule, and the exceptions like Enoch and Elijah only proved the rule. Death was "natural" in the sense that it was universal, but it was lamented, not celebrated.

Mortality was recognized as "a fact of life." Indeed, it had its own consolations. It reminded the people that they "live on borrowed breath,"[4] that they are dependent upon God. And it called them to live wisely. The psalmist acknowledges the limits and troubles of life and draws this lesson:

> So teach us to count our days
>   that we may gain a wise heart.
>
> (Ps. 90:12)

And Ecclesiastes acknowledges mortality (and rejects the possibility of an afterlife; Eccles. 3:18-21), and then observes that a heart of wisdom includes

4. James L. Crenshaw, *Old Testament Wisdom: An Introduction* (Atlanta: John Knox, 1981), p. 198.

delight: "So I saw that there is nothing better than that all should enjoy their work, for that is their lot" (3:22; see also 9:7-9).

Even so, death itself is hardly commended, surely not by Ecclesiastes. In the context of the recognition of mortality, some deaths may be regarded as better than others, but none are regarded as good. A bad death was a premature death, a death, as Hezekiah said, "in the noontide of my days" (Isa. 38:10). A bad death was a death by violence, death "by the sword" (e.g., Amos 7:11). A bad death was a death without an heir (e.g., Ecclesiasticus 44:9). In the death of Absalom all three features of a bad death come together; he died young, violently, and without an heir (2 Sam. 18). In comparison, other deaths are not so bad: death "in a good old age" and "in peace" (as God promised Abraham, Gen. 15:15), death surrounded by one's children (as Jacob in Balaam's praise, Num. 23:10). Such deaths are better by far, but they are not therefore good. The bad death is particularly to be lamented, but no death is simply celebrated.

Life is a gift of God, a gift of the God who gives humans breath and calls them to get a heart of wisdom. To die is to be cut off from God and from the people of God. Hezekiah lamented not only that he was to die "in the noontide of [his] days" but also that his death would separate him from God and from the people of God:

> For Sheol cannot thank you,
> death cannot praise you;
> those who go down to the Pit cannot hope
> for your faithfulness.
> The living, the living, they thank you.
>
> (Isa. 38:18-19)

The dead are no longer able to join the community in pilgrimage to the temple, no longer capable of praise (Ps. 88:10). The dead go to Sheol, to "the land of forgetfulness" (Ps. 88:12), to a place of darkness and silence from which there is no return. Insofar as they could be said to live at all, they live a shadowy existence, cut off from God and from the praise of God.[5] This is about as far from a commendation of death as east is from west.

---

5. George E. Mendenhall, "From Witchcraft to Justice: Death and Afterlife in the Old Testament," in *Death and Afterlife: Perspective of World Religions,* ed. Hiroshi Obayashi (New York: Greenwood, 1992), pp. 67-81, says Sheol "can only be defined as the place the dead are dead" (p. 68). In contrast John W. Cooper, *Body, Soul, and Life Everlasting: Biblical Anthro-*

Israel's hope and consolation were that one day God's faithfulness and grace would bear fruit upon the earth. God would keep God's promises; of that Israel was confident. God's covenant promises, however, were promises for this life and for this world, promises for the life God had given, for the people God had made God's own, and for the world God had created. There was hope, then, for a future time of bliss and blessing, for a time when, as Zechariah said, "old men and old women shall again sit in the streets of Jerusalem, each with staff in hand because of their great age" (Zech. 8:4),[6] but one could only hope to be alive when by the grace and power of God such promises were kept.

The grace and power of God were Israel's hope and consolation. And that grace and power came into conflict with sin and death. The conflict was recognized first, perhaps, in the psalms of lament.[7] It is not that the psalms of lament called the people into conflict with their mortality. Mortality remained a given and both a simple sign of their dependence upon God for every breath and a serious call to wisdom. The conflict was rather with death as a "power" that threatens human beings and that stands as an adversary to God's life-giving Spirit.

There can be little doubt that on this point the psalmists of Israel were influenced by Ugaritic and Canaanite myths, prevalent in the region, that presented death as an adversary. But they did not simply adopt such

---

pology and the Monism-Dualism Debate (Grand Rapids: Eerdmans, 2000), regards Sheol as evidence that "persons are not merely distinguishable from their earthly bodies, they are separable from them and can continue to exist without them" (p. 77). I think Mendenhall's account is to be preferred. However, the Old Testament never gives sustained attention to the question of an afterlife. This strikes many as strange, in part at least because many have come to regard the afterlife as the central motive for religious faith. It was not so for Israel. One may ask, as C. S. Lewis did in his *Reflections on the Psalms,* why God, "having revealed so much of Himself to that people, should not have also taught them [about life in the world to come]" (*Reflections on the Psalms* [New York: Harcourt, Brace and World, 1958], p. 39). His answer, although "only one man's opinion" (p. 42), is instructive. Hopes and anxieties about life after death can be a little overwhelming. They can threaten to displace God from the center; God then becomes important "only for the sake of something else" (p. 40), for the sake of achieving eternal beatitude and avoiding eternal perdition.

6. The quite this-worldly hopes of the prophets included also abundant crops (e.g., Hos. 2:21-22), abundant water (e.g., Isa. 35), peace among the nations (e.g., Isa. 2:4; 9:6), peace among the animals and with the animals (e.g., Isa. 11:6-8), long life (Isa. 65:20, 22), and an intimate covenant fellowship with God (e.g., Jer. 31:31-34).

7. Herman Gunkel said that the psalms of lament are "the place where the religion of the psalms comes into conflict with death" (cited by Christoph Barth, *Introduction to the Psalms,* trans. R. A. Wilson [New York: Scribner's, 1966], p. 49).

myths.[8] The most notable difference is that "death," although regarded as a power and as an adversary, is never given the divine status it had in the myths or regarded as an equal adversary. The cosmic dualism in which life and light stand in conflict with death and darkness does not go all the way down. Only God is God! Moreover, unlike these myths, the psalmists did not speak of deliverance from the power of death by using analogies taken from the natural cycle of life and death. The deliverance from death is not a feature of the natural order of things, laid down from the beginning of time. Nor did they speak of it using analogies to the mythic stories of what had happened outside of or before history. On the contrary, they spoke of the deliverance from death as an event that happens in history, as an event that has happened in history more than once before, when God had, for example, delivered God's people from the death threatened by famine or by war or by sickness. The deliverance hoped for was a historical act of the free faithfulness of God. It was not deliverance from mortality; they will still die. It was not deliverance into some otherworldly bliss. The deliverance hoped for was to be delivered in this history and in this world from the death that threatened to consign them to the "land of forgetfulness." Still, in this conflict with death the faith of Israel and of its psalms would begin to suggest a final triumph of God's steadfast love and power over death.

Considered in this light, a couple of psalms may indeed point toward a life after death. In Psalm 49 the psalmist first considers the universality of death. Rich and poor, the fool and the sage, they all die (v. 10). That rich and foolish oppressors die (vv. 16-20; cf. Isa. 14:3-11), however, is but small consolation in the midst of oppression. But in this psalm the psalmist declares another hope and consolation:

> But God will ransom my soul from the power of Sheol,
>> for he will receive me.

(Ps. 49:15)

Several observations must be made here. The first is the ambiguity of the declaration. Many take it to be simply an expression of confidence that God will provide a rescue within the life of the psalmist from whatever desperate circumstances the psalmist laments. But others quite plausibly take it to be an astonishing declaration of confidence in God's victory over

---

8. See further Brevard Childs, *Myth and Reality in the Old Testament* (Naperville, Ill.: A. R. Allenson, 1960).

the power of death itself. The second observation is that "soul" is a misleading translation of the Hebrew word *nephesh*. We tend to think of "soul" in Platonic terms, as if it were simply a part, the immortal part, of a human being. But *nephesh* is not "soul," at least not in that sense. It might better be translated, "But God will rescue my life [or my self, or simply me] from the power of Sheol." The third observation is that "God will receive me," or as it might be translated, "God will take me up," may refer to the stories of Enoch and Elijah. And the final observation, and the most important, is that death is here construed as having "power," perhaps as being itself a "power," a tyrannical power. The hope is that God will finally rescue us from this "power" and from the ways that it holds us captive and threatens us. Death is not rendered a friend to be welcomed; it is a tyrant to be defeated. Death is not regarded as the liberation of the soul from the body; it is regarded as a menacing power from whose reign we must be liberated.

Something similar is expressed in Psalm 73.[9] Here, too, the psalmist ponders "the prosperity of the wicked" (v. 3). That fact challenges the justice of God and the affirmation that stands at the beginning of the psalm, "Truly God is good to the upright" (v. 1). The psalmist tries as a sage to put the justice of God and the prosperity of the wicked into one coherent picture, but "it seemed . . . a wearisome task" (v. 16). Then, however, he goes "into the sanctuary of God" (v. 17), and there with the people of God he attends to God and to the works of God. There he learns again, and by experience, that God is with him. God holds his hand like a parent walking with an anxious child (v. 23). Then and there the psalmist gives voice to a new confidence:

> You guide me with your counsel,
>   and afterward you will receive me with honor. . . .
> My flesh and my heart may fail,
>   but God is the strength of my heart and my portion forever.
>
> (vv. 24, 26)

Again there is some ambiguity. The psalmist says "afterward," but he does not say explicitly "after death." Perhaps he simply means after this particular episode of his life.[10] The image of a rock and the language of a "portion

---

9. On Ps. 73 see James L. Crenshaw, *The Psalms: An Introduction* (Grand Rapids: Eerdmans, 2001), pp. 109-27.

10. Like Job 19:25-26, where Job hopes for the appearance of his "redeemer" during his lifetime to put the injustice of his suffering right. Handel, of course, read it differently — and quite wonderfully — in the light of the resurrection.

forever," however, at least point in the direction of a relationship that not even death can sever. And again, the source of this ambiguous hope is unambiguous confidence in God's faithfulness. The basis for these little glimpses of hope is not that there is something immortal about a human being but that there is something incredibly gracious and powerful about the God of Israel. Perhaps God's love, at least, is as strong as death (cf. Song of Sol. 8:6).

Perhaps these psalms, which are probably late, had learned to hope for God's triumph over the power of death from the prophets. The prophets too, however, spoke little of a life after death and never of an "immortal soul." Hosea made what was the earliest reference to resurrection when he invited Israel to "return to the LORD" (6:1). If Israel would return to the Lord, he said, then perhaps

> after two days he will revive us;
>> on the third day he will raise us up,
>> that we may live before him.
>
> (6:2)

It was for Hosea a metaphor for the restoration of the nation of Israel, of a new and unlikely national life, after the judgment of God against them. Israel may yet be brought safely through the judgment.

So, too, the magnificent vision of Ezekiel 37. It had been a year or two since the Babylonian army had destroyed Jerusalem, a year or two since the city had been reduced to a heap of rubble; its temple, to a ruin. It had been a year or two of mourning. No pilgrim came to this ruined city for a festival. No priest led any crowd in celebration at this wreck of a temple. David's city! Solomon's temple! The memory and the hope of Israel's glory had been laid waste. God's city! God's temple! The memory and the hope of God's glory had been laid waste, too.

This was not a time for celebration and festival. It was a time for lament and sorrow, for tears and sadness. Still, this was the time an eccentric prophet saw this outrageous vision. The spirit of God set him down in the middle of some godforsaken valley — and the ground was covered with bones. Perhaps some travelers had been caught by a sandstorm. Perhaps some ancient army had been defeated there, and the soldiers left to die, their flesh plundered by scavengers. Perhaps these bones were what was left of Judah's army and of its resistance to Babylon. No matter. Wherever they were going, they never got there. Whatever they were fighting for, they lost. Whatever their hopes and dreams once were, they were dried up along with their bones. It was a desolate place, this visionary valley of dry bones.

Then God asked a silly question: Can these bones live (37:3)? I suspect Ezekiel got a little angry then. There he was — losing sleep again for another sad vision and a stupid question. The answer was obvious: "No! The bones cannot live! Of course not! Let's not be ridiculous!" Any other answer violates human reason and human experience. And it is possible to read Ezekiel's reply, "O Lord GOD, you know" (37:3), as an angry shout, "God, you know as well as I do that these bones cannot live. You *know*." And yet — when one turns to give reply to God — then (and maybe only then) sad and desolate certainty can make room for a little hope, and what began as an angry shout can mellow into a whisper of hope. And it is possible to read Ezekiel's reply also in that way — as a whisper of hope, "O Lord God, *you* know."

Then God told this prophet to be a little ridiculous himself. "Talk to the bones," God said to Ezekiel. "Preach to the dead, Ezekiel." And he did! If he had touched the bones, they might have turned to dust, but he preached to them. Imagine his reaction when the first bone moved a little. Soon enough there must have been an awful racket as bones rattled around, banging into each other mindlessly and fleshlessly — until an ankle bone connected to a shin bone, and a shin bone connected to a knee bone, until that visionary valley was filled with skeletons jumping around stupidly.

Things quieted down some, of course, when muscle and flesh and skin were added to the bone — but it was still just a bunch of moving corpses, until Ezekiel called for the wind, for breath, for the spirit. Then these bones danced, danced in celebration of the mystery of life, danced in joy at a festival of life, danced in the hope of God's good future. It was a splendid vision, a wonderful, funny, ridiculous vision. And Ezekiel didn't have to be a genius to figure it out. But God explained it to him, anyway. "These bones are the whole house of Israel," God said (37:11).

That people, Ezekiel's people, God's people, had just flunked out of history. The destiny and the dream that was Israel had been destroyed. The greatness that was Judah had died. Once God had made them a people and given them a task. God had blessed them and told them to *be* a blessing. As God had heard their cry of pain in Egypt, so they were to listen to the cries of any who hurt. As God had given them the land, so they were to share it and its produce. For a while the people soared — but then they soured. They began to regard God as their servant, not themselves as God's servant.

They ignored the cries of those who hurt, hoarded their goods, neglected justice and kindness. And now they were no people, just the dry bones of a people. Can these bones live? No, these bones cannot live, unless God . . . And the messenger of God whispered hope, "O Lord God, *you* know."

The vision was not about the resurrection of individuals. It was about the resurrection of a people, the renewal of covenant. It was about returning from exile and dwelling in the land again. But it was also about the faithfulness of God, the power and grace of God, the love as strong as death! That was their hope and consolation — and it called them to a faithfulness of their own.

It was not *just* that the people would return to the land, not *just* that Jerusalem would be rebuilt, not *just* that the temple would be restored. It was not simply a nostalgic vision that things would be put back the way they were. Maybe that was the dream of many of the exiles — to go back to Jerusalem again, back to the old life, back to the good old days. Oh, they were ready to promise to do a little better next time — no more messing with Moloch, no more flirting with Baal — they just wanted to go back to the way things were.

Ezekiel's vision, however, was different than that, better than that, and more demanding than that. The people would be made new! God's spirit would make them new! In their dreams and in their deeds, in their character and in their conduct, they would be made new! It was not about turning back to the way things were; it was about being turned forward to God's good future. It was not about an alteration or two, a slightly revised edition; it was about a transformation. It was about resurrection and life in the Spirit.

The last word did not belong to Ezekiel, of course; the best he could do was to look to God and to whisper hope. But the last word did not belong to Nebuchadnezzar or the Babylonians — or to death — either. The last word belongs to God, and to a love as strong as death.

For Ezekiel the resurrection of the dead was still a metaphor for the restoration of the community; he did not yet envision a life after death for the individual member of the community. That would come later. Perhaps it came already in what is frequently called "the Isaiah apocalypse" (Isa. 24:1–27:13). That little section of Isaiah is difficult to date, but it is usually assigned to the postexilic period. Here one finds promised, for the first time perhaps, what will become themes of Jewish apocalyptic literature, a day of universal judgment and of God's cosmic triumph. And here one finds again talk of a resurrection. It is part of the cosmic triumph of God.

On that day God "will swallow up death forever" (25:8; cf. 1 Cor. 15:54). As Sheol swallows up the dead (e.g., Prov. 1:12), so God will swallow up death itself. It will have no escape. God's rule will be established in the earth, not in some spiritual, or heavenly, or other world, and "the Lord GOD will wipe away the tears from all faces" (Isa. 25:8; cf. Rev. 21:4). One may object that this is not yet a promise of resurrection, only of the abolition of death. But the promise of resurrection is not long in coming. In Isaiah 26:19 this promise is given to the people of God:

> Your dead shall live, their corpses shall rise.
> O dwellers in the dust, awake and sing for joy!
> For your dew is a radiant dew,
> and the earth will give birth to those long dead.

By the time the book of Daniel was written (probably during or shortly after the persecution of the Jews by Antiochus IV Epiphanes, 164-167 B.C.E.), the resurrection of individuals was confidently asserted. "Many of those who sleep in the dust of the earth shall awake, some to everlasting life, and some to shame and everlasting contempt" (Dan. 12:2; see also 12:13). Indeed, the resurrection became an article of faith among Jewish apocalyptic writers like the author of Daniel. Born in times of crisis and persecution, Jewish apocalyptic combined despair concerning the present age with the profoundest hope for the future. This world is still God's world, but in the present age it has fallen into the grip of the power of sin and death. The very righteousness of God requires that God act to set the world right, that God restore justice to the world. This present age, in which tyrants usurp God's authority, will not last. The visions of the apocalyptic writers described the course of this age toward its end. Then God will act to end the rule of sin and death and to establish once again God's own cosmic sovereignty. In the age to come God will rule not only over the nations, bringing a reversal of Israel's fortunes, but also over the whole cosmos, shattering the rule of sin and death. No human agency can initiate that good future; it will take an act of God. Little wonder, then, that it comes with cosmic signs and portents, by a judgment against sin and a resurrection from death.

There was no apocalyptic orthodoxy about the resurrection.[11] There

---

11. See the survey by John J. Collins, "The Afterlife in Apocalyptic Literature," in *Death, Life-after-Death, Resurrection, and the World to Come in the Judaisms of Antiquity,* ed. Alan J. Avery-Peck and Jacob Neusner (Leiden: Brill, 2000), pp. 119-39.

were, for example, diverse views about who would be raised from the dead. Sometimes just the righteous would be raised, with the sinners left in Sheol (e.g., the Similitudes of Enoch, *1 Enoch* 46:6). And sometimes all the dead would be raised, the righteous to blessedness and sinners to perdition (e.g., the Apocalypse of Ezra, 2 Esdras 7:3-36). There were diverse views also about the nature of the resurrected body. Sometimes the emphasis fell on the continuity of the risen body with the former body (e.g., 2 Maccabees 14:46). Sometimes the emphasis fell on a transformation of the former body. In the Similitudes of Enoch, for example, those who are raised will be clothed "with garments of glory" (*1 Enoch* 62:15). And in the *Apocalypse of Baruch* the dead are raised without change in their form, but subsequently they are transformed into the splendor of angels (*Apocalypse of Baruch* 50:2–51:10). In spite of the diversity, however, resurrection was always the power and righteousness of God at work. The resurrection of individuals was always part of a larger hope, a hope for the whole cosmos and for the community. It was always the resurrection of bodies, even if the emphasis sometimes fell on transformation. And, while it enabled Jewish martyrs to face death with courage and reminded them all that there were things worse than death, it was never a commendation of death; it was always an affirmation of God's power to abolish death.[12]

There were also diverse accounts of the intermediate state, the state of the dead after death and before the resurrection. It was a commonplace in apocalyptic literature that God would restore the original Paradise at the end of time, and it became a common view (but by no means a consensus) that there was in the present time "a hidden Paradise," a place of rest and blessing in which the righteous awaited the resurrection.[13]

The hope that God would act to end the rule of sin and death, that God would bring this present evil age to an end and establish God's good future on the earth by judgment and resurrection, was the hope that shaped Jewish thought in the first century. To be sure, not all Jews shared this hope. The Sadducees did not, but they were evidently in the minority. The Sadducees accepted only the Torah, and they claimed not to find any evidence in Torah of such a hope. They were also, however, among the po-

12. See Richard Bauckham, "Life, Death, and the Afterlife in Second Temple Judaism," in *Life in the Face of Death: The Resurrection Message of the New Testament,* ed. Richard N. Longenecker (Grand Rapids: Eerdmans, 1998), pp. 80-95.

13. See Joachim Jeremias, *"paradeisos,"* in *Theological Dictionary of the New Testament,* ed. G. Kittel and G. Friedrich, trans. G. W. Bromiley, 10 vols. (Grand Rapids: Eerdmans, 1964-76), 5:767.

litical and economic elite, having protected their vested interests in and around Jerusalem by a policy of accommodation and collaboration with the ruling powers. Perhaps because they had accommodated tyrants, they resisted this apocalyptic hope that God would set the cosmos right and raise the dead.

Jesus ben Sirach, writing around 180 B.C.E., held to the older view of death and the dead. There is no coming back from death, he said (Sirach 38:21), and the dead are cut off from the praise of God.

> Who will sing praises to the Most High in Hades . . . ?
> From the dead, as from one who does not exist, thanksgiving
>   has ceased.
>
>   (17:27-28)

His work circulated, of course, in the first century, and there must have been some besides the Sadducees who still held the older view. Still, it had evidently become the minority view.

Another alternative was suggested by some writings in circulation among the Jews in the first century that had borrowed the language and ideas of Hellenistic philosophy for consolation rather than the indigenous apocalyptic language of resurrection. The Wisdom of Solomon and 4 Maccabees, for example, both spoke of the righteous as if they only seemed to die (Wisdom of Solomon 3:1-4; 4 Maccabees 7:19; 16:25). They adopted the concept of the immortality of the soul. Even here, however, immortality is not a characteristic of the human soul itself but a gift of God (e.g., Wisdom of Solomon 1:12-15; 4 Maccabees 18:23).

Many rabbis of the first century evidently shared the apocalyptic hope for the restoration of the world and for the resurrection of the body. The talmudic literature, which put to writing rabbinic traditions that survived the destruction of the temple in 70 C.E., surely did. Indeed, George Foot Moore, an eminent scholar of this literature in the last century, called the resurrection of the body "the primary eschatological doctrine of Judaism."[14] Hillel and Shammai, rabbis roughly contemporaneous with Jesus, famously disagreed about many questions, but they agreed about the resurrection of the body.[15] The rabbis even insisted that the resurrection of the

---

14. George Foot Moore, *Judaism in the First Centuries of the Christian Era* (Cambridge: Harvard University Press, 1944), II, p. 379.

15. *Genesis Rabbah* XIV and *Leviticus Rabbah* XIV, cited by Pinchas Lapide, *The Resurrection of Jesus: A Jewish Perspective* (Minneapolis: Augsburg, 1983), p. 57.

body had been taught in the Torah, and their confrontations with those who denied the resurrection of the dead may remind Christian readers of the confrontation of Jesus and the Sadducees (Mark 12:18-27). I give just one example of many: "Our masters taught, 'I kill and I make alive' (Deut. 32:39). One might think that one person would experience the killing and the other the making alive as it is customary in the world; but the text says 'I wound and I heal' (Deut. 32:39). As wounding and healing applied to one and the same person, so also killing and making alive applied to one and the same person. This provides an answer for those who say that the resurrection of the dead cannot be proved from Torah (Sanhedrin 91b)."[16]

Whether the resurrection of the body could be "proved from Torah" or not, it was "an intelligible development of the faith contained in the Hebrew Scriptures."[17] Jewish confidence in God was bound by its own integrity to move in the direction of such a hope. While it is different from the earlier view of death, it stands in continuity with Israel's earlier faith.

Israel's faith in God and in the faithfulness of God finally required it. There was one God to whom loyalty was due (the Shema, Deut. 6:4). And this one God is Lord of all. Other gods, other powers, were not regarded as worthy of worship. This one God was the Creator, who separated the light from the darkness, gave life to every living thing, and made of dust a human person. If that is so, then the same God surely has the power to re-create the world, to restore the cosmos, and to make the dust a human being again.[18] This one God was sovereign over the creation; the Baalim that claimed to be at work in natural processes were no match for this God (1 Kings 18:1-46). More than that, this one God made a people for himself out of what had been no people. He called Abraham and Sarah out of Ur and promised to bless them. When a bunch of slaves cried out to high heaven against the oppression of Egypt, he heard their cries and answered them. He had compassion for them and rescued them, led them to Sinai and covenanted with them. That covenant with its promises and that compassion, God's readi-

---

16. Cited by Labide, *The Resurrection of Jesus*, p. 57. He gives several other examples. See also more recently the important book by Jon D. Levenson, *Resurrection and the Restoration of Israel: The Ultimate Victory of the God of Life* (New Haven: Yale University Press, 2006).

17. Bauckham, "Life, Death," p. 84.

18. Bauckham, "Life, Death," p. 86: "The Old Testament God — the Creator, the Source of life, and the Lord of life — undoubtedly *could* raise the dead. That he *would* do so only became clear once death was perceived as contradicting God's righteousness and God's love."

ness to hear the cries of those who hurt, would be the basis of Israel's common life and of its hope. It was the basis also for the confidence of the sick in psalms of lament that God would hear their cries and rescue them from premature death. And because it was a hope in God who was Lord of all, it was the basis also finally for a hope that would spill over to include all the nations and the whole cosmos — and the dead. The hope for a world set right and for a resurrection from the dead was born of Israel's confidence in God's power and compassion. God's faithfulness to God's own character and covenant — and that alone — required and enabled such a hope.

This hope stands in continuity with the tradition it had received also by taking death seriously. Death is not denied in this tradition. Death is real. It is not just an appearance of death that leaves the real person untouched. And death is an evil. It is not the greatest evil, but it is an evil just the same. It is not commended as a liberation of the soul from its corporal prison. Death sunders human beings from their own flesh, from the community of praise, and from God. Death is a power that threatens, and in the face of which the people of God cry out to God and against God, for death is finally here a power that threatens also the faithfulness of God to God's promises.

This hope is consistent also with the anthropology of the Old Testament. Unlike the Platonic tradition of anthropological dualism, where a human being is one part mortal body and one part immortal soul, in the Jewish tradition a human being is a psychosomatic whole. Human persons are not Platonic souls caught in bodies with their passions (nor Cartesian ghosts in a machine); a human person is, as Paul Ramsey used to like to say, "an embodied soul or ensouled body."[19] Human persons are neither merely bodies nor merely minds. They are neither merely biological organisms nor merely their capacities for understanding and choice. They are the coinherence of mind and body, the unity of body and soul. The Hebrew word *nephesh* is, as we have seen, sometimes translated as "soul," but it might better be translated as "a living being." In the creation story, by God's breath and gift the dust was made *nephesh*, "a living being" (Gen. 2:7). We are created from the dust as embodied creatures, and the hope for resurrection is the hope that, by the same power of God, we may be recreated from the dust as embodied creatures.

That creation story may be used to call attention to another feature

19. See, for example, Paul Ramsey, *The Patient as Person: Explorations in Medical Ethics* (New Haven: Yale University Press, 1970), p. xiii.

of Jewish anthropology important to apocalyptic hope. After Adam was created, God said something quite unusual in the creation story. God said, "It is not good. . . ." What was "not good" was "that the man should be alone" (Gen. 2:18). The same point had been made differently, of course, in the first creation story. There, when God makes humankind, he makes community; "male and female he created them," and God said it was "very good" (Gen. 1:27, 31). We are not solitary individuals; we are persons-in-relation. Relationships are not just part of our flourishing as individuals; they are intrinsic to our identity as persons. We are born and live and die as persons-in-relation. One threat of Sheol was the awful silence that cuts us off not only from the praise of God but also from our relationships. We are created as communal creatures, and the hope for resurrection is the hope not just for the new creation of a solitary individual but for the new creation of persons-in-relation, the re-creation of community, indeed, for the renewal of the creation upon which we all depend and with which we are intimately related. This hope was a hope for the people, for the cosmos, and a hope that by God's grace we might have a share in that good future of God's people and God's creation.

A third feature of Jewish anthropology should yet be mentioned. The *nephesh* is *basar;* the living creature is "flesh." Whole selves — embodied and communal selves — are "flesh" in their contrast to God and in their dependence upon God, in their creatureliness, in their weakness and mortality. Whole selves — including their quite remarkable capacities to think and choose, to trust and hope, to "have dominion" — are "flesh." They are not God; they may and must rely on God. The *nephesh* is *basar,* and without God human weakness and mortality would make their inevitable way toward death. Without God human sociality would turn to enmity, blame, and shame. Without God great human powers would demonstrate their weakness, their "flesh," by their inability to preserve the cosmos from tilting back toward chaos. From the beginning without God there is just death. But from the beginning, it is the case not only that the *nephesh* is *basar* but also, by God's grace, that the *basar* is *nephesh;* it is *not* without God. The flesh, too, is from God, and it is good. The flesh is created by God to be with God. Whole selves — embodied and communal selves, mortal and dependent, creative and powerfully gifted with reason and will — are flesh, and it is good. Human weakness and mortality find their answer, the answer to their longing, in God. *Nephesh* and *basar,* human beings may and must trust and hope — not in some immortal soul, not in some divine spark of reason, not in the human capacities to think and choose and have "dominion," not even in their capacities to trust and hope — but in God. The apocalyptic hope found the answer to the human longing for life in God and in the power of God to give life to the dead, to make the dust *nephesh*, "a living being," again. God's love is stronger than death. God and the power of God, that was "Israel's strength and consolation" in the face of sin and death. God and the power of God, that was not only Israel's hope but also the "hope of all the earth," the "dear desire of every nation," and the "joy of every longing heart."[20]

The Resurrection of Jesus

Israel's apocalyptic hope was that God would act to defeat the powers of sin and death and to establish God's unchallenged sovereignty in what is, after all, God's world. It would be signaled by resurrection and judgment. It was, as we have said, an intelligible development of Israel's faith, but it also provided the convictions and hope in terms of which the significance of Jesus was intelligible.

He came announcing the good future of God, "the kingdom of God," and he made that future both known and present by his works of healing and his words of blessing. He was the "long-expected" one, the one who would bring God's rule, the one who would establish God's future. Or so it seemed, at least, until the power of empire put him to death, until the power of death made mockery of the claims implicit in his words and deeds and mockery of the faith of those who followed him. He was dead — and the hope that he was the one in whom God's faithfulness and power would finally be displayed was dashed (e.g., Luke 24:21). Their hope was gone, dead — unless God . . . Then on that ordinary day at the opening of an ordinary tomb came the extraordinary message, "He is not here. He has been raised."

Hope for resurrection was an intelligible development of Israel's faith, and apocalyptic hope provided the background of intelligibility to Jesus' life and ministry, but was the resurrection of Jesus rendered intelligible by this hope? To that question the answer has to be yes and no.

The answer has to be no because, although many expected a resurrection at the end of time, no one expected the resurrection of one person in the middle of time. Jesus had come announcing the good future of God

20. The phrases come, of course, from the second verse of Charles Wesley's wonderful hymn "Come, Thou Long Expected Jesus."

and already making its power felt in his words of blessing and his works of healing. Disciples gathered around in the expectation that he might be the one to usher in the end, to restore Israel, to set right the nations and the cosmos. They knew well enough what he meant when he talked of the resurrection at the end of time. When he said that at the end of the age "the righteous will shine like the sun in the kingdom of their Father" (Matt. 13:43), they probably heard the echo of Daniel 12:3. They surely took his side in that confrontation with the Sadducees about the resurrection (Mark 12:18-27). Jesus evidently shared the hope of the first century about the resurrection of the body as an eschatological event that would signal God's victory over the powers, including the powers of death and sin — and so did they. But when he talked about his own death and resurrection,[21] they didn't get it. They could not endure the thought of his death; this project was supposed to end in triumph, in a victory celebration at Pilate's abandoned palace, not in disaster, not in death. But they also could not understand Jesus' talk of his own resurrection as if it were to precede the general resurrection at the end of time. When, after the transfiguration, Jesus had told them not to tell anyone what they had just seen "until after the Son of Man had risen from the dead," Mark reports that the disciples were "questioning what this rising from the dead could mean" (Mark 9:9, 10). They didn't get it, and little wonder. That was not in the apocalyptic picture. And when he had been put to death, they did not expect that he would be raised in a few days.[22] They thought their hopes for him and for Israel and for God's world had been dashed. The apocalyptic literature had not envisioned the resurrection of just one before the end.

But the answer must also be yes. The resurrection of Jesus is rendered intelligible by this apocalyptic hope because his resurrection was an eschatological event. It was a new thing, of one piece with the resurrection at the end of time. Jesus was the "first fruits of those who have died" (1 Cor. 15:20, 23). Paul uses, of course, an image from harvest time; the "first fruits" were the first of the harvest, offered to God in a sacrifice to acknowledge that

---

21. Whether he really did, of course, is a matter of considerable scholarly debate. Many think the words were put on the mouth of Jesus by the church after the events. N. T. Wright, *The Resurrection of the Son of God* (Minneapolis: Fortress, 2003), has argued forcefully, however, that they make perfectly good historical sense as the words of Jesus himself.

22. This may be the best argument for thinking that the predictions of passion and resurrection are put on the mouth of Jesus by the church as they remembered his story after the resurrection. Even if N. T. Wright is right, however, and the predictions were uttered by Jesus himself, the disciples did not (and could not) understand them until after the events.

the whole harvest belonged to God and to give thanks to God for his gifts of the land and its produce. The image makes the point that the resurrection of Jesus is part of the resurrection at the end of time and yet distinguished from it in time. The whole argument in 1 Corinthians 15 insists on this connection between the resurrection of Jesus and the final resurrection. There is no affirmation of Christ's resurrection if one does not also accept the resurrection that is to come (e.g., vv. 12-13, 15-16). There is no understanding the significance of Jesus' resurrection apart from the background of intelligibility provided by Jewish apocalyptic hope.

Some in Corinth evidently denied that there was a resurrection to come. They were either ignorant of the Jewish tradition that gives the resurrection of Jesus its intelligibility as an eschatological event, or they had simply lost touch with it. They evidently understood the resurrection of Jesus to be connected not to the resurrection to come but to some kind of spiritual transcendence over the body and over the world to which the body ties us. Such an understanding had its roots in dualism. And from the same root grew several other problems in Corinth. That dualism permitted some to draw libertine conclusions. Since the body has no spiritual significance, what you do in the body (or to the body or with the body) has also no spiritual significance. But Paul reminded them of the resurrection of Jesus and of their solidarity with him (even if his resurrection precedes their own). "The body is meant not for fornication but for the Lord, and the Lord for the body. And God raised the Lord and will also raise us by his power. . . . Therefore glorify God in your body" (1 Cor. 6:13-14, 20). The same dualism prompted others to asceticism. Because the body is evil, the spiritually elite claimed transcendence over the body, claimed that they were already angels, and insisted on the practice of celibacy or "spiritual marriages." But Paul reminded them of the "not yet" character of their existence, warned them against temptation, and encouraged sexual relationships of mutuality and equality within marriage. He acknowledged celibacy as a "gift" but not the sort of "gift" that allowed one to boast about being already fully spiritual, and he refused to make it a duty or a sign of being among the spiritually elite (1 Cor. 7:1-7). Their dualism also nurtured their spiritual elitism, their claim to spiritual transcendence not only over their bodies but also over the social body. They asserted their independence from Paul and from the church. They boasted about their spiritual gifts and neglected their solidarity with the poor and with the church. But Paul reminded them of their baptism, their initiation into the cross and resurrection of Christ and into the one body of Christ. "In the one Spirit we were all baptized into one body . . ." (12:13). The Spirit gives gifts to each, not that any may boast but that each may minister to the common good (12:4-31). "Prophecies," "tongues," "knowledge," and all the other spiritual gifts about which they boasted "will come to an end," but "love never ends" (13:8). It is love that characterizes the good future of God, not the pride of those who think of themselves as spiritually elite. And the clincher for all these arguments in 1 Corinthians — against libertinism, asceticism, and elitism — is the resurrection of the body at the end of time, the resurrection that is of one piece with the resurrection of Christ's body but separated from it in time (1 Cor. 15).[23]

Whenever the church loses touch with this Jewish tradition of the resurrection of the body or is inhospitable to it, dualism threatens to distort its gospel into a promise of spiritual transcendence over the body and its faith into some esoteric knowledge possessed by the spiritually elite. Then we may find ourselves alienated from our own bodies and alienated from our solidarity with the body of Christ, the church that finds its birth and its hope in solidarity with this crucified and risen Christ.

The Jewish hope and consolation render the resurrection of Christ intelligible as an eschatological act of God. By raising Jesus from the dead God acted to establish the good future Jesus had promised and made present by his works of healing and his words of blessing. By this act God vindicated God's own righteousness, God's own faithfulness. God is indeed the one who loves justice and sets the world right. God is indeed the compassionate one who hears the cries of those who hurt and who makes and keeps his promise of blessing. By this act God vindicated Jesus as the Christ, as God's own agent to establish the good future of God. He is indeed the one who made God's reign present among us, whose words and deeds displayed God's way and cause. In spite of the cross, that Roman sign that Caesar is in charge, in the resurrection Jesus has been made Lord and Christ (Acts 2:36). The resurrection vindicated Jesus as the crucified Messiah.[24]

---

23. Karl Barth, *The Resurrection of the Dead,* trans. H. J. Stenning (London: Hodder and Stoughton, 1933), p. 113: "[T]he discourse of the whole Epistle proceeds from a single point and harks back again to this same point," namely, the resurrection of the body.

24. See the excellent study by Nils Alstrup Dahl, "The Crucified Messiah," in his *The Crucified Messiah and Other Essays* (Minneapolis: Augsburg, 1974). The essay argues that "the basic historical fact in the life of Jesus is his death by execution as an alleged king of the Jews. The conviction that the crucified Messiah was vindicated by God who raised him from the dead marks the beginning of Christianity and the central theme of New Testament theology in all its complexity" (p. 8).

The cross becomes a sign not only of Caesar's tyranny but also of God's love, a love that is stronger than death; it becomes a sign of Christ's love and faithfulness, a sign of his solidarity with those who are beaten down and crushed, a sign of his solidarity with the suffering and dying, and a paradigm for a Christian's faithful living and dying. We have learned to call that Friday "good" not because it commends death but because it commends a life of steadfast love and faithfulness. It is a sign that, in spite of appearances, God is in charge, and that in spite of death, God is the great life-giver. *[handwritten: good Friday]*

Six centuries after Ezekiel had seen a vision promising that the last word would not belong to Nebuchadnezzar, the resurrection made it clear that the last word did not belong to Herod or to Caesar or to Pontius Pilate — or to death — either. The last word belongs to God, and God has spoken it. It was an apocalyptic event. When the powers of death and doom had done their damnedest, God raised this Jesus up. When Jesus of Nazareth was crucified, dead, and buried, if some voice from heaven had raised that same silly question God put to Ezekiel, "Can these bones live?" the best one could possibly have done would be to whisper hope, "O Lord God, *you* know." It is impossible, unless God . . . And God raised this Jesus up in apocalyptic power. God raised him up in our history and in our world, and our history and our world have — happily — no escape. God had the last word that day, and it was — and is — a shocking, ridiculous, hilarious "Yes!" "Yes, these bones can live!" "Yes, God gives life where death ruled!" "Yes, God raises up the humiliated and oppressed!" "Yes, God sets the world right!" "Yes, God cherishes the world God made!" "Yes, God makes all things new!" The last word is God's yes upon the whole creation. *[handwritten: The last word]*

This is no commendation of death. This is a celebration of God's love and power, the love that is stronger than death, the power that defeated death. Death was swallowed up in an eschatological victory. As the Apocalypse of Ezra put it, "The earth shall give up those who are asleep in it, and the dust those who rest there in silence" (2 Esdras 7:32).

The Hope of the Church

Pilate, of course, was back in his office on Monday, trying to exercise a little damage control, putting some spin on the rumors that Jesus had been raised. And Caesar probably had little inkling of the apocalyptic events that had just occurred in a troublesome outpost of his empire. And people still died. It looked like the same old world. Many Jews did not believe that

Jesus had been raised, not just because "the dead are dead," but also because, if he had been raised, then everyone else should have been raised with him. If he had been raised, it should be already "the age to come."

Many, however, did believe. They had heard the stories of an empty tomb. They had heard the witnesses of his appearances. And the Spirit was poured out — as Joel had promised:

> In the last days it will be, God declares,
> that I will pour out my Sprit upon all flesh. . . .
>
> (Acts 2:17-21, citing Joel 2:28-32)[25]

That, too, was an eschatological event. As Christ was the "first fruits of those who have died" (1 Cor. 15:20, 23), so in the power of that resurrection the Spirit was the "first fruits" of God's good future (Rom. 8:23). The Spirit was the *arrobon* of that future, the "first installment" of that future (2 Cor. 1:22), the "guarantee" of that future (2 Cor. 5:5), and the Spirit made its power felt in the life of the community. It made its power felt in Jerusalem with a quite extraordinary ability to communicate across language barriers; it was a reversal of Babel and of its curse (Acts 2:4-11; cf. Gen. 11:1-9). But the Spirit also made its power felt in the quite mundane sharing of the community's possessions; it was a fulfillment of covenant and a token of God's good future. The promise of Deuteronomy 15 was fulfilled; "there was not a needy person among them" (Acts 4:34; cf. Deut. 15:4). And the good future was revealed in friendship, in *koinonia;* they "were of one heart and soul," everything "was held in common" (Acts 4:32).[26] Little

---

25. The story of Pentecost is, of course, found only in Luke-Acts, but the association of the Spirit with the resurrection is affirmed elsewhere. In John's Gospel it is the risen Lord who "breathed on [the disciples] and said to them, 'Receive the Holy Spirit'" (John 20:22). And in Matthew's Gospel, although the Spirit is not mentioned, the risen Christ promises, "I am with you always, to the end of the age" (Matt. 28:20). The Spirit is the presence of Christ in his absence. In both cases, moreover, as in Acts, the Spirit empowers the church's mission in the world.

26. Acts alludes here not to the Hebrew Scripture but to Greek proverbial wisdom. Aristotle already had cited "'[friends have] one soul,' 'friends hold in common what they have,' 'friendship is equality'" as proverbial wisdom (Aristotle, *Nicomachean Ethics* 9.8.1168b, trans. Martin Ostwald, Library of Liberal Arts [New York: Bobbs-Merrill, 1962], p. 260). Moreover, according to Martin Hengel, *Property and Riches in the Early Church* (Philadelphia: Fortress, 1974), p. 5, the Gentiles told stories of communities that "held all things in common" and distributed "to each according to their need" as expressions of a dim memory and a dimmer hope. The work of the Spirit gave a token in Jerusalem not only of the fulfillment of Jewish hopes but also of human hopes.

wonder that between these two verses Acts reminds the reader of the resurrection. This was "Easter in ordinary."[27] This was the power of God that raised Jesus from the dead and would raise the dead at the end of time, making its power felt in this world and in this history. The power of God was not assigned a little place of its own, perhaps a little place in the past or a little place in the future, but in either case exiled from the present. It was not assigned a place in some other world, exiled from this one. No, here and there, now and again, and frequently in the commonplace practices of reconciliation and forgiveness, and of course in "love, joy, peace, patience, kindness, generosity, faithfulness, gentleness, and self-control," the "fruit of the Spirit" (Gal. 5:22), the good future of God made its power felt.

Still, the old age continued. The powers of sin and death continued to assert their doomed reign. Jesus had been raised, but it was not yet the age of God's unchallenged sovereignty. There were tokens of God's good future, but the "first fruits" only made one eager for the harvest. The church learned to live in the time between the resurrection of Jesus and the general resurrection at the end of time. It meant life in the Spirit, and therefore it also meant resistance to the continuing powers of sin and death. It meant celebration of God's great victory over all that hurts and harms, over the tyrants, over the powers of sin and death, and it also meant waiting and watching and praying for God's good future. It meant life under the signs of the cross and resurrection; it meant lament and hope.

Perhaps the quintessential sign of the Spirit's presence is that it prompts us to cry "Abba! Father!" (Gal. 4:6; Rom. 8:15-17). That was the language Jesus used in prayer — and notably in the Garden of Gethsemane (Mark 14:36).[28] It was an invocation, Joachim Jeremias argued, that displayed the intimacy of Jesus with the Father.[29] When by the Spirit we cry

27. The title of one of Nicholas Lash's books, *Easter in Ordinary: Reflections on Human Knowledge and the Knowledge of God* (Charlottesville: University Press of Virginia, 1988). Lash created the phrase by combining phrases from poems by George Herbert and Gerard Manley Hopkins. See Lash, pp. 195-96.

28. It is likely that the Aramaic *abba* is behind the prayers of Jesus in which he addresses God as "father" (Greek *pater*), but the Aramaic form is found in the Gospels only in the prayer at Gethsemane.

29. Joachim Jeremias, *New Testament Theology*, trans. John Bowden (New York: Charles Scribner's Sons, 1971), pp. 61-68. See also Jeremias, *The Prayers of Jesus* (London: SCM, 1967), pp. 57-65. Although Jeremias's claim was widely accepted and often repeated, it has been challenged by some, notably James Barr, "*Abba* Isn't Daddy," *Journal of Theological Studies* 39 (1988): 28-47. Even if "*abba* isn't daddy," however, the invocation suggests not submission to patriarchal power but reliance upon the love of a parent.

"Abba! Father!" we, like Jesus, invoke the one upon whose parental love and care we finally depend, and the Spirit assures us "that we are children of God, and if children, then heirs, heirs of God and joint heirs with Christ" (Rom. 8:16-17). As Paul reminds us in Romans 8 (and as Gethsemane itself makes clear enough), we may cry "Abba! Father!" in the midst of suffering, both the world's suffering and our own. "We know that the whole creation has been groaning in labor pains until now; and not only the creation, but we ourselves, who have the first fruits of the Spirit, groan inwardly while we wait for adoption, the redemption of our bodies" (8:22-23). In the midst of an un-Eastered world the Spirit "helps us in our weakness" and "intercedes with sighs too deep for words" (8:26). And by the Spirit we share those sighs, those inarticulate longings for a future we only know in part and dimly. By the Spirit we have caught a glimpse of God's good future, and by the Spirit we ache for that future and mourn that it is not yet, still sadly not yet. By the Spirit we hope, but our hope too lives under the sign and the sigh of the cross.

That hope, Jesus' hope, the hope we share by the gift of the Spirit, was cosmic in its scope. It was a hope, after all, that the world would be put right. It was hope for "new heavens and a new earth, where righteousness is at home" (2 Pet. 3:13). That would require the justice and judgment of God; the world would not be put right without judgment. But on the far side of that judgment the mercy of God will restore and renew "all things" (Eph. 1:10; Rev. 21:5). Then "death will be no more" (Rev. 21:4).

That hope, Jesus' hope, the hope we share by the gift of the Spirit, was not, however, less personal by being cosmic. Each Christian hopes for the good future of God — and to share in it. We may hope to participate in the resurrection of Christ. We may hope for "the redemption of our bodies" (Rom. 8:23) along with the renewal of the whole creation, in solidarity with both Christ and any who weep because that future is not yet.

In what was probably the first of Paul's letters to the churches, he responded to a little crisis of hope in the church at Thessalonica. Some members of that community had died, and others worried that they had lost out on the promises of God. Paul does not respond by commending death or by assuring them that their immortal souls are now happily free from their bodies. That is not Paul's strategy, and that is not Paul's gospel. He appeals rather to the tradition he had handed down to them: "Since we believe that Jesus died and rose again, even so, through Jesus, God will bring with him those who have died" (1 Thess. 4:14). That is the basis of their hope, the resurrection of Christ as an eschatological event, as an

200

event that is of one piece with the general resurrection at the end of time, their own resurrection. Because Christ has been raised, the Thessalonians may be confident that their dead friends will be raised as well. The dead will be no worse off than the living on the day of Christ's coming, his parousia (4:15).

"Parousia" was a term used when rulers visited a colony over which they ruled. Since Thessalonica was the capital of the province of Macedonia, the term was probably a familiar one for a visit by the emperor. It was customary (and prudent) to go outside the city before he arrived to meet the emperor, to welcome him, and to usher him into the city with proper respect. How much the more when the Lord comes! At his coming "the dead in Christ will rise first. Then we who are alive . . . will be caught up in the clouds together with them to meet the Lord in the air; and so we will be with the Lord forever" (4:16-17). The point is not that we stay "in the air" somehow. The point is rather that we go to meet the Lord, to welcome him, to say we had been hoping he would come, to report that we had been praying *Maranatha* ("Our Lord, come"), and with proper respect to usher him back to the earth he rules.[30]

With this hope for the world and for the dead, with this hope we have by the resurrection of Jesus, is how the Thessalonians are to encourage and console and exhort each other. This is the hope that gives them courage and comfort. It is no otherworldly hope. It is no commendation of death or of a disembodied immortality. Death remains a cause of sorrow and grief. The Spirit will help in our grief with sighs too deep for words, but when such sighs find words, those words are likely to echo *Maranatha*. We will still grieve, but we need not grieve as if there were no hope. There is hope, even for the dead, and the basis of that hope is the power of God that raised Jesus from the dead. That resurrection on an ordinary day in Jerusalem is of one piece with the general resurrection on "the day of the Lord" (5:2). Paul invites the Thessalonians to shout into the graves of their friends, "Death will not have the last word. This life belongs to God."

Paul's words to the Thessalonians can hardly be confused with either a Platonic doctrine of the immortality of the soul or the Stoic consolation

---

30. The passage is full of conventional apocalyptic imagery. The shout, archangels, the trumpet, and clouds are all frequent images of apocalyptic literature (e.g., Dan. 7:13; 10:6; 2 Esdras 4:36; 6:23; *1 Enoch* 14:8; 20:1-8; Rev. 1:10; 14:2; 19:6). The language is poetic, not a prosaic description of exactly the way things will happen. It is not to be read as stage directions for the future.

literature. It is God's power to raise the dead, not the human soul's immortality, to which he points. And unlike the Stoic consolation literature, he does not tell the grieving to use their reason to restrain their grief; he tells them to "encourage one another with these words [the gospel of Jesus' resurrection and that of the dead]" (4:18).

Hard on the heels of this consolation and encouragement to the Thessalonians Paul sets his remarks about "the times and the seasons" (5:1). Appropriately so, for the apocalyptic hope for the resurrection of their beloved dead, even if it is assured by the resurrection of Jesus from the dead, still raises that typical apocalyptic question, "When will this be?" (Mark 13:4; cf. Dan. 12:6). Paul does not claim to know "the times and the seasons" (1 Thess. 5:1) of God's salvation, and he does not think any human can claim to know them. Jesus himself did not know them (Mark 13:32) and, if he is to be trusted, no one does (Acts 1:7). But Paul does know the power of God that raised Jesus from the dead, and that power is the true source of the comfort, encouragement, peace, and security of the Thessalonians. God will have the last word, and God has already spoken it. That is the church's hope and certainty. Alive or dead, we are in the hands of God. Paul will say it quite clearly in Romans: "If we live, we live to the Lord, and if we die, we die to the Lord; so then, whether we live or whether we die, we are the Lord's. For to this end Christ died and lived again, so that he might be Lord of both the dead and the living" (Rom. 14:8-9). It is enough to know that God has raised Jesus from the dead and that by the same power God will give life to the dust. Worry and speculation about "times and seasons" are foolishness. Without claiming to know more than human beings can know, the Thessalonians — and the rest of us — are to "encourage one another and build up each other" (1 Thess. 5:11). Dying well and grieving well do not require knowing when "the day of the Lord" will come, but they do require a community.

Some have found a hint in this passage that not only the living but also the dead have some foretaste of God's good future, that even the dead have already some taste of the triumph of God over death. When Paul says, "God has destined us not for wrath but for obtaining salvation through our Lord Jesus Christ, who died for us, so that whether we are awake or asleep we may live with him" (5:9-10), he is probably, I think, simply referring again to our solidarity with Christ in the resurrection to come, but perhaps he is suggesting that by the power of the life-giving Spirit the dead are somehow "with him" already.

Whether that suggestion is made in Paul's consolation to the

Thessalonians or not, it does seem to be made elsewhere in the New Testament. It is never given as an alternative or substitute for the hope of resurrection. It is consistent not with a Platonic commendation of death but with the accomplished — and expected — victory of God over death. In the resurrection of Jesus that victory has come into the present, and — so we may hope — also for those who have died, even if the resurrection of the body is still future. The hope is that those who have died in this (long) interim may already, by the grace and power of God, share in some way in that victory. They are, after all, "with Christ" (Phil. 1:23; 1 Thess. 5:10). But if they, with the living, have already some share in Christ's victory over death, they also share with the living the longing expectation of the last day (Rev. 6:9-11). They share with the living both the already and the not-yet character of God's good future.

The Intermediate State

We must be careful, of course, about claiming to know more than we do. This "intermediate state" of the dead, the state of the dead after death but before the final resurrection, like the apocalyptic "times and seasons," has been the subject of much fruitless debate and speculation. The New Testament never treats it as a topic in its own right — unless 2 Corinthians 5:1-10 is read as an account of the intermediate state. There are a number of difficult exegetical problems in this passage, and widely divergent interpretations have been proposed. Some take the "longing to be clothed with our heavenly dwelling" (2 Cor. 5:2) to be fulfilled at death when the dead are provided with "spiritual bodies"; others take the fulfillment of that longing to await the parousia, when the dead are raised. Both seem to ignore the claim of the first verse that "we have [present tense: already now] a building from God, a house not made with hands, eternal in the heavens." The image is one of solidarity with the risen Christ, the temple "not made with hands" (cf. Mark 14:58). The image is not anthropological and individualistic; the image is eschatological and corporate. It is a participation in Christ's death and resurrection marked already by baptism, and it is a participation that awaits the final resurrection; it is already and not yet. Again, some read the "groaning" to be a longing for deliverance from the burden of our physical bodies, a deliverance provided by death. (The reading lens for such an interpretation has been ground by Platonists.) Others take the "groaning" of verse 4 to be prompted by an anxiety that we will die before the parousia. And still others take the "groaning" to be a longing for the parousia, prompted by the burdens of suffering we bear in these bodies and in this age. The last seems best, given our solidarity with the groaning creation. We groan for "the redemption of our bodies" (Rom. 8:22-23). We could mention many other exegetical quarrels with respect to this passage. But this much at least seems clear: 2 Corinthians 5 represents no radical departure from Paul's consistent emphasis on a hope that is founded on the resurrection of the crucified Jesus, that reaches into the whole creation, and that calls each of us to live in ways that glorify God (v. 9).[31] The passage is set in the context, after all, of the confession of faith: "we know that the one who raised the Lord Jesus will raise us also with Jesus, and will bring us with you into his presence" (2 Cor. 4:14).

How the dead already participate in God's good future, what it means to be "with Christ" after death — these are questions the New Testament does not address. They are questions we do well to leave to God. Nevertheless, we are curious, of course, as curious as the Thessalonians were about "times and seasons." Only let our curiosity not prompt us to say more than we can know, more than Scripture itself suggests. Too often reflection on the "intermediate state" has deflected attention away from the power of God to make things new. Too often it has surrendered the hope of resurrection to Platonic notions of the "immortality of the soul." Too often it has sacrificed the cosmic and corporate hope of the church to satisfy a concern for otherworldly and individual bliss. Too often our eagerness to console those who grieve has prompted us, if not to commend death, then to deny it.

But if speculation about "the intermediate state" can run such risks, we do not escape them by speculative dismissals of such a state. Karl Barth sought ingeniously to eliminate the intermediate state by taking the resurrection of the dead out of time. In *The Resurrection of the Dead* he argued that because ordinary time has no hold on the God who made both space and time and because it no longer has any hold upon the dead, the dead are

---

31. On this difficult passage I have found E. Earle Ellis, *Paul and His Recent Interpreters* (Grand Rapids: Eerdmans, 1961), pp. 35-48, the most helpful. Among those who take Paul here to be concerned with the intermediate state (and moving toward Hellenistic notions of an individual and immortal soul), see L. Cerfaux, *The Christian in the Theology of St. Paul* (London: Chapman, 1967), pp. 191-212. For the claim of fundamental consistency with the rest of Paul's "resurrection thought," see Richard Longenecker, "Is There Development in Paul's Resurrection Thought?" in *Life in the Face of Death*, pp. 171-224.

immediately raised to newness of life in God's eschatological kingdom.[32] The transformation of the body happens, according to Barth, immediately after an individual's death, for the dead are not in time. I admit that I have trouble wrapping my mind around this idea, but the problems go deeper than my own feeble theological imagination. It seems to me to run counter to the assumptions of the New Testament that the dead are still in time. Surely the very problem that Paul addresses in 1 Thessalonians 4 presupposes that the dead are still in time, and so does Paul's answer. Paul does not say, "The dead have already been raised"; rather, he says that, when Christ returns, "the dead in Christ will rise" (1 Thess. 4:16). Revelation, too, assumes that the dead are still in time; at least the martyrs are envisioned as crying out, "How long?" (Rev. 6:10).

Moreover, the account of God's being and activity in Scripture does not suggest a timeless God. God's eternity is not timelessness.[33] Timeless-

---

32. See Barth, *Resurrection of the Dead*, pp. 217-22. He is followed in this by Jürgen Moltmann, *The Coming of God: Christian Eschatology* (Minneapolis: Fortress, 1996), p. 103, and most recently by Thomas Long, *Accompany Them with Singing — the Christian Funeral* (Louisville: Westminster John Knox, 2009), pp. 51-54. Joel Green, *Body, Soul, and Human Life* (Grand Rapids: Baker Academic, 2008), also eliminates the intermediate state, pp. 140-48, in favor of an immediate resurrection, by eliminating time; his argument is at once exegetical and motivated by a commitment to "non-reductive materialism," but he fails to give an account of the timelessness his argument requires, and he sacrifices the connection of the resurrection of the body with the cosmic renewal with which it is associated in apocalyptic (and early Christian) hope.

33. See Nicholas Wolterstorff, "God Everlasting," in *God and the Good: Essays in Honor of Henry Stob*, ed. Clifton Orlebeke and Lewis Smedes (Grand Rapids: Eerdmans, 1975), pp. 181-203. Barth himself is not, as I read him, anyway, fully consistent on the relation of God and time. He says (especially in his early writings) that God simply transcends time in an "eternal *Now*" (e.g., *The Epistle to the Romans*, trans. Edwyn C. Hoskins [London: Oxford University Press, 1933], p. 437) but later rejects this understanding of eternity. "Eternity is not merely the negation of time. It is not in any way timeless. On the contrary, as the source of time it is supreme and absolute time, i.e., the immediate unity of past, present, and future" (*Church Dogmatics* III/1, trans. J. W. Edward et al. [Edinburgh: T. & T. Clark, 1958], p. 67). It is difficult to know what this "unity of past, present, and future" means, but if Christ reveals it to us (as for Barth he must), then his life in time as a coherent life is the clue. Jesus was in time; his life moved from past to present to future with the coherence of faithfulness. He did not try to — or need to — disown his past. He lived with faith in God toward the future. He could therefore live every moment fully and faithfully. In him there was "peace between origin, movement, and goal, between present, past, and future" (*Church Dogmatics* II/1, trans. T. H. L. Parker et al. [Edinburgh: T. & T. Clark, 1957], p. 62). Such an understanding of the unity of past, present, and future, however, does not seem to me to warrant the claim about an immediate resurrection.

ness, too, has roots more Platonic than biblical.[34] If God is a God who has acted in creating the world and in response to the human actions that are responses to his actions, if God is an agent, and if God has a cause for God's people and for God's creation, then God is not timeless but supremely temporal.

To eliminate the intermediate state by eliminating time runs the same risk that some speculation about the intermediate state encounters, namely, minimizing the significance of a cosmic hope, a hope for the whole creation (with its time) that God made and loves. It runs the risk, moreover, of theological triumphalism, of ignoring the "not yet" character of our existence and that of the dead. In its rush to Easter it runs the risk of neglecting Holy Saturday, that day of mourning; it runs the risk of denying the reality of death and its evil.

It seems better to me to stick closer to biblical images. The image of "sleep" is one such image, found joined to talk of resurrection in Daniel 12:2, "Many of those who sleep in the dust of the earth shall awake," in 1 Thessalonians 4:14, and in Ephesians 5:14. The sleeping are not conscious of time, of course, but those who sleep remain in time. A related image, of course, is rest; in Revelation 14:13, for example, those who "die in the Lord" are promised "rest from their labors." It is a blessed rest, a resting in peace and in the promise of God, no longer afflicted with sin or suffering. We have mentioned the assumption found in some Jewish texts — and evidently shared by some Christian texts (notably Luke 23:43) — of a "hidden paradise," a place of repose and blessing where the righteous dead await the resurrection. Still, the martyrs of Revelation 6:10 are not envisioned as sleeping but as waiting, watching, hoping, praying for the final triumph of God's cause against the tyrants, and crying out, "How long, O Lord?" The image at once the most modest and the most consoling is that the dead are "with Christ" (e.g., Phil. 1:23). And Christian baptism is enough to remind us that "if we have been united with [Christ] in a death like his, we will certainly be united with him in a resurrection like his" (Rom. 6:5).

The reserve with which the New Testament approaches this topic of the intermediate state may be compared with the fact that it fairly thunders with the message of resurrection. That is the victory of God over

---

34. See Plato, *Timaeus* 37-38. And see also William Kneale, "Time and Eternity in Theology," *Proceedings of the Aristotelian Society* (1961), who argues that Christian theology was influenced by classical Greek philosophy when it began to regard God's eternity as timelessness (cited by Wolterstorff, "God Everlasting," p. 183).

death, and that message echoes in the confidence that God's power and grace protect and care also for those who have died. The New Testament never orients believers toward the private bliss of an individual "immortal soul"; it always orients believers toward God's good future, in which by God's grace they have already — and forever — a part. It never underestimates the reality of death or characterizes it as anything but an "enemy" (1 Cor. 15:26). It is ready to affirm that somehow that future is present also for the dead, but we stammer and stutter when we attempt to describe that present reality. And if Paul's topic in 2 Corinthians 5 was the intermediate state, he seems to stammer a bit himself, mixing metaphors of clothing and habitations. One need not be embarrassed by such stammering in the face of the mystery of divine protection in and through and beyond death, but such stammering should not hide the awful reality of death, the basis for hope in the victory of God over death, or the cosmic scope of the hope of the early church.

Resurrection Bodies

Of course, we stammer and stutter also when we attempt to imagine resurrection bodies. This, too, has been a topic of much fanciful and sometimes self-indulgent speculation. Still, if the resurrection of Jesus from the dead governs our imagination, there are some things that can be said in the narrow space between saying nothing and fantasy. Jesus remains the paradigm; there is no other. The risen Jesus is the first fruits of God's good future, the beginning and the promise of a new creation. So, we do well to consider the Gospel stories of his appearances as the risen Lord.

In those stories there is both continuity and discontinuity between Jesus before his resurrection and after it. Both the continuity and the discontinuity are striking, and both are instructive, but they do not always fit easily into a coherent picture. Consider the continuities first. The one the disciples encountered after Easter is the same one they had encountered when he called them to discipleship. It is the same person, the same body. And that it is the same body is the critical mark that it is the same person, the critical mark of continuity. In more than one of the stories in the Gospels, he was recognized as the same Jesus because of his body. When he appeared to the disciples in Luke's Gospel (Luke 24:36-43), for example, the disciples were at first "startled and terrified, and thought that they were seeing a ghost," but Jesus called attention to his body, indeed to the wounds inflicted upon his body on the cross. "Look at my hands and my feet," he said. "See that it is I myself. Touch me and see; for a ghost does not have flesh and bones as you see that I have." And then, as if to confirm the reality of that body, he ate a piece of fish. In John's Gospel, too, when he appeared first to the disciples, he "showed them his hands and his side" (John 20:20). Thomas was not there on that Easter night, and he earns the epithet "doubting Thomas" by his refusal to believe the story the disciples told unless he could see the wounds in his hands and touch the marks left by the nails in his hands and the sword in his side (20:25; cf. 19:31-37). When Jesus appeared again, he offered Thomas the opportunity he had demanded, and Thomas promptly made the climactic confession, "My Lord and my God!" (20:28). And when Jesus appeared to the disciples a third time in John's Gospel, at the Sea of Tiberias, he ate with them (21:1-14). The body, the real, material body, is the fundamental mark of continuity between Jesus before and Jesus after the resurrection.

There are also, however, some discontinuities, some transformation. Jesus is not simply a reanimated corpse. The resurrection is not simply resuscitation. The body of the risen Christ is evidently not an ordinary body. It seems the risen Lord can appear and disappear suddenly. On more than one occasion he enters a room through doors shut tight (John 20:19, 26). And he is not always recognizable from his body alone; Mary Magdalene does not recognize him until he calls her by name (John 20:14-18), and the disciples on the way to Emmaus do not recognize him until he has taught them the scriptures, received their hospitality, and broken bread with them (Luke 24:13-35). It is a body, to be sure, the same body, but somehow transformed, "glorified," capable of things one just cannot expect from an ordinary body.

Without appealing to such stories of Jesus, Paul nevertheless seems to take them as paradigmatic when he faces the questions, "How are the dead raised? With what kind of body do they come?" (1 Cor. 15:35). He seems a little impatient with the question, but he moves quickly to an emphasis on the transformation of the body. Our bodies need transformation if they are to be no longer subject to death and suffering, but resurrection bodies are still bodies. Christians hope not for liberation from their bodies, but for "the redemption" of their bodies (Rom. 8:23).

In answering the question of the Corinthians Paul uses the analogy between seed and its fruit and contrasts our perishable, dishonored, and weak bodies with resurrection bodies, "imperishable," "raised in glory," and "raised in power" (1 Cor. 15:36-43). The continuity is there. It is still a body that is raised, still the same person, the same body, but transformed, "glorified," redeemed.

One mark of its transformation is that it is now "imperishable." Paul's point is clearly not that the soul is immortal; the point is rather that by the power of God this person, this body, will not and cannot perish. It is still, if you will, mortal, still dependent upon God for its life; it is by God's faithfulness and power that it lives; it is only by the life-giving Spirit of God that it is "imperishable." As Paul says in Romans, "If the Spirit of him who raised Jesus from the dead dwells in you, he who raised Christ from the dead will give life to your mortal bodies also through his Spirit that dwells in you" (Rom. 8:11).

A second mark of this transformation is that it is no longer a body of "dishonor" but "raised in glory." Paul's point cannot be that embodiment itself is dishonorable, as if it held the soul or reason captive to the passions, for then the body could hardly remain the fundamental mark of continuity. The point is rather, I think, something like the point Paul makes earlier in 1 Corinthians when he is talking about the body of Christ, the church. There he says that the church puts on display the good future of God when it treats its members with love, when we "clothe with greater honor" those that we think less honorable (1 Cor. 12:23). It is the way God works, Paul says (v. 24), and the outcome is that "members may have the same care for one another. . . . If one member is honored, all rejoice together with it." There is no place in God's good future for boasting or elitism, for creating little hierarchies of rank and honor. If death is the great leveler by bringing us all down to the dust, the resurrection will be the great equalizer by bringing us all to "glory." The "glory" is not ours by our accomplishments, as if we could boast. This transformation "comes from the Lord, the Spirit" (2 Cor. 3:18). It is ours by participation in Christ's body, in the new humanity, in Christ's glorified humanity. Each person, each body, "raised in glory," will be honored, and "all will rejoice together with it." This transformation of the body, of course, requires a transformation of community as well. Our embodiment, even when transformed, is a sign of our sociality.

A third mark of this transformation of the body is that it is no longer weak but "raised in power." Surely the risen Jesus is Paul's paradigm here. When Jesus was raised the "Son of God with power" (Rom. 1:4), he was no longer subject to the powers of sin and death or to any of the powers that would usurp God's dominion and destroy God's creation. Perhaps the best sign of this transformation in the Gospel stories and in Jesus' own body is his wounds. They remain, as we have said, evidence of the continuity between Jesus before and after the resurrection. Still, a transformation takes place. The nail prints in his hands and feet had been displays of Caesar's power when they were inflicted. They were evidence of the weakness of Jesus against the tyrannies of death and empire. But after the resurrection, what once was the display of the power of Caesar and of death became the display of God's power and faithfulness, the display of Jesus' faithfulness and love. By God's power the humiliated, dishonored, and weak Jesus was raised, and his wounds were raised with him. His body with its wounds was glorified, exalted. The one they counted last was made first. The power of God was at work when God raised Jesus from the dead, but to raise him from the dead was to exalt him to sovereignty over the powers, to "put all things under his feet" (Eph. 1:22; cf. Ps. 8 and its account of humanity). Christ remained dependent upon the power and faithfulness of God, but the transformation of his resurrection included the establishment of his own power and authority (cf. also Matt. 28:18), which he exercises not in competition with the power of God but in accord with the cause of God. And in the life that is ours by being raised with him, sharing in that new humanity, we will continue to depend upon the power of God and of Christ and the Spirit, but the risen body will have, by the grace of God, powers of its own, powers to relate to others, to the renewed cosmos, and to God. Those who have been raised with Christ will not exercise these powers in competition with the power of God or Christ but freely in accord with the sovereignty of God and of God's Christ. Our embodiment, even transformed, sets us in relation to God and to the cosmos.

Paul continues to consider the question about the kind of body the dead will have when they are raised by making one more contrast. Unfortunately, the NRSV gives a misleading translation. There the contrast is between "a physical body" and "a spiritual body" (1 Cor. 15:44).[35] One might infer from that translation that the discontinuity centers upon the transformation from material to spiritual, but that is not Paul's point. Paul's adjectives are *psychikon* and *pneumatikon*, which are better translated "natural" and "spiritual," or perhaps better still "soul-ish" and "spirit-ish." Moreover, both adjectives modify *soma*. *Soma*, "body," is not something immaterial here; it cannot be thought of as something ethereal, and it is the basic marker of continuity. The discontinuity is not a transformation from material to spiritual but a transformation in what gives life to the

35. See Wright, *The Resurrection*, pp. 348-56.

body. The *pneumatikon soma,* the "spiritual body," is a real embodied and communal self fully enlivened by the Spirit of God, the first fruits of God's good future.

Although we have focused on the body itself, the continuity and transformation of the body have pointed us toward a resurrection existence that cannot be reduced to the physical existence of an isolated individual. Our embodiment, even in this age, inevitably involves us in relationships — to other human beings, to the cosmos, and to God. To be embodied is to be in relationship, and that remains the case with resurrection bodies.

Consider again the Gospel stories. The body of the resurrected Jesus is the same body that walked the dusty roads of Galilee and was executed by Caesar. The continuity marked by that body, however, is also marked by his relationships to other people. The risen Christ appears to those he has known and loved, and he knows and loves them still. He appears to the women who have followed him (Matt. 28:9-10), to Mary Magdalene (John 20:14-18), to Peter (Luke 24:34), to the disciples (Matt. 28:16-20; Luke 24:13-51; John 20:19–21:23). Forgiveness and fellowship and service were characteristic of his relationships to others before the resurrection, and after it as well. Surely forgiveness is signed in the appearances, in greeting the disciples with his peace, and in blessing them. The fellowship meals so characteristic of his ministry are also characteristic of his visits with the disciples after the resurrection. And there he is, not now washing the feet of his disciples, but fixing them breakfast on the shore of the Sea of Tiberias. There is continuity also in the nature miracle of the Sea of Tiberias (cf. John 21:1-14 with its parallel in Luke 5:1-11). And there is continuity also in his relation with God. He lives again, as he lived before, because God gives life. He is now, as he was, dependent upon God's love and faithfulness. The faith in God and in the faithfulness of God, the trust in God and the loyalty to God's cause, that marked his life from the beginning, that marked his journey to the cross and his endurance of it, is characteristic also of this risen one.

Together these continuities disclose that, although death threatened to sunder this Jesus from his body, from his community, and from God, by the power of God death failed to make good on its threats. God had — and will have — the last word.

The relationships of Jesus to other people, to the earth, and to God are also qualified by his resurrection. The lives of others and of the earth remain, of course, marked by the not-yet character of this age, and the full transformation of these relationships awaits the general resurrection. Still, there are discernible changes. God's good future has dawned, and the Spirit is poured out as the first fruits of it. Jesus still knows and loves those he knew and loved before — and many more — but there is also transformation. He relates to them now as the risen one, the exalted one, the one to whom all authority has been given, the one who will come again in the final triumph over sin and death. He is present to them in this interim between his own resurrection and the general resurrection by the Spirit. As he promised, "I am with you always, to the end of the age" (Matt. 28:20), he continues to relate to people and to be present in a great variety of ways, ways consistent with the ways of Jesus before the resurrection but transformed. He still calls people to repentance, but now as the risen Christ. He still commands obedience, but now as Lord of all. He still greets them with his peace. He still forgives them and blesses them. He still comes in the breaking of the bread. He still heals. He still comforts. He still weeps with those who weep. He still sends people out in service to God's cause. But he does this now as the risen Lord by the Spirit that is at work in the church and in the world.

At the end of the age, when he appears again in his glorified body, when we too are raised, Christ's relation to us will doubtless be qualified again, "glorified." There will be no more need to call us to repentance. Our obedience will not need to be commanded because it will be so freely offered. There will be no sickness that needs healing or tears that need comforting. But there will be greeting and blessing and love and joy and peace. And at the end of the age, our own relationships with others will be healed. Our embodied identities are social identities, and there will be both continuity and transformation, a transformation wrought by mutual forgiveness and reconciliation, a transformation already signaled in this age now and again by the power of the Spirit.

The relation of Jesus to this world created and sustained by God is also obviously qualified by his resurrection. He loved it and he loves it still, but he is even more clearly Lord over it after his resurrection. He does not violate it by his resurrection; he draws it toward its own transformation and renewal. The creation, too, needs transformation if it is to be released from its bondage to decay (Rom. 8:21). The pattern of continuity and transformation should guide our imagination concerning the new creation as well. Utilizing that pattern, the pattern of the resurrection of Christ, John Polkinghorne says, "[T]he new creation does not arise from a radically novel creative act *ex nihilo*, but as a redemptive act *ex vetere*, out of the old."[36] That new creation, that old creation made new, will be the "ecological niche" for resurrection bodies.[37]

There is also, of course, both continuity and transformation in the risen Jesus' relation to God. If the cross had rendered doubtful the hope that this one might be the Messiah of Israel, the chosen one of God, the resurrection vindicated that hope. If the cross had put to the test both God's faithfulness and the faithfulness of Jesus, the resurrection vindicated both God and Jesus. By the resurrection this Jesus is exalted to God's right hand. The continuity allowed, indeed required, the church to see and to say that the risen one is the same one who walked among us and did signs and wonders, that the vindicated one is the same one who was crucified. The continuity allowed, indeed required, that the church affirm the incarnation, that this Jesus was the Word made flesh at his birth, but the incarnation was an inference required by the resurrection. (The resurrection was a part of the original proclamation and a part of all four Gospels; the birth of Jesus was not.) Our own relation to God will also be transformed. If the threat of death and suffering renders doubtful the hope that we, too, are to be counted among the children of God, our own resurrection will put that doubt to flight. The continuity entails, of course, that we are already the children of God, but even that relation will be "glorified."

The continuities and transformations between Jesus before and after his resurrection may and should mark our imagination concerning our own resurrection bodies. Still, we should be careful about claiming to know more than we can. We should be wary of self-indulgent fantasies. Such caution is required also by the first epistle of John: "what we will be has not yet been revealed" (1 John 3:2). Such caution, however, need not prevent us from celebrating the embodied and communal life that God gives and will give, a resurrected life to be lived in "the ecological niche" of

36. John Polkinghorne, *The God of Hope and the End of the World* (New Haven: Yale University Press, 2002), p. 116. It is a wonderful book. It grew out of the consultations of a group of scientists, biblical scholars, and theologians at the Center of Theological Inquiry at Princeton. Another product of those consultations is John Polkinghorne and Michael Welker, eds., *The End of the World and the Ends of God: Science and Theology on Eschatology* (Harrisburg, Pa.: Trinity, 2000). The authors included in that book also consistently invoke the pattern of continuity-discontinuity to think and talk about cosmic eschatology. It contains some speculation, to be sure, but the speculation is consistently disciplined by science and by Scripture.

37. David H. Kelsey, *Eccentric Existence: A Theological Anthropology* (Louisville: Westminster John Knox, 2009), 2:1020. His account of "eschatologically fully consummated living human personal bodies" (1:552-57) is excellent.

God's renewed cosmos. "Beloved, we are God's children now; what we will be has not yet been revealed. What we do know is this: when he is revealed, we will be like him, for we will see him as he is" (1 John 3:2).

In this interim between Jesus' resurrection and our own, one other continuity in the resurrected life of Jesus should be briefly mentioned. As Jesus had called the disciples to faith and faithfulness and had sent them out in service to God's cause, so he sends them out again as the risen Lord (Matt. 28:16-20; Luke 24:47; John 20:21). These commissions are each worded in the distinctive language of the different Evangelists, but each reprises a distinctive emphasis in the respective Evangelist's portrait of Jesus before the resurrection. So, for example, John's commission, "As the Father has sent me, so I send you" (John 20:21), repeats an earlier motif in John (cf. John 17:18). And in the words of the risen Christ to Peter in John's Gospel there is again, as there had been before, the recognition that, although life is a good gift of God, worthy of celebrating and toasting, in faith and faithfulness one's own survival may not be made the law of one's being (John 21:18-19).

Life Is Good — but Not the Greatest Good

We have commended life, celebrated life, as the gift of God. Life — embodied and communal life — and its flourishing belong to the creative and redemptive cause of God. The signs of God's intention were — and are — breath and a blessing, a rainbow, a commandment, a healing ministry, and, finally and decisively, an empty tomb. To remember the biblical narrative is to recognize and celebrate life and its flourishing as goods, as goods against which we may not turn without turning against the cause of God. They are to be received with thanksgiving and used with gratitude. Acts that aim at death and suffering do not fit the story, do not cohere with devotion to the cause of God or gratitude for the gifts of God. Death and suffering are not to be intended, not to be commended.

All the more remarkable, then, that Jesus "set his face to go to Jerusalem" (Luke 9:51). He walked steadily and courageously a path that would lead to his suffering and to his death. And he called his disciples to follow him. To remember this story, to heed this call, is not suddenly now to regard death and suffering as goods after all, to commend them as good in themselves. It is rather to acknowledge that we may not live as though our survival or our ease were the law of our being; it is to acknowledge that life and its flourishing are not the ultimate goods, not "second gods."[38] Sometimes life must be risked, let go, given up. Sometimes suffering must be endured or shared for the sake of God's cause in the world. A refusal ever to let die and the attempt to eliminate suffering altogether are not signs of faithfulness but of idolatry. And if life and its flourishing are not the ultimate goods, neither are death and suffering the ultimate evils. They need not be feared finally, for death and suffering are not as strong as the promise of God. You need not use all your resources against them. You need only to act with integrity in the face of them.

beautiful

A story-formed community tries to capture this posture toward life and death by making distinctions between killing and allowing to die, between suicide and accepting death, between inflicting suffering and enduring it.[39] And it honors the story of Jesus, who "set his face to go to Jerusalem," not only by theories of atonement but also by practices of faithful living and faithful dying.

the limits of self-care

---

38. Karl Barth, *Church Dogmatics* III/4 (Edinburgh: T. & T. Clark, 1961), p. 392.

39. The moral significance of those distinctions may be harder to defend publicly when the story in which they are embedded is denied or ignored. See Gilbert Meilaender, "The Distinction between Killing and Allowing to Die," *Theological Studies*, September 1976, pp. 467-70. And see Allen Verhey, *Reading the Bible in the Strange World of Medicine* (Grand Rapids: Eerdmans, 2003), pp. 321-24, for an account of the contemporary challenges to the distinction in the context of utilitarianism and an emphasis on autonomy. The previous two paragraphs are drawn largely from that section of my earlier work.

CHAPTER TWELVE

The "Instruccion": Remember and Follow Jesus

Late hym remembre hym and thynke on the passion off Cryste, for therby all the deuylles temptacions and gyles be moste ouercome and voyded.

Crafte and Knowledge For To Dye Well[1]

"Let the dying remember Jesus and think about the passion of Christ." The *Ars Moriendi* tradition took the death of Jesus to be the model for a Christian's faithful dying. That little self-help handbook *Crafte and Knowledge For To Dye Well* surely did. There the crucial piece of advice to Moriens to help him die well and faithfully was the "instruccion" to "remember" Jesus and his passion, to "thynke on" it. The death of Jesus was paradigmatic for a Christian's dying. The *Ars Moriendi* had that right, I think, and it is time to take that cue.

Cautions

We should, however, be a little cautious about taking this cue. There are several reasons for caution. For one thing, it was a horrible death. Jesus'

---

1. *Crafte and Knowledge For To Dye Well* (hereafter *Crafte*), in *The English* Ars Moriendi, ed. David William Atkinson, Renaissance and Baroque Studies and Texts, vol. 5 (New York: Peter Lang, 1992), p. 11. Page references to this work will be placed in the text.

death was a death by violence, the result of an act of judicial murder by a tyrannical government. It was the premature death of a man "in the noontide of [his] days" (Isa. 38:10). It was a dying made worse by friends who forsook him and enemies who abused him, made worse by abandonment, torture, and pain. It was not the sort of death we would wish for ourselves, not the sort of death we should wish for anyone. In that sense we should surely not take Jesus' death as paradigmatic for anyone's death. Still, given that caution, his faith and his faithfulness, his hope and his patient love, his humility and his courage are all on display in his dying, and surely these are paradigmatic for a Christian's dying.

We should be cautious about taking this cue also because, when we remember the stories of Jesus' death as somehow paradigmatic for our own dying, it is easy — and more than a little dangerous — to shift attention from Jesus to ourselves. It is tempting to read the story as if it were simply about us. It is about us, to be sure, but only because by God's grace we share in it. It remains, first of all, the story of Jesus' death. Jesus was the Christ, the Son of the living God. We are not. His suffering and death have a cosmic significance that our sufferings and deaths simply do not have. It is not simply that Jesus provides an example of some facts about the human condition that exist independently of him; it is rather that he transforms the human condition. Because Jesus was Jesus the Christ, we may live and die in faith and not in fear. Given that caution, it remains the case that, because he was with us and for us in his death, because he is "the pioneer and perfecter" of our faithfulness (Heb. 12:2), it is altogether appropriate that we look to Jesus as a paradigm of faithful dying. It is altogether appropriate that, remembering the story of Jesus' dying, we set the stories of our own dying alongside that story so that our stories can be challenged, corrected, made new, sanctified.

Another note of caution should also be sounded. It is sometimes said that religion is a good thing because it can console people in the face of death. I suppose, but we should be careful about corrupting Christianity by making it "useful" to our own projects. People have frequently tried to "use" God for their own agendas, but God is God and will not be "used." It is God's agenda that we must serve, not God who must serve our agenda.[2]

2. The mystical theology of Bernard of Clairvaux and Jean Gerson acknowledged that we might begin with loving God as a means of loving ourselves, but they insisted that we get to the point of loving ourselves as a means of loving God. In Bernard's account of love, the first degree is to love self for one's own sake, the second degree is to love God for one's own sake, the third degree is to love God for God's sake, and the fourth degree is to love self for

We should not attend to the story of Jesus because it may be "useful" for dying well; we should rather attend to the story of Jesus because it reveals the truth about our world and about living and dying in it. When the test becomes what is "useful," the church too often accommodates a cultural agenda. Then a Platonic culture can prompt the church to tell a story of world-denial and hospitality to death. Or then again, a secular culture can prompt the church to tell a story emptied of transcendence and God's action. Moreover, the "useful" consolations of religion can sometimes be false and can distort not only dying but also living. It seems to me that the Platonic dualism that has plagued the church has been guilty of that. When death is commended by deriding the body and the world God made, living is distorted and the awful reality of death is not faced honestly and truthfully. Then religion can become, as Freud insisted it was, a form of denial. Then there is more wisdom among those ancestral mothers who "refused to be consoled." Still, given that caution, the truth can be "useful." At least it is not prudent or wise to deny it or to resist it; it is prudent rather to struggle to conform to it. So it is altogether appropriate to revisit the story of the cross as the story where the truth about our world was nailed and as the paradigm for our own truthful dying.

It is difficult to know where to begin to tell the story of the cross and how to limit it. *Crafte* first cited Gregory the Great to the effect that every deed of Christ is for our instruction. Then it insisted that "suche thynges as Cryst dyd dyinge on the crosse the same shulde euery man do att hys last ende" (p. 11). And finally it mentioned just five things, that he prayed, cried out to God, wept, commended his soul to God, and gave up his spirit. That little list did not prompt it to reconsider its commendation of death, but it should have, and I propose we start again with it — and with Gethsemane. There, according to Hebrews 5:7 at least, we find the first four items on that little list of five; "Jesus offered up prayers and supplications, with loud cries and tears, to the one who was able to save him from death."

To start with Gethsemane, however, requires two additional notes of caution. The first is a warning against disconnecting the story of Jesus' passion and death from the rest of the story of Jesus. We must not forget the full, if short, life that had gone before his death. We must not forget that Jesus came announcing that the good future of God was at hand, that God

God's sake. See Bernard of Clairvaux, *On Loving God, with an Analytical Commentary*, ed. Emero Stiegman, Cistercian Fathers Series 13B (Kalamazoo, Mich.: Cistercian Publications, 1995), pp. 25-31.

was about to act to end the rule of sin and death. We must not forget that Jesus made that good future present and real in his works of healing and in his words of blessing. When he healed the sick, when he restored the possessed to self-control and community, when he raised the dead, the good future of God made its power felt already. When he preached good news to the poor, when he exalted those who had been humiliated, when he forgave sinners, the good future of God made its power felt. The passion that fueled his life and work was his longing for the reign of God. If we disconnect the story of his dying from the story of his ministry, we risk disconnecting the passion story from his passion for the reign of God. And then we will fail to appreciate the faithfulness of the cross and its significance for our own salvation, reducing it to the price paid for the passage of our souls to bliss.[3]

One final cautionary word is important as we turn our attention to the stories of Jesus' death — and to Gethsemane. All four Gospels tell the story of Jesus death, but there are important differences in the ways in which they tell it. They all have the passion narrative, and in each case it begins with the plot to kill Jesus, but by additions and omissions and by modifications within common material, each Gospel speaks with its own distinctive voice about the death of Jesus. John, for example, omits the story of Gethsemane. The church decided wisely not to choose just one Gospel or to accept Tatian's early harmony of the Gospels.[4] And we, too, should not simply choose one or homogenize the four into one. We must, of course, make some decisions about which stories to consider, but in considering any of the stories we will try to hear the distinctive voice of the Evangelist.[5] We may be confident that each is instructive not just concerning the death of Jesus but also concerning a Christian's dying. So we will begin, for example, by considering not just Gethsemane but also John's telling of the story without it.

3. This caution against an exclusive focus on the death of Jesus when considering atonement and salvation has recently been made by theologians from quite different theological perspectives. See, for example, J. Denny Weaver, *The Nonviolent Atonement* (Grand Rapids: Eerdmans, 2001), and Rita Nakashima Brock and Rebecca Ann Parker, *Proverbs of Ashes: Violence, Redemptive Suffering, and the Search for What Saves Us* (Boston: Beacon Press, 2002).

4. See Oscar Cullmann, "The Plurality of the Gospels as a Theological Problem in Antiquity," in *The Early Church: Studies in Early Christian History and Theology,* ed. A. J. B. Higgins, abridged edition (Philadelphia: Westminster, 1966), pp. 37-54.

5. For an account of the death of Jesus that is both comprehensive and attentive to the distinctive voices of each Evangelist, see Raymond Brown, *The Death of the Messiah: From Gethsemane to the Grave* (New York: Doubleday, 1994).

Gethsemane

Jesus is on his way to his death. He knows it. But he does not welcome it as one would a "welbeloued and trusti frende" (*Crafte*, p. 3). He is "distressed and agitated" (Mark 14:33; "grieved and agitated," Matt. 26:37), and he says to Peter and James and John, "I am deeply grieved, even to death" (Mark 14:34; similarly Matt. 26:38).[6] He knew the hymns appropriate to the conclusion of the Passover meal; they had just sung one (Mark 14:26). But he also knew the laments, and his words to Peter and James and John echo the words of Psalms 42–43,

> Why are you cast down, O my soul,
>   and why are you disquieted within me?
>
> (Ps. 42:5, 11; 43:5)

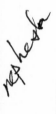

It is probably not necessary to repeat again that "soul" in both this story and in the Psalms is not some Platonic soul, not some immortal part of the person held captive by the body and its passions. It is the *nephesh*, the whole person, embodied and communal and dependent upon God, who is troubled. It is in his viscera as well as in his "soul" that Jesus is distressed by the prospect of his death.

Asking his disciples to wait, to "watch," to stay awake while he goes off to pray, he goes a little farther into the garden. He asks them to stay awake, I think, because although he wants to be alone to cry out to God, he does not want to be alone, he does not want to be abandoned by his friends. Then he falls on the ground, and prays to the one whose cause he serves to save him from death. It was a familiar enough request in the lament psalms. "Abba," he cries, "for you all things are possible; remove this cup from me" (Mark 14:36). It takes only a little imagination to think that those words were accompanied by some "sighs too deep for words" (Rom. 8:26).

Oscar Cullmann famously contrasted this scene to the scene of Socrates' death in Plato's *Phaedo*.[7] And it is a stunning comparison: On the

---

6. Luke also has the Gethsemane story, but he presents Jesus as much more composed on his way to his death. He does not characterize Jesus as "agitated" or provide these words of Jesus. And later in the story Luke reports that, instead of falling to the ground, as in Mark and Matthew, Jesus simply kneels. Luke — or at least a later copyist of Luke's Gospel — does add the story of the visitation of an angel who comforts and strengthens Jesus in his agony and takes note that "his sweat became like great drops of blood" (Luke 22:43-44).

7. Oscar Cullmann, "Immortality of the Soul or Resurrection of the Dead?" in *Im-*

one hand, there is Socrates discoursing dispassionately about immortality, transcending the passions through reason, welcoming his death. On the other, there is Jesus, troubled at the prospect of his death, anxious about the possibility of being forsaken by friends and by God, crying out to God in agony and in anguish. He does not respond to the prospect of his death with an attempt to rise above his passion by means of Platonic contemplation. He does not respond with Stoic resignation. And he does not welcome death.

In Gethsemane we see the sorrow and distress of Jesus, his fear and agony, in the face of death. None of that is denied any more than the reality of death is denied. But we see not just fear; we also see the courage of Jesus. Courage is not the absence of fear; it is doing what must be done in spite of fear. We see not just his agony; we see also the faith and the faithfulness of Jesus. Faithfulness is not a denial of this world's sadness; it is quite capable of lament; but it lives — and dies — in loyalty to God and to the cause of God and in the reckless confidence that God should and will have the last word in this world. We see, then, not despair, but courage and faithfulness. When Jesus asked, as so many psalmists had, to be delivered from death, he may have hoped simply to be spared from a premature death. He knew, as so many psalmists had said, that God's promise was life. But he also knew, as many other psalmists had said, that death was real and a real evil. He knew, as many apocalyptic seers had seen, the power of death and sin. When he said, at the end of the prayer that begins with the invocation of Abba, "yet, not what I want, but what you want" (Mark 14:36), he subordinated his wants, his hopes, to the cause of God. He expressed his readiness to endure the terrors of death if the cause of God in the world required it. That cause was a good more weighty than his own survival. It is not that he thought that the will of God was arbitrary, willing life one moment and

---

mortality and Resurrection: Death in the Western World; Two Conflicting Currents of Thought, ed. Krister Stendahl (New York: Macmillan, 1965), pp. 9-54. In the same volume Harry A. Wolfson, "Immortality and Resurrection in the Philosophy of the Church Fathers," pp. 54-97, provides an essay that is critical of Cullmann's position, but it attends very little to Scripture, appealing to the church fathers to suggest that Cullmann's account of the New Testament position needs correction. With Cullmann I take the lines of authority and correction to go from Scripture to theology. Much later James Barr, The Garden of Eden and the Hope of Immortality (Minneapolis: Fortress, 1993), criticized Cullmann and argued for a more positive account of "immortality" than Cullmann gave. He focused on Gen. 2 and 3 and on the durability of the nephesh. The argument, however, seems unsuccessful to me; he himself admits that "our story does not speak of 'life after death'" (p. 19) or of the immortality of the soul, and he reports that he is "not opting for immortality" (p. 41).

death the next, but that he would be faithful to God the life-giver, even if it meant his death.

At the end of the story it will finally be made clear that the God of all hope is also faithful to him. God is trustworthy. The verse in Hebrews 5:7 that begins "Jesus offered up prayers and supplications, with loud cries and tears, to the one who was able to save him from death," ends with this astonishing claim: "and he was heard because of his reverent submission." God heard his cry and answered it. God saved him from death. God did not save him from a premature dying, but God saved him from the power of death. God took him from the dead, lifted him up, gave him life, and highly exalted him.

This is one of those places it is important to remember that we are not the Christ. Our deaths do not have the sort of cosmic significance that his did, nor is the "necessity" of our death quite the same as the unique necessity of his.[8] Because his resurrection precedes ours, we are not now free from the universal necessity of our own deaths, but because his resurrection is of one piece with our own, we may face that necessity with hope and courage. Without denying the uniqueness of Christ's agony, we may still learn from Christ in Gethsemane that, in the face of death, it is fitting to lament, to cry out to God, to ask that we be spared from death. We may also learn from Christ in Gethsemane, however, that our survival is not the only good or even the chief good to be considered, whether in our living or in our dying. We may learn from Christ to trust the one who will finally save us, not necessarily from a premature death, not from the universal necessity of death, but finally from the power of death.

No Gethsemane: The Difference John Makes

There is no Gethsemane in John's Gospel. Indeed, although John seems to know the tradition, he deliberately does not include it. In John's Gospel Jesus says, "Now my soul is troubled. And what should I say — 'Father, save me from this hour'? No, it is for this reason that I have come to this hour. Father, glorify your name" (John 12:27-28).

In John Jesus' cross is his "glory." He is "lifted up" on the cross (3:14; 8:28; 12:32-34). Early in John's passion narrative, Jesus announces that "the hour has come for the Son of Man to be glorified" (12:23). This is the

8. This is so regardless of the way different theories of atonement construe the unique necessity of Jesus' death.

"hour" — and the glory — that all the "signs" in John had pointed toward. John's narrative of the passion not only omits Gethsemane but also transforms the arrest scene to put Jesus in charge (18:11-14). In John Jesus even carries his own cross (19:17).

But we read John badly if we think that death itself is glorified in it.[9] It is not death that is commended in John's Gospel but life. The Gospel was written "that you may come to believe that Jesus is the Messiah, the Son of God, and that through believing you may have life in his name" (20:31). Jesus came "that they may have life, and have it abundantly" (10:10).[10] Jesus is a life-giver, not a death-dealer. Within John's Gospel, moreover, the reader is never allowed to separate the significance of the death of Jesus from his resurrection. Already in the story of Jesus cleansing the temple (2:13-22), John makes it clear that Jesus will be raised. When Jesus is asked for a sign of his authority to act the way he did in the temple, he says, "Destroy this temple, and in three days I will raise it up" (2:19). Those who heard it did not understand it at the time, but John makes sure that his readers do. "He was speaking of the temple of his body. After he was raised from the dead, his disciples remembered that he had said this; and they believed the scripture and the word that Jesus had spoken" (2:21-22). From the beginning, then, the reader knows that Jesus will be raised, and the resurrection is allowed to shine its light on the whole story of Jesus, including the story of his death. It is not his death considered by itself that is his glory, but his life and death considered in the light of the resurrection.

The cleansing of the temple is by no means the only occasion on which John reminds the reader of the resurrection. Following the healing miracles in John 4:46–5:18, Jesus claims that the Father has given to him the power and the authority to raise the dead and to render judgment (5:19-29). These are, of course, the events of the last day, but they are already making their power felt in Jesus. The resurrection of the last day is still future; "the hour is coming when all who are in their graves will hear his voice and will come out" (5:28-29). But already those who believe in Jesus share in his life; "the hour is coming, and is now here, when the dead will

---

9. In an otherwise perceptive book Douglas J. Davies, *A Brief History of Death* (Oxford: Blackwell, 2005), states that "Christianity glorified death" (p. 7). If he was thinking of the Gospel of John, then he should have said that John "glorified" the self-giving love that was ready to endure even death for the sake of others. If he was thinking about the *Ars Moriendi*, he should have said that a Platonized theology had "glorified death." But as a statement about either Scripture or Christianity, his claim is simply wrong.

10. It is also worth observing that John uses the term "life" thirty-six times.

hear the voice of the Son of God, and those who hear will live" (5:25). That was the deeper significance of the healing miracles. The passage from death to life that is already experienced is "an anticipation of — but not a substitute for — the physical resurrection."[11] The life Jesus promises, the life the Word made flesh grants, is not simply a "spiritual" life (of the sort the Gnostics or other dualists might envision); it is an embodied and communal life (of the sort the Creator had intended).

Other references underscore the point (6:39, 40, 44, 47-51; 10:17-18), but the story of the raising of Lazarus (11:1-44) clinches it. In that seventh and climactic sign Jesus joins Mary and Martha in their grief. This is no celebration of death, no commendation of death. Grief is appropriate. Jesus himself is "greatly disturbed in spirit and deeply moved" (11:33); he weeps (11:35). But death does not have the last word. Jesus has the last word. Jesus *is* the last word, and the last word is "resurrection and life" (11:25). He calls to Lazarus to come out of the tomb — and he does (11:43-44). The dead Lazarus in his grave hears the voice of the Son of God, and he comes out (cf. 5:25, 28-29). And they see "the glory of God" (11:40).

It was not yet the final resurrection, of course; Lazarus was raised still a mortal man, still vulnerable to death. He would die again (12:9-11); his sisters would grieve again. But in anticipation of that final resurrection, Lazarus came out of that tomb. And by the power and authority of Christ over death he and his sisters — and the readers — may be assured both that the dead will be raised "on the last day" (11:24) and that in the meanwhile nothing can separate us from Christ's love and presence. It is a love stronger than death. Death remains an awful and painful reality, but the power and authority — and the love — of Christ are also a reality, and finally a more powerful reality. In Christ the power of death has met its match and will be overcome.

John links the death and resurrection of Lazarus to the death and resurrection of Jesus. Like all the "signs," it points ahead to the hour of Jesus' glory, but this one is most clearly linked to the passion narrative in John. Hard on the heels of Lazarus coming out of the tomb comes the plot to kill Jesus (11:45-53) and the rest of the passion narrative. John, moreover, inserts reminders of this episode with Lazarus into that narrative (12:1-2, 9-11). But the story of Lazarus is also linked to the resurrection narrative in John. In both stories there is a tomb and a stone that must be moved (11:38;

---

11. Andrew T. Lincoln, "'I Am the Resurrection and the Life': The Resurrection Message of the Fourth Gospel," in *Life in the Face of Death: The Resurrection Message of the New Testament,* ed. Richard N. Longenecker (Grand Rapids: Eerdmans, 1998), p. 128.

20:1). In both stories the grave clothes are mentioned (11:44; 20:7). But whereas Lazarus came out of the tomb still "bound with strips of cloth" (11:44), at the resurrection of Jesus the grave cloths were lying in the tomb (20:5). Lazarus had been raised still vulnerable to death (12:9-11), but Jesus came from the tomb triumphant over death.

It should be clear, then, that John does not glorify death itself. It is not death that is glorified but Jesus. It is not death that is glorified but "life in his name." The resurrection of Christ still precedes our own, but John underscores our participation in it already. And in John's Gospel the mark of that participation, the mark of "life in his name," the mark of "glory," is love. That is why the cross is the "hour of his glory." We see his glory, glory as of the only-begotten of the Father, the Father who so loved the world that he gave his Son (3:16), on the cross, in the self-giving love of the cross. And this is the glory that Jesus shares with those who follow him (17:22). They may and must abide in the life Jesus gives; they may and must abide in his love and keep his commandments (15:9, which are in John just faith and love). They, too, are "lifted up" to acts of self-giving love.

It is not surprising, then, that John adds to the passion narrative his stunning scene of the foot washing at the Last Supper (13:1-20) with its instruction that the disciples should "wash one another's feet" (v. 14). Jesus is teacher (v. 13) and example (v. 15) here, but both his teaching and his paradigmatic significance are set in the context of his glorification, his vindication as the one in whom the Father's love is made known and real. We are not the Christ, but we can learn from him and follow him, participate in his life and glory, his self-giving love, even as we are dying.

Jesus was not a victim of death in John. He took the prospect of his death as the occasion for a definitive disclosure of his identity. We are not the Christ, but we need not simply be victims of death either. We, too, can take the occasion of our dying to be a time for the definitive disclosure of our Christian identity. That will not be done by stoically keeping a stiff upper lip. That will not be done by Platonic contemplation of some other world. It will be done by quite mundane acts of fidelity and love, of gratitude and forgiveness, of truthfulness and care. And it will be done in ways that honor, and do not deride, our embodied life and our relations with others. (It is striking that in John's passion narrative Jesus acknowledges his thirst as he is dying [19:28], secures safe passage for his disciples from the garden [18:8], and makes arrangements for his mother's care from the cross [19:26-27].) Then, even on the way to our death, something of God's triumph over death may be revealed.

Whether we follow John's narrative and regard the passion as the "hour" of his "glory" or that of the Synoptic Gospels and regard his passion as the "hour" of the tyrants, of death, and of "the power of darkness" (Luke 22:53), both lead us to the cross.

The Words from the Cross[12]

"My God, My God, Why . . . ?"

Mark and Matthew provide a single word from the cross, this terrible cry of anguish, "My God, my God, why have you forsaken me?" (Mark 15:34; Matt. 27:46). Both report that Jesus cried out again just before his death, but they do not tell us what he said. This terrible cry of anguish brings to a climax the horrors of his death. On the way from Gethsemane to Golgotha death had made its power felt again and again. Death threatens, as we have said, alienation from our own flesh, alienation from our communities, and alienation from God. Death made its power felt in Gethsemane already when disciples failed to "watch," failed to stay awake, would not or could not keep vigil with Christ.[13] It made its power felt when one disciple betrayed him, when another denied him, when they all forsook him and fled. It made its power felt when the council of his own people condemned him and when Pilate sentenced him. It made its power felt when the soldiers tortured him. It made its power felt in crucifixion, the most deliberately degrading and painful form of capital punishment that the Roman tyrants could inflict.[14]

---

12. The seven sayings from the cross are usually given in this order: Luke 23:34; Luke 23:43; John 19:26-27; Mark 15:34 (Matt. 27:46); John 19:28; John 19:30; and Luke 23:46. That traditional order is sensible enough; it results from a harmonization of the four Gospels. Harmonization, however, as we have said, can be dangerous, diluting the distinctive voice of each Evangelist. It ought to be remembered that only one of these sayings appears in more than one Gospel. Or, to put it differently, three different sayings are "the last words" of Jesus in the four Gospels. The order followed here treats the saying that appears in Mark and Matthew first, then the three sayings from Luke's Gospel, and finally the three sayings from John.

13. The threefold failure to "watch" reflects the threefold call to "watch" at the end of the apocalyptic discourse in Mark 13, which was addressed not just to the disciples but finally "to all" (v. 37). The readers of Mark's Gospel were called to watchfulness, too.

14. Mark underscores the horror of death by crucifixion by using the term "crucified" eight times between 5:13 and 16:6. On the horror and scandal of death by crucifixion (and its use primarily on the "lower class"), see Martin Hengel, *Crucifixion* (Philadelphia: Fortress, 1977).

But the greatest threat was the threat of alienation from God, and on that cross death made its power felt when it seemed God had forsaken him.

This is hardly a commendation of death. This is awful stuff. No one should die like this. It must have been the strangest, most dreadful day of his life on earth. There was the torturing pain of pierced hands and feet, the painful difficulty of so simple a bodily task as breathing. And there was the aloneness! To be sure, a crowd was there, but they were mostly mocking him and taunting him; in the middle of this crowd he was alone, abandoned by his friends. But most of all, there was that sense of God-forsakenness, that worry that the one to whom he had cried out in Gethsemane had abandoned him after all, had denied him, had betrayed him. Darkness fell upon the land at noon. It was strange but fitting. The light is supposed to overcome the darkness, but on this day the darkness seemed to overcome the light, to put it out — and with it, hope. It was Sheol, "the land of gloom and deep darkness" (Job 10:21).

For three hours in that darkness Jesus suffered, mute. And then he cried this cry: "My God, my God, why have you forsaken me?" What could he have meant? At the moment of his death, had Jesus lost his faith? Could it be that he had thrown himself on the wheel of God's purpose in the world only to be crushed by it? Could it be that his hope had been an illusion all along and only recognized as such at this dreadful end of it? Could it be that he *was* abandoned, and that this awful cry simply reveals that abandonment? Could it be that death has the last word, and that Jesus finally knew it? More than one reader of Mark and Matthew has asked these questions. And more than one theologian has answered yes.[15]

Good Jew that he was, Jesus knew the Psalms. He knew that songbook of the second temple. He knew the great hymns of Israel's faith, those songs of praise that invited all the nations and all of nature to join in Israel's praise of God. But he also knew the laments, those great cries to God in sickness and in sorrow, in catastrophe and in grief.[16]

15. See Albert Schweitzer, *The Quest of the Historical Jesus* (New York: Macmillan, 1961), pp. 370-71, for the account of Jesus as "crushed" by the wheel of God's purpose. See Jürgen Moltmann, *The Crucified God: The Cross of Christ as the Foundation and Criticism of Christian Theology* (Minneapolis: Fortress, 1993), for an account of Jesus as abandoned by God.

16. There are more laments than hymns in the Psalms. On the biblical lament see the following: the collection of Walter Brueggemann's writings on the Psalms in Patrick D. Miller, ed., *The Psalms and the Life of Faith: Walter Brueggemann* (Minneapolis: Fortress, 1995); Walter Brueggemann, *The Message of the Psalms: A Theological Commentary* (Minneapolis: Augsburg, 1984); Patrick Miller, *They Cried to the Lord: The Form and Theology of*

The psalms of lament were not dirges. In the dirge, at least in David's dirge at the deaths of Saul and Jonathan (2 Sam. 1:19-27), the decisive feature is the contrast between past glories and present misery. In its refrain and conclusion there is a sharp and total contrast to the remembered glories of Saul and Jonathan: "How the mighty have fallen!" *Once* they were "beloved and lovely"; once "they were swifter than eagles, . . . stronger than lions"; *now* "how the mighty have fallen." The reversal that marks the dirge has been called the "tragic reversal"[17] — it moves from glory to shame, from strength to powerlessness. It is, I suppose, suffering finding voice — but not hope. In lament, however, suffering finds a voice addressed to God. The laments look heavenward and find hope. The distress and powerlessness and anger and sorrow are still there, still finding voice, but the laments finally share Israel's faith that the saving reversal — and not the tragic reversal — is the plot of their story with God. Lament reverses the reversal; it moves from distress toward wholeness, from powerlessness toward certainty, from anger toward confidence in God's justice, and from sorrow toward hope in God. There is no pretense in lament, no denial, no withdrawal to some otherworldly realities. To look to God is not to look away. Lament unflinchingly acknowledges that life is beset by betrayal, loneliness, bewilderment, anxiety, anger, anguish, suffering, and finally death. It calls upon God to be faithful, to set things right, and it is confident that God is faithful and will set things right.

Jesus knew the Psalms. He knew the sad songs of lament. And he knew Psalm 22. In his agony on the cross he made the lament of Psalm 22, a "psalm of David," his own. He made David's cry his own: "My God, my

---

Biblical Prayer (Minneapolis: Fortress, 1994); and Claus Westermann, *Praise and Lament in the Psalms* (Atlanta: John Knox, 1981). To this list may be added works in practical theology that focus on lament, notably, Kathleen D. Billman and Daniel Migliore, *Rachel's Cry: Prayers of Lament and Rebirth of Hope* (Cleveland: United Church Press, 1999); Emilie Townes, ed., *A Troubling in My Soul: Womanist Perspectives on Evil and Suffering* (Maryknoll, N.Y.: Orbis, 1993); Nicholas Wolterstorff, *Lament for a Son* (Grand Rapids: Eerdmans, 1987); and Sally Brown and Patrick D. Miller, eds., *Lament: Reclaiming Practices in Pulpit, Pew, and Public Square* (Louisville: Westminster John Knox, 2005). See also the recent essay by John Swinton, "'Why Me, Lord?': Practicing Lament at the Foot of the Cross," in *Living Well and Dying Faithfully: Christian Practices for End-of-Life Care,* ed. John Swinton and Richard Payne (Grand Rapids: Eerdmans, 2009), pp. 107-38. My own previous attention to lament may be found in Allen Verhey, *Reading the Bible in the Strange World of Medicine* (Grand Rapids: Eerdmans, 2003), pp. 114-40.

17. Norman Gottwald, *Studies in the Book of Lamentations,* Studies in Biblical Theology 14 (Chicago: Alec R. Allenson, 1954).

God, why have you forsaken me?" He knew Psalm 22, and good Jew that he was, he knew the whole psalm. He knew it continued (for eight more verses) in desperate complaint, "Why are you so far from helping me?" But he also knew that Psalm 22 moved from this terrifying cry of anguish to a trusting plea for help:

> Do not be far from me. . . .
> Deliver my soul from the sword,
>   my life from the power of the dog!
> Save me from the mouth of the lion!
>
> (vv. 11, 20-21)

He knew that Psalm 22 shifted again, and suddenly, to the praise of God's faithfulness and to the certainty of a hearing:

> [God] did not despise or abhor
>   the affliction of the afflicted;
> [God] did not hide his face from me,
>   but heard when I cried to [God].
>
> (v. 24)

And he knew as well that that certainty of a hearing grew into a song of thanksgiving and a hymn of praise and that it flowered in a vision of the cosmic triumph of God.

> You who fear the LORD, praise the LORD! . . .
> All the ends of the earth shall remember
>   and turn to the LORD;
> and all the families of the nations
>   shall worship before the LORD.
> For dominion belongs to the LORD,
>   and the LORD rules over the nations.
> To the LORD, indeed, shall all who sleep in the earth bow down;
>   before the LORD shall bow all who go down to the dust,
>   and I shall live for the LORD.
> Posterity will serve the LORD;
>   future generations will be told about the Lord,
> and proclaim the Lord's deliverance to a people yet unborn,
>   saying that the Lord has done it.
>
> (vv. 23, 27-31)

Jesus was in agony, but not in despair. If Jesus knew the whole psalm — and he did — then it may be confidently said that he had not lost his faith or his hope.

Surely the Evangelists, too, knew the whole psalm. Only Mark and Matthew record this word from the cross, but all the Gospels cite Psalm 22 in one way or another. All of them report, for example, that the soldiers cast lots for Jesus' clothing (Ps. 22:18; Mark 15:24; Matt. 27:35; Luke 23:34; and John 19:23-24). Indeed, in John this is explicitly regarded as a "fulfillment" of the psalm. Again, Mark and Matthew use the language of Psalm 22:7 to describe the mocking derision of those who passed by "shaking their heads" (Mark 15:29; Matt. 27:39). Indeed, the very taunt of the mocking crowd in Matthew's Gospel echoes Psalm 22:4 and 8 (Matt. 27:43). And these references by no means exhaust the parallels between this psalm and the death of Jesus. There is the darkness (Ps. 22:2), the thirst (v. 15), the company of evildoers (v. 16). The second cry in Matthew and Mark just as Jesus died (Matt. 27:50 and Mark 15:37) may well be a reference to Psalm 22:24, "[God] heard when I cried to him." Hebrews 2:12 puts Psalm 22:22 on the very lips of Jesus:

> I will proclaim your name to my brothers and sisters,
>   in the midst of the congregation I will praise you.

The early church evidently considered this psalm to be "the Psalm of Christ."[18]

Nevertheless, Psalm 22 remains a lament, and Jesus' word from the cross remains a cry of anguish. Neither David nor Jesus celebrated death; neither celebrated human suffering; neither made death or suffering good. If the whole psalm makes it clear that Jesus had not lost his faith or hope, it also makes it clear that there is no contradiction between faith and lament, no inconsistency between hope and lament. Indeed, hope is displayed in lament, in the aching acknowledgment that it is not yet God's good future, still sadly not yet God's good future.

Something like the dawn of an Easter morning must have broken in on David's night of anguish. There is no other way to explain the sudden shift in Psalm 22 from complaint to its vision of the triumph of God. But Easter morning had not yet dawned for Jesus, and it would not until this Friday had been spent in agony and that Saturday was spent in the silence

18. Chad Walsh, *The Psalm of Christ: Forty Poems on the Twenty-Second Psalm* (Philadelphia: Westminster, 1963).

of death. We must hear Jesus' word as lament. We should not rush past the terrifying cry of anguish to the certainty of a hearing, neglecting or discounting or effectively silencing the voice of suffering. Jesus had not lost faith, had not lost hope, but the lament was real. And if Jesus is the paradigm for faith and hope in the face of death, his lament is also paradigmatic. Lament is fitting in the face of death. Jesus made this human cry of anguish his own cry. And so may we. It is the Psalm of David and the Psalm of Christ, and it may be our psalm, too.

We have answered one of the questions prompted by this cry of anguish. On the basis of Psalm 22 it is clear that Jesus had not lost his faith or his hope. But there remains that other, no less frightening set of questions. Had Jesus in faith and hope thrown himself on the wheel of God's purpose in the world, only to be crushed by it? Had his hope been an illusion, only recognized at death? Did God finally forsake him, abandon him? And the answer to all these questions, too, is no.[19] No, God did not abandon him! The psalm can be cited again. God "did not despise or abhor / the affliction of the afflicted" (Ps. 22:24). But the best evidence is that Easter morning. God rescued the one in whom he delights (cf. Ps. 22:8 and the taunt of the mockers in Matt. 27:43). God would not let death have the last word.

And if and when in the face of death we make this psalm our own, we may be sure that we are not and will not be abandoned. We may be sure that Christ is with us. He knows the dark recesses of our caverns of gloom; he was there first. Into whatever pit of loneliness we fall, Christ can find us. It does not make suffering a good, but we may be at least assured that we do not suffer alone. It does not make death a good, but we may trust and hope that not even death can separate us from the love of God finally. We may cry out to God in anger and in hope, in anguish and in faith, joining the sad complaint that it is not yet God's good future to a sure confidence in the faithfulness of God. We may lament.

"Father, Forgive Them"

In Luke's Gospel the first word from the cross is a prayer, "Father, forgive them; for they do not know what they are doing" (Luke 23:34).[20] Again,

---

19. See further William Stacy Johnson, "Jesus' Cry, God's Cry, and Ours," in *Lament*, pp. 80-94.

20. Many manuscripts of Luke's Gospel, including the oldest, do not contain this

cautions are in order. We are not Jesus. His death had a sort of cosmic significance that ours cannot claim. His death was the basis, on certain theories of atonement at least, for the divine forgiveness of human sins. Moreover, our deaths are seldom the result of another's transgression. To be sure, death can result from violence, from a drunken driver, from a missed diagnosis, or even simply from secondhand smoke. Even so, we are not Jesus; not even the martyrs or the victims of state torture and murder can claim to be Jesus.

We should be careful also about shifting attention from Jesus to ourselves, as if this were simply about us. It is about us, of course, but only because the story is about Jesus. The story is not told that we can have some easy peace of mind about our little moral failings. It is not told simply as an illustration of the human condition that is obvious enough without Jesus. It is not told, for example, simply because Jesus' forgiveness is a good example of the prudence of forgiveness. Jesus does not just illustrate the human condition; he transforms the human condition. He transforms our condition, even as we are on our way to death.

Jesus transformed the human condition by making real and present the future judgment and forgiveness of God the Father. The cross, too, along with the resurrection, was an eschatological event. The darkness at noon (Luke 23:44; cf. Amos 8:9; Joel 2:31) signaled its significance; this was indeed the Day of the Lord, a day of judgment. It's the crowning irony in Luke's story of the crucifixion, so full of irony. There is irony in the fact that those who scoff at Jesus all speak the truth in the titles they use to mock him (Luke 23:35-39). There is irony in the truth of the taunting inscription on the cross (Luke 23:38). But no irony is greater than this one, that this Jesus, condemned to die by the verdict of an unjust judge, prays that his Father, the judge of all the world, should forgive those whom

---

prayer. The external evidence would seem to argue against its inclusion. Moreover, ordinarily the shorter version should be preferred. On the other hand, the internal evidence strongly supports its inclusion. Luke emphasizes prayer as a practice of Jesus; he is, for example, the only Evangelist to report that Jesus was praying at his baptism (Luke 3:21) and at the transfiguration (9:29). In Luke Jesus frequently invokes God as "Father" (e.g., 10:21; 11:2; 22:42; 23:46). In Luke the risen Jesus sends the disciples out into all the world with a message of the forgiveness of sins (24:47). Moreover, the prayer finds an echo in the prayer of Stephen (Acts 7:60). It is, however, hard to imagine why it would have been omitted by a later scribe; perhaps the destruction of Jerusalem prompted some to think that the prayer was not effectual. It is, I think, impossible to know whether it was a part of the original Gospel or added by a later scribe. But if it was added by a later scribe, that scribe well understood both Jesus and Luke.

God's justice might rightly condemn. There on that cross was already the final judgment. On that cross Jesus made real and present both God's truth and God's grace in judgment. In Jesus and in his word of forgiveness we may recognize that we are sinners, that all those gathered around this cross and around this story are condemned by it.[21] In this righteous and crucified Christ we are all brought into judgment. We, like Judas, have betrayed this Jesus. We, like Peter, have denied him. This truth hurts; but condemned by this gracious word, we may repent. And then we may taste another future, for in Jesus and in his word of forgiveness we have a little foretaste of a future on the far side of that judgment. In this righteous and crucified Christ and in his word of forgiveness we are brought safely through the judgment to God's grace; we are already brought safely through the future judgment and enter already a world where God's mercy and forgiveness are the rule.

In this word of forgiveness we see Jesus as the true Son of his Father. Surely the readiness to forgive was characteristic of God already in the Old Testament. Any reading of Hosea should be enough to make that clear (see, e.g., not just the relation of Hosea to Gomer but also Hos. 11:1-9). The readiness of God to forgive was the assumption in the practice of the rituals of Yom Kippur, the Day of Atonement (see Lev. 16:29-34). A sacrificial atonement for the sins of the people rendered those sins forgiven on that day. God's readiness to forgive did not, of course, render particular injustices or the infidelities in the common life of the people a matter of indifference to God. Sin was — and is — condemned, but that condemnation is neither the first nor the last word in the Old Testament. God's readiness to forgive was displayed in God's readiness to embrace the people in spite of their infidelities, in God's readiness to embrace the sinner, in God's readiness to let go the (righteous) indignation that was prompted by injury or insult for the sake of the renewal of a relationship. God's readiness to forgive meant that forgiveness — and a renewed relationship with God — was possible for the people and for anyone who turned to the Lord in re-

---

21. The Gospel of Luke adds to the narrative of the cross two accounts of lament. On the way to the cross a crowd follows Jesus "beating their breasts," wailing and lamenting for him (Luke 23:27). And after Jesus had died, the crowd who had gathered to see the sight "returned home, beating their breasts" (Luke 23:48). It is hard to know quite what to make of this. At the very least it suggests a throb of compassion in that crowd from Jerusalem in response to the suffering and death of another. But perhaps it is something more, something like repentance, something more like the act of that tax collector in the temple who, "beating his breast," said, "God, be merciful to me, a sinner!" (Luke 18:13).

pentance (e.g., Ezek. 18:25-32). That repentance required restitution for injustices against other human beings (e.g., Lev. 6:1-7); it required seeking their forgiveness and righting the wrong.

One more point about God's readiness to forgive in the Old Testament: there grew a hope for an eschatological forgiveness, for the renewal of covenant identity and community by the mercy and forgiveness of God, for a renewed relationship with God (e.g., Jer. 31:31-34; Isa. 65:17-25). That hope provides the context for Jesus' announcement that God's good future is at hand and for his performance of that future also in his readiness to forgive. Christ, the Son of his Father, made and makes already real and present God's eschatological forgiveness. He still calls for repentance, to be sure (e.g., Mark 1:15), but to repent is to welcome that good future and to be formed by it. The focus falls not on sackcloth and ashes, not even so much on restitution (which is, however, not forgotten), but on the joyful renewal of broken relationships between God and the people and between members of this community. God's good future — and its grace — makes its power felt in the variety of ways in which Jesus performs forgiveness: in his friendship with sinners, in his healing them, in his fellowship with those whom the "righteous" had forced to the margins of the community, and in his refusal to participate in the human cycles of vengeance and violence.

Jesus' performance of the Father's readiness to forgive finds climactic expression on the cross and in the words of forgiveness that he managed to speak from it: "Father, forgive them . . ." (Luke 23:34). Jesus transforms the human condition by making real and present the future judgment and forgiveness of God the Father. In him we are already brought safely through the future judgment and enter already a world where God's mercy and forgiveness are the rule. We die well and faithfully when we are assured by this word of God's readiness to forgive and to embrace us. It is the point underscored by *Ars Moriendi* and its attention to the cross. Following Bernard, it had urged Moriens to see the readiness of God to forgive in the disposition of Christ on the cross; "take hede and see," it said, "his armes spredde to cylppe the [his arms spread to embrace you]" (*Crafte*, p. 6). We may die assured of God's embrace.

In Jesus and in this word of forgiveness we are not only assured of God's forgiveness but also brought through the judgment into a future in which God's love and mercy are the rule. By that same grace, then, we are called to the forgiveness of others, called to establish already in this world a little foothold for that future. Accordingly, although the cautions remain, Luke evidently does intend this word to be paradigmatic for Christians and, indeed, paradigmatic for dying Christians. It is hardly accidental that he puts this prayer also on the lips of Stephen at his death (Acts 7:60). Stephen, of course, was the first Christian martyr, but all who are dying can bear witness *(martus)* to the cross by forgiving others.

The readiness to forgive is a mark of dying well and faithfully. It is resistance to the rule of sin and death in the face of death. Death and sin make their power felt in the sundering of relationships, in alienation from those we love and ought to love. Death and sin make their power felt in the nursing of grievances, in the desire for revenge, in the self-serving insistence that justice be done and that any offense against us be punished. The human condition is one long story of keeping score of offenses, real or imagined, responding tit for tat, reacting to offenses by some effort to "get even." But of course, we never do. Our efforts to "get even" will inevitably seem offensive to another, will seem excessive or unjust, and can prompt another round of reactions and retaliations. The story of retribution seems endless. And it is so even if, instead of retaliation, we choose "passively" to nurse our grievances, to hold our grudges. Past sins, whether ours or another's, seem to determine our present and our future in this vicious cycle, and we seem as destined to alienation and enmity as we are to death.

But the story is *not* endless. The final judgment has been revealed on the cross. In Christ's word of forgiveness, spoken as the Son of his Father and as a prayer to his Father, the cycle of vengeance and retaliation is broken, and relationships are restored. Christ transforms the human condition by this word of forgiveness. The new life in Christ makes its power felt in forgiveness, in the readiness to embrace, in reconciliation. To die well and faithfully is not to take grudges to the grave. It is not to nurse little grievances while we lie dying. It is to forgive. It is to seek to be reconciled with those we have counted as enemies. This is no "straight-line dues-paying morality."[22] This is a common life formed by the grace of God. And it is to be performed also in our dying and in our care for the dying.

The virtue of forgiveness is the readiness to embrace the one who did us wrong, to let go the indignation of an injury or an insult, the indignation that, whether "righteous" or not, can be as much at fault for the brokenness of our relationships as the injury or insult itself. The readiness to forgive has its basis and its inspiration in God's forgiveness. The practice of forgiveness in the church ("Whenever you stand praying, forgive"; Mark 11:25) makes that obvious enough. But it is, of course, precisely what Ephe-

---

22. Lewis B. Smedes, *Forgive and Forget* (San Francisco: Harper and Row, 1984), p. 124.

sians says, "Put away from you all bitterness and wrath and anger and wrangling and slander, together with all malice, and be kind to one another, tenderhearted, forgiving one another, as God in Christ has forgiven you" (Eph. 4:31-32).[23]

The gospel of God's forgiveness is, as Matthew's parable of the unforgiving servant (Matt. 18:23-35) makes quite clear, both gracious and demanding. To receive such grace is to be enabled and permitted to live — and to die — in accord with it. It is not that we earn forgiveness by being forgiving ourselves. It is no calculating "works righteousness," not even at the endings of our lives. It is rather that we are made new, made a part of transformed humanity in which kindness, compassion, mutual love, and forgiveness are the rule. That is good news indeed.

Let it be said again, however, that neither God's readiness to forgive nor this virtue of forgiveness among Christians denies the claims of justice. Indeed, forgiveness assumes justice and affirms justice in the very act of forgoing the claims that one might rightly make against another. Forgiveness does not render sin a matter of indifference to either God or to the community. If sin were a matter of indifference to God, God would not have to forgive sins but could simply ignore them. And a community called to the readiness to forgive is not called simply to ignore injury and injustice. The readiness to forgive, the eagerness for renewed relationships, provides the context for communal discipline, not a substitute for it. (See Matthew 18, which sets communal discipline in the context of the charge to protect "the little ones" and the duty to forgive.)

And let it be said again that we are not the Christ. We not only forgive others; we need to be forgiven by others. We die well and faithfully not only by a readiness to forgive and embrace but also by a readiness to repent, to apologize, to make things right. The readiness to repent is also inspired by this prayer from the cross. It is as the Son of his Father that he prays it, and he reveals by it and makes real by it God's readiness to embrace. By it we are brought safely through the judgment. And if so, then we need not be fearful of the judgment. The good news of God's forgiveness, of God's readiness to

---

23. The phrase "forgiving one another, as God in Christ has forgiven you" (Eph. 4:32), might also be translated "be gracious to one another, as God in Christ has been gracious to you." The word used in this phrase to name both the act of God and the human activity is *charizomai*, a word that may include forgiveness but might also be translated more broadly as "to be gracious." The aorist tense for God's act suggests an action in the past, an action once for all, and the present tense for the participle used to name the human activity suggests a continuing activity, a virtue.

embrace, frees us to recognize ourselves as sinners, to repent. It makes possible new beginnings and reconciliation. When the risen Christ appeared to the disciples, to those who had denied him and abandoned him, he did not come to them to punish them. He forgave them. He blessed them with his peace. He opened possibilities of reconciliation, and he called them to begin again to follow him in anticipation of God's good future. That good future was marked as the rule of God's mercy and forgiveness not only by this word from the cross but also by his very appearance to them. The crucified and risen Lord assures us that for as long as repentance and forgiveness are possibilities we are not fated by our past but free to begin again, to restore relationships, even as we are dying.

To be sure, these new beginnings may be complicated and difficult. And, of course, reconciliation takes two; the readiness of just one of the estranged to embrace the other does not accomplish reconciliation. But if the readiness and desire of one to embrace the other is announced, it is an invitation that may end in an embrace. Reconciliation is frequently complicated by the truth. Isn't everything? Sometimes the readiness to embrace is announced as contingent upon an apology framed in precisely the way an offended party sees the offense. The embrace of Christ should help us to endure the truth, to acknowledge the truth of our own faults in the breaking of relationships, to apologize. But our readiness to forgive and to embrace others should not be made contingent upon a willingness of others to admit their faults in precisely the way in which we see their faults. Rather, both the readiness to embrace and the willingness to accept that embrace must accept a future that is not determined by the way either party has kept score up to now. We are not the Christ. Our claims to innocence are as frequently self-deceptive as truthful. Reconciliation almost always involves acknowledging the solidarity in the sins of the past. In restored relationships the hold that sin has had on each and all of us in this present evil age is acknowledged and broken.

Reconciliation will sometimes require the help of the community, of faithful friends, and it is no small part of helping one to die well. And sometimes it will require of the community considerable discernment to know whether the truth requires of the readiness to forgive and of the eagerness to renew broken relationships also an apology or some restitution. But always that truth and deliberation about it must be set in the context of God's greater forgiveness and the gift and task of reconciliation.

A father who had effectively disowned his gay son learned that his son had AIDS. The person who brought him this news also insisted that he visit his son and be reconciled to him. When the father arrived, he was moved, but he did not know exactly what to say. "I forgive you," he finally said. His son was also moved by his father's visit, but he was curious about his father's remark. "For what?" he asked. "For being gay, I guess," his father replied. "Oh," said the son, and after a moment he added, "and I forgive you too." "For what?" asked the father. "For being my dad!" Words of forgiveness like these can sometimes sound very much like accusations, and the accusations can reopen old wounds, adding one more offense to the tally. It was not a promising opening conversation, but the friend saw promise in the readiness to embrace, and with a little help, that readiness to embrace, to be reconciled, led to another conversation and eventually to a genuine embrace. They still had some things to work out together, some truths to endure together, but the context was no longer the past reckoning of offenses but the readiness to embrace, the eagerness to begin again a relation of father and son. Eventually the son went to his father's house to die. There he was cared for by his father. The son died a little later — but he died a little better. When the son died, the father said that he died a little, too — but the life he lived was better, too, for the reconciliation with his dear son.

Jesus embraces the world, and in that embrace we have a new reality of relationships not based on a "dues-paying morality" — also with the members of our own family. The art of dying does not call us to love them less but to love them better, to love them in ways appropriate to the love of God for them. The art of dying does not call us to neglect them but to ask forgiveness for the ways we have neglected them in the past. The art of dying does not call for the renunciation of "carnal" relationships but for the renunciation of the little grudges we may carry against them. The art of dying demands the readiness to embrace them, to forgive them and to be forgiven by them, to be reconciled.

"Today You Will Be with Me in Paradise"

Each of the Gospels reports that Jesus was crucified with two others, but only Luke includes their conversation. As Luke tells the story, one of those condemned to die added his voice to the taunts of the leaders and the soldiers. The leaders had scoffed at Jesus, "If you are the Christ of God, the chosen one, save yourself!" The soldiers had mocked him: "If you are the King of the Jews, save yourself!" And then one of those crucified derided him: "If you are the Christ, save yourself and us!" (see Luke 23:35-39). Ironically, of course, they all spoke the truth in the titles they used to taunt Jesus, but it was mockery and a torment. Perhaps this criminal thought to curry the favor of the soldiers; perhaps he simply wanted there to be one person more miserable than he was. The second condemned man, however, did not join his voice to the taunts; indeed, he rebuked the first man. "Do you not fear God?" he asked, and reminded the first that he too was condemned to die (v. 40). How could he dare go to his death mocking and taunting another human being — and an innocent one at that? How could he dare go to his death adding to the torment of another dying man? Even as he suffers his way toward his own death, this second criminal rebukes the injustice of the taunt; on his own way toward death he does justice and loves mercy and walks humbly with God. And he recognizes not only that Jesus is innocent, but that he is indeed the Christ, the chosen one, the rightful King of Israel. He says to Jesus, "Jesus, remember me when you come into your kingdom" (v. 42). Luke does not pause to explain how this condemned man knows so much, but he makes the request of a believer, a request that would later appear on the gravestones of some early Christians.[24] He believes that God will vindicate this Christ, and he hopes and prays that the vindicated Christ will share with him his triumph over the powers — including the power of death.

This thief made an appearance in the *Ars Moriendi*, it will be remembered, a model of the repentant sinner (and the best evidence of the authenticity of a deathbed confession). Luke surely intends him to be a paradigmatic figure. He is indeed a paradigmatic repentant sinner, the lost sheep who is found at last, the prodigal child who comes home. But he is also a paradigm of righteousness in his justice, mercy, and humility before God. Like Jesus, he dies a horrific death, a premature and violent death, but by his faith and hope, by his refusal to be self-absorbed in his dying, by his concern for those who also die, by his devotion to the cause of God, he is a paradigm of dying well and faithfully.

To the request of this thief Jesus replied with this word from the cross: "Today you will be with me in Paradise" (v. 43). The thief had asked to be remembered when Jesus came into his kingdom, presumably on the last day. But Jesus, evidently confident that God would vindicate him, promised the thief that "today," presumably the day of his death, he would

---

24. E. Earle Ellis, *The Gospel of Luke*, rev. ed., New Century Bible Commentary (Grand Rapids: Eerdmans, 1981), p. 268.

be "with Christ" in that hidden Paradise where the righteous await the resurrection and God's final triumph.[25] Here, as regularly in Luke, "today" serves to mark a kind of promissory note, a down payment on God's good future. The future remains future, but it makes its power felt already now, already "today."

When, for example, in Luke's Gospel Jesus opens his public ministry by reading Isaiah 61 in a Nazareth synagogue, he says, "Today this scripture has been fulfilled in your hearing" (Luke 4:21). To be sure, Jesus announces "good news to the poor," and in that announcement the good future of God reaches into the present, but it remains a promissory note on the good future of God to which both Isaiah and Jesus pointed. Again, when in Luke's Gospel Jesus visits the home of Zaccheus and learns of his promise to practice justice and generosity, he says, "Today salvation has come to this house" (Luke 19:9). Zaccheus's promise points toward the fullness of God's salvation; it hardly exhausts it. It is a mark that God's future reign of justice and mercy has broken into the present and is already real. And here in this word to the thief the promise of Jesus is not a substitute for what the condemned man requested; it is the promissory note on that future. The future remains future, but it makes its power felt already now, already "today," even for the dead.[26] The dead criminal, like the living, already has a part in the victory of God over death, but it is not yet the final resurrection or the day of Christ's coming. Death does not have the last word because it *will not* have the last word.

This word did not make that condemned man's suffering or his death suddenly good. This word was hardly a commendation of death. But it surely did alleviate his suffering some to know that he was not abandoned in it. I imagine he died a little more peacefully, no longer needing to hang on desperately and hopelessly to life as if death would have the last word over him.

---

25. See N. T. Wright, *Surprised by Hope: Rethinking Heaven, the Resurrection, and the Mission of the Church* (New York: HarperOne, 2008), pp. 150-51.

26. Once again the promise of the intermediate state is simply that the thief will be "with" Jesus. But one might ask, of course, where Jesus was on the Friday after his death around three o'clock or on that Saturday following his death. Was he in that hidden Paradise awaiting his own resurrection? Or was he in Hades, preaching to the dead? Or was he simply in the tomb, in the silence of Sheol, cut off from the praise of God? Luke evidently has no interest in such questions. But he is sure of the victory of God over death, and in his Gospel he has Jesus assure this dying man of a share in it "today."

"Father, into Your Hands I Commend My Spirit"

Luke has a third word from the cross, spoken as Jesus "breathed his last" (Luke 23:46). It is in Luke (and in the traditional order of the words from the cross) Jesus' last words before his death. Again it is a prayer, and again it is taken from a psalm of lament, Psalm 31. Unlike Jesus' use of Psalm 22:1 in Mark and Matthew, however, this verse (Ps. 31:5) is not part of the lament itself (vv. 11-13). It is rather part of the prayer for deliverance and an expression of confidence and trust.

Psalm 31 twice draws a contrast between falling "into the hand of the enemy" (vv. 8, 15) and resting in the hand of God (vv. 5, 15). In Psalm 31 the enemies "plot to take [the] life [of the psalmist]" (v. 13) and slander him, treating "the righteous with pride and contempt" (v. 18). Given the litany of taunts that Jesus had just endured in Luke's Gospel, the lament of Psalm 31 seems altogether appropriate, even if the curse on the enemies (vv. 17b, 18) hardly fits with Jesus' earlier prayer that his enemies be forgiven. At any rate, we need not here reiterate what we noted above about the appropriateness of lament and about its coherence with faith and hope. Here it is legitimate to abstract this prayer from its context in lament. Indeed, this verse was frequently used independently of the psalm within which it is found as the evening prayer of a pious Jew.[27]

As Jesus prepared to die, he said the same prayer that many other pious Jews repeated as they prepared to sleep. Of course, to express confidence in God as one prepares to die is a more profound display of faith than to express such confidence when one is simply getting ready for bed. But it is the same confidence. It is the same God. And it is the same prayer. The pious practice of this evening prayer trains one for confidence at the end of life. To trust in God to care for and to keep one's life may be harder at the end of life, but such trust then is made easier by the habit of attending regularly to God and to the faithfulness of God. To die well and faithfully is easier if one has lived well and faithfully.

Perhaps Jesus had prayed this prayer many times before. We do not know. But we do know, given especially Luke's account of Jesus, that Jesus engaged in the practice of prayer. From the time of his baptism (Luke 3:21)

---

27. I. Howard Marshall, *The Gospel of Luke* (Grand Rapids: Eerdmans, 1978), p. 876. Ethelbert Stauffer, *Jesus and His Story,* trans. Richard Winston and Clara Winston (New York: Knopf, 1960), p. 142, observes the same point and suggests that it was the ninth hour, the conventional time for the evening prayer.

forward, Luke had frequently noted that Jesus was praying. Now at the time of his death Jesus prays again. To pray, to attend to God, gives new courage for both daily life and for death. The virtues of an honest prayer, among which may be counted faith and hope and love and humility and gratitude, are also the virtues of living well and faithfully — and of dying well and faithfully. One does not pray in order to achieve those virtues. They are not formed when we use prayer as a technique. But they are formed in simple attentiveness to God, and they spill over into new virtues for daily life — and for dying and caring for the dying.

The *Ars Moriendi,* as we have noted, emphasized the significance of prayer to dying well and to caring well for the dying. Later we will take another cue from the *Ars Moriendi* on the place of prayer in faithful dying. Here we simply note that Jesus' prayer as he is dying is paradigmatic. When Stephen dies, he makes this prayer his own, addressing Jesus rather than the Father: "Jesus, receive my spirit" (Acts 7:59). And so may we, letting ourselves go into the hands of God, confident that God can and will deliver us from the hands of that enemy, death.

"Woman, Behold Your Son!"

The Gospel of John gives three other words from the cross. We have already noted that John tells the story of the cross quite differently. There is no Gethsemane agony. In John Jesus' cross is his "glory." He is "lifted up" on the cross (3:14; 8:28; 12:32-33). It is not that death itself is glorified, or suffering itself. It is rather "the Resurrection and the Life" that is celebrated. In the light of Jesus' triumph over death, his cross is the definitive disclosure of his self-giving love, and of the Father's self-giving love. And "life in his name" is to be marked by that same self-giving love in community. That is the glory he shares with those who follow him.

Given John's Gospel to this point, with its emphasis on the cosmic contest of light and darkness, truth and the lie, life and death, when the reader comes to "the hour of his glory," the reader may well expect some profoundly spiritual words from Jesus on the cross. The powerful and creative Word of God described in the prologue, the Word that "in the beginning . . . was with God, and . . . was God" (John 1:1), the life-giving Word without whom "not one thing came into being" (1:3), the Word that was life and light (1:4), this Word "became flesh" (1:14a). The world God made had alienated itself from God and from the Word, but God loved the world, and the Word "became flesh." The powerful and creative Word identified with human embodied life with its vulnerability to suffering and to death. We would behold "his glory, the glory as of a father's only son, full of grace and truth" (1:14b) upon a cross. We would behold his glory, and the father's glory, in the self-giving love of the cross, in sharing human suffering and death. It was clear already in the prologue that death could not hold him, that the darkness could not overcome the light and the life (1:5). Risen and ascended, he will still be the incarnate Word, still identified with human beings in their weakness and vulnerability. His wounds will be raised with him (20:27). So what words does this creative and powerful Word find on the cross? "Woman, behold your son!" "I thirst!" and "It is finished." These three words from the cross in John are surprisingly mundane, prosaic even.

But we should not be disappointed by these words. On the contrary, these three words in their very earthiness are theologically profound. At the very least, these words from the cross spell defeat for any attempt to read John's Gospel as if it were a Gnostic gospel or any attempt to construe Jesus' death as a Docetic death. It stands in sharp contrast, for example, to the *Gospel of Peter*.[28] There the divine power of Jesus evidently left him before his suffering and death (*Gospel of Peter* 5:19), and there, even so, on the cross Jesus "was silent, as if having no pain" (*Gospel of Peter* 4:10). In John Jesus is still identified with the human condition, still the powerful and creative Word made flesh. And these "fleshy" words signal the awful threats of death. Death threatens to separate us from our own flesh, from our communities, and from God. And Jesus responds to these threats in ways at once mundane and faithful. His death was real and awful, but in the way he met those threats he is a paradigm for dying well and faithfully. To die well and faithfully requires not some kind of Platonic transcendence but quite mundane acts of fidelity. It requires that we honor, and do not deride, our embodied life and our relations with others.

John reports that Jesus was crucified on Golgotha with two others, that Pilate put the title on the cross, "Jesus of Nazareth, the King of the

---

28. The *Gospel of Peter* was mentioned by Eusebius, who noted that Bishop Serapion of Antioch in the second century worried about its Docetic tendencies. Docetism is the view that Jesus' body, and especially his suffering, was not real but only an "appearance" (from *dokeo*, "to seem"). The book itself, however, was not known until a fragment was discovered in the late nineteenth century. For an English translation of the Greek fragment, see Raymond Brown, *The Death of the Messiah — from Gethsemane to the Grave: A Commentary on the Passion Narratives*, vol. 2 (New York: Doubleday, 1994), pp. 1318-21.

Jews," that the soldiers "cast lots" for the tunic of Jesus to fulfill the scripture (John 19:24; cf. Ps. 22:18). Then he — alone among the Gospels — notes that Jesus' mother was there. She stood "by the cross" with her sister and some other women, including Mary Magdalene.[29] John, "the disciple whom he loved," was with them, also standing near (John 19:25-26). Their simple presence must have brought some respite from the threat of death, that it sunders us from those we love. And their presence allowed the dying Jesus to respond to that threat of death by caring for them and by instructing them to care for one another after his death. He said to his mother, "Woman, behold your son!" and to John, "Behold your mother!" (John 19:26-27 RSV). And the Gospel notes that "from that hour the disciple took her into his own home" (v. 27 NRSV).

It is an earthy word, a son concerned about his mother after his death, making what provisions he could for her security and well-being. Perhaps it is little wonder that some commentators have searched for a deeper, more "spiritual" meaning. To be sure, John's Gospel is full of passages that have a deeper meaning than the surface significance of the words, but the deeper meaning is usually quite clear to the readers.[30] In this case, however, it seems to me that the efforts to find a more "spiritual" meaning range from the curious to the bizarre. Marian piety sometimes takes the episode to be "a proclamation of Mary's spiritual motherhood of the faithful, as the new Eve, . . . a figure of the Church."[31] Rudolf

29. The other Gospels report that women who had followed Jesus, including Mary Magdalene, were there, but "looking on from a distance" (Mark 15:40-41; Matt. 27:55; Luke 23:49).

30. There are usually verbal hints for the reader. Perhaps here the fact that Jesus addresses his mother as "woman" might prompt us to remember the other story in John in which Jesus addresses his mother in this way, in John 2:4. It is the story of the wedding at Cana, where Jesus changes water into wine, the first of the signs. The deeper significance of that sign is spelled out in the narratives and discourses that follow it. The old is changed into something new and better. The temple is replaced by the risen Christ (2:13-21). Nicodemus, who understood the old things quite well, is told of the Father's love for the world, of the Christ being "lifted up," and of a new birth by the Spirit (3:1-21). John the Baptist gives place to the new (3:22-30). The Samaritan woman learns of new water, a new worship in spirit and in truth; indeed, the very presence of this figure in the story, a woman and a Samaritan and a sinner, suggests that something wonderfully and strangely new is happening (John 4:1-42). It is true that this sign, like all the others, points ahead to the cross and resurrection, and it is altogether plausible that John reminds us of it by the way Jesus addresses Mary. But it does not provide a deeper meaning for this first word of Jesus from the cross.

31. Bruce Vawter, *The Four Gospels: An Introduction* (Garden City, N.Y.: Doubleday, 1969), 2:259.

Bultmann, on the other hand, suggests that Mary represents Jewish Christianity and John represents Gentile Christianity, that Gentile Christianity is here charged to honor Jewish Christianity as the mother from whom it has come, and that Jewish Christianity is charged to be "at home" within Gentile Christianity.[32] Well, maybe. But I think C. H. Dodd would find these interpretations as "singularly unconvincing" as he finds every other effort to find a symbolic meaning of this passage.[33] It is hard to disagree with him.

Perhaps we should be content with this mundane word. Perhaps, indeed, we should celebrate it. It discloses a Word made flesh who not only shared human susceptibility to death but also showed concern for those who would grieve for him. He had no money to will to them. His clothes had just been seized by the soldiers. But Jesus charged his mother and the disciple whom he loved to receive and to take care of each other. Perhaps that does point to a deeper meaning, to the sort of mutual love that marks "life in his name." But that love is itself quite mundane, or better, that love is quite spiritual without ceasing to be mundane. In this word Jesus shows one facet of a faithful dying. Dying well and faithfully includes provision, as one is able, for the well-being of the survivors.

"I Thirst"

The next word from the cross in John's Gospel comes hard on the heels of the instruction to Mary and John, and it is even more mundane. "I thirst," Jesus said. He was thirsty. It is not surprising. Exposure on the cross on an afternoon on Golgotha would almost certainly have caused not only exhaustion but also dehydration. This is the Word made flesh, and a body needs water, craves water, delights in water when thirsty. And he was thirsty. It does not get more mundane than that.

Death threatens to sunder us from our own flesh, but the good future of God makes its power felt a little in the face of death when the needs of the body and the delights of the flesh are not neglected or forgotten. "I'm thirsty," he said, and thank God for the humanity of those who gave him

32. Rudolf Bultmann, *The Gospel of John: A Commentary,* trans. G. R. Beasley-Murray et al. (Oxford: Blackwell, 1971), p. 673.

33. C. H. Dodd, *The Interpretation of the Fourth Gospel* (Cambridge: Cambridge University Press, 1953), p. 428.

something to drink, even if it was just the sour wine soldiers drank. It is another mundane facet of dying well and faithfully, that we need not and should not disdain or deride the flesh, its comfort or its delights, while we are dying.

It is shocking to some. This is the one who promised the Samaritan woman "living water," promised that if she would drink it, she would "never be thirsty" again (John 4:10, 14). Now the one who promised that water thirsts! But Jesus was evidently thirsty on that day at Jacob's well, too. At least he asked the woman for a drink. He was flesh on that day — and on the cross. The "living water" is not a substitute for drinking water. The "spiritual" water is not in competition with the delights of a drink on a warm day in Samaria or on Golgotha. The need for water points toward our dependence on the creation and on the Creator. The delight in water points toward the gifts and grace of the Creator, who loved the world and gave his Son for its life. Faith and faithfulness do not require and do not permit disdaining the body, even as we are dying.

John observes that in this cry there is a fulfillment of scripture. Perhaps he was thinking of the lament of Psalm 22 again (as he clearly was a few verses before when he cited that psalm in connection with the casting of lots for Jesus' tunic; John 19:24). There the psalmist complained that

> my mouth is dried up like a potsherd,
>   and my tongue sticks to my jaws;
>   you lay me in the dust of death.
>
> (Ps. 22:15)

More likely, John sees the whole episode as in accord with Psalm 69:21: "for my thirst they gave me vinegar to drink."[34] Psalm 69 is another psalm of lament. It is remarkable that each Gospel makes use of the psalms of la-

---

34. The opening words of Ps. 69 strikingly combine the images of drowning and thirst.

> Save me, O God,
>   for the waters have come up to my neck.
> I sink in deep mire,
>   where there is no foothold;
> I have come into deep waters,
>   and the flood sweeps over me.
> I am weary with my crying;
>   my throat is parched. (vv. 1-3)

ment.[35] It is clearly not inconsistent with faith or faithfulness in the minds of the Evangelists.

Once before John had cited Psalm 69. At the cleansing of the temple the "disciples remembered that it was written, 'Zeal for your house will consume me'" (John 2:17). That citation of Psalm 69:9 comes just before the demand to see a sign and Jesus' reply, "Destroy this temple, and in three days I will raise it up" (John 2:19). Evidently John was already thinking of Psalm 69 as another "psalm of Christ." The psalmist suffers his way toward death, and he suffers not least from the taunts of his enemies. He complains to God and cries out to God to rescue him from death and from his enemies.

> At an acceptable time, O God,
>   in the abundance of your steadfast love, answer me. . . .
> Let me be delivered from my enemies
>   and from the deep waters.
> Do not let the flood sweep over me, . . .
>   or the Pit close its mouth over me.
>
> (Ps. 69:13b-15)

Then the psalm moves to the certainty that "the LORD hears the needy" (v. 33) and to an invitation to "heaven and earth" and to "everything that moves in them" to join in the psalmist's praise of God (v. 34).

Psalm 69, however, does not quite fit the story of the cross. For one thing, the psalmist admits that he is not altogether innocent (v. 5) even while he protests the injustice of his suffering. For another, whereas John

---

35. Paul, too, makes use of the psalms of lament. Ps. 69:9 is attributed to Christ in Rom. 15:3. Ps. 18:49 is very likely also to be understood as the voice of Christ in Rom. 15:9. 2 Cor. 4:13-14 may well allude to Ps. 116:10, "I kept my faith, even when I said, / 'I am greatly afflicted.'" See Richard B. Hays, "Christ Prays the Psalms: Israel's Psalter as the Matrix of Early Christology," in *The Conversion of the Imagination: Paul as Interpreter of Israel's Scripture* (Grand Rapids: Eerdmans, 2005), pp. 101-18. Hays examines Paul's use of these and other psalms along with the use of the lament psalms by the Gospels and by Hebrews (Heb. 2:10-12; 10:5-7) and argues persuasively that there was an exegetical tradition older than the New Testament itself that read the lament psalms (especially the royal lament psalms, those attributed to David) with their movement from suffering to hope as providing a hermeneutical key to understanding the death and resurrection of Jesus. Indeed, Hays suggests cautiously that the ancient confession that Jesus died and was raised "in accordance with the scriptures" (1 Cor. 15:3-5) may be a reference to the royal lament psalms (p. 107 n. 20).

has just reported the presence of those who love Jesus at the cross, the psalmist

> looked for pity, but there was none;
> and for comforters, but [he] found none.
>
> (v. 20)

And whereas the offer of sour wine in John seems motivated by human kindness, it is the psalmist's enemies who give him poison for food and vinegar for drink (v. 21). Finally, this is an imprecatory psalm; it curses the enemies and prays to God for their destruction. "Let them be blotted out of the book of the living" (v. 28). That hardly fits the word in Luke's Gospel about forgiveness. It may fit John's insistence early on and consistently that God will bring judgment (e.g., John 3:18-20), but that judgment is early on and consistently set in the context of God's love for the world and of God's intention not "to condemn the world" but to save it through Jesus (e.g., John 3:16-17). John's use of Psalm 69 leaves us with the question whether this form of lament, the imprecatory psalm, the complaint joined to a curse, is ever appropriate for the dying. Perhaps we would be wise simply to judge that this is one of the ways in which the psalm is *not* a "psalm of Christ" or fitting for those who would be faithful to him in their own dying. But, as we have said, forgiveness itself presupposes judgment. The cross discloses both the self-giving love of God and of God's Christ and the terrible truth about the human condition and about some deaths.

Some people, as Jesus himself did, die as a result of horrible injustice. Some people are still victims of state violence. Some people — some children — are murdered. Some die because of random violence. Some die because of the woeful negligence of others. The list of deaths due to injustice would be a long one. And the poverty of the mantra of the death awareness movement, "death is natural," and the ideal of acceptance are nowhere clearer than in such contexts. It is not death then which is "natural" but rage. It is not simple acceptance that is called for but protest. The injustice and horror of such deaths cannot be papered over with talk of death being "natural," and the legitimacy of an angry protest should not be denied by demands for either Stoic *apatheia* or Christian forgiveness. The imprecatory psalms at least allow that lament, that protest, that anger in the face of injustice. They insist that the truth be disclosed and that justice be done. They take right and wrong quite seriously. The imprecatory psalms express their anger and protest not just because the psalmist is a victim of injustice but because these things ought not to be, because these things are wrong, because these things are hateful not only to the psalmist but also to God. And that points to another feature of the imprecatory psalms that must not be overlooked. They look to God. They look to a righteous and faithful God to set things right. They do not take vengeance into their own hands; they leave it to God. The imprecatory psalms turn judgment over to God, putting both one's self and one's enemies into the hands of God. They do not presume to take God's justice into their own hands. That God delays setting things right is also a matter of protest, but not an excuse for returning evil for evil. But do the imprecatory psalms provide a model for the dying or the grieving?

Any affirmative answer to that question must be surrounded by cautions. One obvious caution is the human tendency to self-righteousness. It is a human tendency that can be exacerbated by religious pride. But another caution, and the more important caution, is the reminder that Psalm 69 is here set in the context of the cross. The imprecatory psalms, with their protest against injustice, against the wrong, must be set in the context of self-giving love, set in the context of forgiveness and a readiness to embrace the enemy. Otherwise they risk being captured by that vicious cycle of retaliation and revenge, simply reinforcing the human condition. But Jesus, as we have said, transformed it. Without denying the significance of right and wrong, indeed while insisting on it, he did not curse his enemies but blessed them. When he was reviled, he did not return the insult. He did not return evil for evil. So, let there be angry protest against injustice, but let it look to God. Let it look to God's self-giving love. Let it look to Christ's forgiveness. We will still pray that the kingdom will come, that the world will be set right, but we will not curse but bless the enemy. It is not easy, of course, to join the demands of justice with the readiness to forgive, but it must be done if the cross is to be honored. It must be done lest justice be an excuse for revenge and lest forgiveness be cheapened.

Matthew and Mark also note that someone by the cross gave Jesus a drink (Mark 15:36; Matt. 27:48) but without including this word from the cross. Earlier in those Gospels, moreover, Jesus had been offered "wine mixed with myrrh" (Mark 15:23; cf. Matt. 27:34), evidently intended as a sedative. Jesus refused it. He evidently wanted to be clearheaded for his dying. We have already insisted that faithfulness does not require disdaining the body. It is not that Jesus refused a sedative because he celebrated suffering or pain. But he was willing to endure pain for the sake of preserving the possibility of thinking and speaking coherently on the cross. A Christian may make a similar decision, refusing sedation for the sake of a clear-headed visit with friends or family, enduring some pain for the sake of another opportunity to express gratitude and forgiveness.

The last word here, however, is to repeat what we said first. This mundane word, this this-worldly word, acknowledges Jesus' embodiment and our own. It responds to the threat of death that would alienate us from our own flesh by legitimate attention to the needs and delights of the body, even as we are dying.

"It Is Finished"

The last word of Jesus from the cross in John's Gospel is the announcement that "It is finished." His dying is done. His life is complete. The work given to him by the Father is completed (cf. 17:4). It is all accomplished and consecrated. This is a cry of victory, of accomplishment. He has died well and faithfully. His death was indeed the moment for the definitive disclosure of his identity as the self-giving love of the Father, this identity as the powerful and creative Word made flesh.

And having said these words, "he bowed his head and gave up his spirit." One is reminded, of course, of Luke's Gospel and of Jesus' use of the evening prayer of Psalm 31:5: "Into your hands I commend my spirit." Having lived his life and died his death faithfully, he surrenders his life into the hands of God.

We are not Jesus. Neither our lives nor our deaths have the cosmic significance that his had. Nevertheless, this Jesus teaches us how to live well and to die well. We may hope that our deaths complete and consecrate our lives as faithful followers of this Jesus. Our lives are full of incompleteness, of brokenness, of ragged edges, and of flawed accomplishments, but we may nevertheless hope that we, too, can take the occasion of our dying to be a time for the definitive disclosure of our Christian identity. That will not be done by stoically keeping a stiff upper lip. That will not be done by Platonic contemplation of some other world. It will be done by quite mundane acts of fidelity to our own bodies, to our friends and families, and to God, in quite mundane works and words of love and care, of gratitude and forgiveness.

Then we, too, may lay down our heads as if to sleep and let ourselves go into the loving hands of God, confident that the powerful and creative Word can raise us up by the same power that made the dust a *nephesh* and called Lazarus from the dead.

Remembering the Caregivers

We have taken a cue from the "instruccion" to remember Jesus, to think on his passion and death. But we should not leave the story of Jesus without noting the stories of those who were present to Jesus and cared for him. To be sure, many abandoned him. Friends betrayed him, forsook him, and would not share in the burden of his dying. Mark's Gospel especially emphasized this point. The disciples forsook him on his way to his death; it was part of the way in which death made its power felt even before he died; it was part of the horror of his death that he died alone.

Nevertheless, all the Gospels, even Mark's, contain stories of those who cared for Jesus on his way to his death and shared the burden of his dying. The passion narrative begins with the story of the plot by the elite to kill Jesus, but hard on the heels of that report comes the story of a woman who lavishes Jesus with care.[36] The woman, who is left nameless in Mark and Matthew (although they insist that the story will be told as long as the good news is proclaimed "in memory of her") and identified as Mary, the sister of Martha and Lazarus, in John, anointed the body of Jesus with a costly ointment. It was a lavish act, and it prompted the disciples to accuse her of wasting resources that could be used for the poor. Jesus defended the woman and her generous attention to him, saying to the disciples, "Let her alone; why do you trouble her? She has performed a good service for me. For you always have the poor with you, and you can show kindness to them whenever you wish; but you will not always have me" (Mark 14:6-7).

The story is often read as if Jesus here elevated spiritual concerns above bodily needs, as if concern for the poor were at best a secondary concern for the church. But that is a poor reading because, in the first place, as Jesus' citation of Deuteronomy 15:11 makes quite clear, care for the poor remains an obligation of covenant and a test of communal fidelity.[37]

---

36. The story is found in this location in three Gospels: Mark 14:3-9; Matt. 26:6-13; and John 12:1-8; the parallel story in Luke is set much earlier, Luke 7:36-50.

37. In Deut. 15 the covenant law gave the community the responsibility to eliminate poverty and to correct injustice. The blessing of God would follow upon the community's obedience; then there will be "no one in need among you" (Deut. 15:4). The very presence of poverty was enough to call forth God's judgment, enough to condemn a community's grudging tightfistedness toward the poor. But God is patient; and the presence of the poor, the fact that "you always have the poor with you," is the occasion for the continuing invitation to "open your hand to the poor and needy neighbor in your land" (Deut. 15:11). In this passage Jesus rebukes the disciples, to be sure, but not for their concern about the poor. Rather, he re-

And in the second place, the care this woman provided for Jesus was quite attentive to the needs and pleasures of the body. The thoughtful host would provide an anointing as a part of hospitality. The oil could soothe and the aromas could please a weary body (see Prov. 27:9 and Eccles. 9:8). Whether she anointed his head (Mark and Matthew) or his feet (John), it seems clear enough that Jesus appreciated it. To be sure, anointing was also used to consecrate prophets and priests and kings in Israel, and this anointing is surely a reminder that this Jesus whom the elite plotted to kill was the Christ, the "anointed one." But in the story Jesus made another association: he said, "She has anointed my body beforehand for its burial" (Mark 14:8; cf. Matt. 26:12; John 12:7). Whether the woman knew Jesus would soon die or not, it was interpreted as an act of caring for the body of the one on the way to death and the tomb, and Jesus received such care graciously. Without such care and such caregivers it is more difficult to die well and faithfully.

Another helper on the way to his death was Simon of Cyrene (Mark 15:21).[38] He was evidently a stranger, simply "a passerby" coming into Jerusalem at the same time the soldiers were making their way with the condemned out of Jerusalem toward Golgotha. (Perhaps he was coming to Jerusalem for the Passover.) The soldiers ordered him to carry the cross of Jesus, who was evidently too weak to carry his own cross. He did not volunteer his help, but he did help. And the help he provided to this condemned man made his own life different. The fact that Mark assumes his children's names are known to his readers suggests that Simon not only helped Jesus with the burden of his cross but also came to share that death by baptism.

Some years ago, at a physician-clergy breakfast at the Institute of Religion in the Texas Medical Center, I asked the group what biblical story had most shaped their respective ministries. Many replied, as I expected they would, with references to the Good Samaritan and to Matthew 25. But Dr. Andy von Eschenbach, who was then an oncologist at M. D. Anderson,

---

bukes them for their rebuke of this woman's carefree generosity when caring for the poor is a communal responsibility. In the absence of Jesus, such generosity will be — or should be — turned toward the poor. For further reflection about the economic implications of this story, see Allen Verhey, *Remembering Jesus: Christian Community, Scripture, and the Moral Life* (Grand Rapids: Eerdmans, 2002), pp. 273-75.

38. The story is also found in Matthew (27:32) and Luke (23:26) but not in John. In John Jesus carries his own cross (19:17). Once again, as he had by omitting the Gethsemane agony, John underscores that the death of Jesus is his glory.

told the story of Simon of Cyrene. I had not anticipated a reference to this story, so I asked him to explain. He said something like this: "I meet people every day who are on their way to their death. I am a stranger to them. But I am compelled and called and blessed to be present to them on their journey and to help them a little with their burden." Thus Simon of Cyrene became a paradigm for a doctor.

Two times Jesus was offered wine. The first was "wine mixed with myrrh" (Mark 15:23).[39] It was regarded as a sedative to ease the pain of the dying. Jesus refused it, evidently because he wanted to remain clearheaded, but it was surely not wrong to have offered it. Mark does not say who offered it, but it is a good bet it was not the soldiers. If pious Jews offered it to the condemned on the basis of Proverbs 31:6, "Give strong drink to one who is perishing," then the context of that passage may provide another and different reason for Jesus' refusal. "It is not for kings to drink wine," it says (31:4). It is the duty of kings to

> speak out for those who cannot speak,
> for the rights of all the destitute.
>
> (31:8)

Jesus, as the inscription on the cross said, was "the King of the Jews" (Mark 15:26), and when he made the cry of Psalm 22 his own, he gave voice to the lament and protest of the destitute. The second offer of wine was a caring response to Jesus' thirst (Mark 15:36; Matt. 27:48; John 19:29). The crowd of bystanders was largely hostile, but at least one person in that crowd responded with compassion and gave the dying Jesus a drink. It would not save his life, but it did provide a little relief from his thirst. The passion narrative takes note of the caregiving of strangers and, by recording it, honors it.

In John's Gospel Mary, the mother of Jesus, some other women, and John were present at the cross. They were present to the dying Jesus, sharing the pain of that cross, caring for him to the last as well as they could. There was not much they could do, of course, but they could be there. And that was — and is — no small gift to the dying.

All the Gospels note that Joseph of Arimathea tended to the proper burial of Jesus (Mark 15:42-47; Matt. 27:57-61; Luke 23:50-56; John 19:38-42; John notes that Nicodemus also came to help). The Evangelists note this

---

39. Matt. 27:34 also mentions this offer of wine, but he changes it to wine "mixed with gall" in order to allude to Ps. 69:21.

not just because it proves Jesus was truly dead but also because he lived and died as an embodied person and because the respect and care shown to the body, also the dead body, is an appropriate sign of the respect and care due the person. To be sure, persons may not be reduced to their bodies. But neither may bodies be reduced to mere meat, consigned to the realm of mere things. We are not in our bodies the way Descartes's ghost was presumably in the machine. We are embodied selves, and communal selves as embodied. To be sure, because persons may not be reduced to their bodies, there is discontinuity between persons and their "mortal remains." But because persons may not be reduced to minds or ghosts or disembodied souls, there is also continuity between persons and their "mortal remains." Jesus did not just "seem" to be a body, as Docetism insists. Caring attentiveness to the "mortal remains" is a token of care and respect both for the one who has died and for those who grieve. The person is dead; the body will decay; relationships are broken; communities are dismembered. But the body was once — and is still — identified with the person who has died. The body was once — and still is — the medium by which we display the affection, loyalty, and honor due the person.

There were a few who cared for Jesus on his way to Golgotha and the tomb — some friends, some strangers, some family. Everyone who would die well and faithfully, even Jesus, needs such caregivers. The *Ars Moriendi* made the same point in its way; it called attention to the importance of faithful friends to dying well. But in the *Ars Moriendi* the faithful friends were attentive only to the soul of Moriens, urging upon him the separation from and disdain for his body and his "worldly attachments," his carnal relationships. The biblical story, however, suggests the significance of care for the dying person precisely as an embodied and communal self, not simply as a disembodied soul.

CHAPTER THIRTEEN

The Virtues for Dying Well

*This preparation for death must be practiced through our whole
life, and the spark of faith must be continually fanned so that it
grows and gains strength. Love, joined to it, will attract hope,
which gives no cause for shame. None of these things, however,
comes from us; rather they are gifts of God to be sought by contin-
uous prayers and petitions if we lack them; if they should be present, they must be strengthened so that they grow. The stronger is
our faith, accompanied by love and hope, the more diminished is
our fear. . . . [A]n action continually repeated will become a
habit, the habit will become a state, and the state become a part of
your nature.*

Erasmus, "Preparing for Death"[1]

We broke with the *Ars Moriendi* tradition by beginning not with a commendation of death but with a celebration of life. That different starting
point was required by the biblical narrative. From creation to eschaton the
Bible commends embodied and communal life. From the gift of breath at
the beginning of the story to the gift of an empty tomb at the center of it to

1. Erasmus, "Preparing for Death" (1553), in *Collected Works of Erasmus: Spiritualia
and Pastoralia*, ed. John W. O'Malley (Toronto: University of Toronto Press, 1998), pp. 392-
450, 398, and 421.

God's final triumph at the end, life is good. It may not be the greatest good, but it is good. Mortality may be a simple sign that we depend on God for every breath, but death itself is not commended.

Nevertheless, we followed the "instruccion" of the *Ars Moriendi* tradition to remember Jesus and to "thynke on the passion off Cryste."[2] That "instruccion" is fundamental to the effort to imagine a contemporary *ars moriendi*. So we considered the story of Jesus' death as paradigmatic for a Christian's faithful dying. We are ready now to take another clue from *Ars Moriendi* and to revisit the virtues it regarded as essential to dying well and faithfully. Without celebrating death, we may nevertheless learn from the story of Jesus' dying; we may learn faith, hope, a love that is patient, humility, serenity, and courage. When we are formed by the story of Jesus, these virtues will also be formed in us. They are, as Erasmus insisted, "gifts of God," but the gifts of God can be demanding, and as Erasmus also insisted, they must be "sought" by prayer and "strengthened" by practice. By prayer and practice these virtues may become, by God's grace, "a part of your nature."

Faith

Faith is first on this list of virtues for dying well and faithfully. It is, as *Ars Moriendi* said, the primogenitor of all the virtues, and the faithfulness of Jesus is the paradigm for a Christian's faith in the face of death.

There is always some faith in the face of death. Indeed, dying is frequently the occasion for the definitive display of one's real faith, whatever formal creed one otherwise expresses. And anyone who would die in ways that are fitting to the creed by which he or she has tried to live will put faith and faithfulness first on the list of virtues for dying well and faithfully. It is not only Christians who want to die well and faithfully, after all. The very meaning of dying well and faithfully, however, will vary according to one's faith. Epicureans, for example, die well and faithfully when they take delight in whatever pleasures are available up to the moment of death, indulging their desires until that time when they and their desires will simply be no more. This is no easy matter in the face of death; it requires considerable strength of Epicurean character. Buddhists, on the other hand, die

---

2. *Crafte and Knowledge For To Dye Well* (hereafter *Crafte*), in *The English* Ars Moriendi, ed. David William Atkinson, Renaissance and Baroque Studies and Texts, vol. 5 (New York: Peter Lang, 1992), p. 11. Page references to this work will be placed in the text.

well and faithfully when they rise above all desire, for desire lies at the root of suffering. The way of Buddhist enlightenment surrenders all craving for permanence in a world of flux and gives up the struggle against death itself, that sign of impermanence and oblivion. In this way the Buddhist may achieve *anatman* (or nonself) and Nirvana, which is the perfect extinction of self. This too, obviously, is no easy matter; it requires disciplined concentration to empty the mind of self and desire. Even the secularist may provide an example of the point. Those secularists who have put their faith and confidence in science and technology die well and faithfully, I suppose, when their "medicalized" dying bears witness to that faith by their confidence that the latest piece of medical wizardry will yet deliver them from their mortality.

There is always some faith, then, in the face of death. How could it be otherwise? Dying reminds us that we are radically dependent creatures. It reminds us that our existence is contingent and that we are not in control of our own existing. Santayana made the point quite elegantly:

> We say conventionally that the future is uncertain; but if we withdrew honestly into ourselves and examined our actual moral resources, we should feel that what is insecure is not merely the course of particular events but the vital presumption that there is a future coming at all, and a future pleasantly continuing our habitual experience. We rely in this, as we must, on the analogies of experience, or rather on the clockwork of instinct and presumption in our bodies; but existence is a miracle, and morally considered, a free gift from moment to moment. That it will always be analogous to itself is the very question we are begging. Evidently all interconnections and sequences of events, and in particular any consequences which we may expect to flow from our actions, are really entirely beyond our spiritual control. . . .
>
> What is the result? That at once, by a mere act of self-examination and frankness, the spirit has come upon one of the most important and radical of religious perceptions. It has perceived that though it is living, it is powerless to live; that though it may die, it is powerless to die; and that altogether, at every instant and in every particular, it is in the hands of some alien and inscrutable power.[3]

---

3. George Santayana, "Ultimate Religion," in *Obiter Scripta*, ed. J. Buchler and B. Schwartz (New York: Charles Scribner's Sons, 1936), pp. 283-84, cited by H. Richard Niebuhr, *The Responsible Self* (New York: Harper & Row, 1963), pp. 113-14. My account of faith as confidence and loyalty is indebted to H. Richard Niebuhr.

To be sure, it is possible to attempt to avoid this insight, to avoid a response to that "alien and inscrutable power." There is not much one can do about the contingency of our existence, after all, and it can be painful to acknowledge it. And to be sure, there are plenty of distractions, plenty of little decisions over which we do seem to have some control. Distracted we may be, but not without faith. For in avoiding or denying our dependency, we pretend to be in control of our own existence, trusting our own autonomy, or else we lose our self in the machinery that surrounds us, trusting in Bacon's project to deliver the human condition — us — from our vulnerability to death.

If and when such faith in ourselves or our technology is broken, if and when we acknowledge the truth of our own contingency, the truth that we are finally "in the hands of some alien and inscrutable power," then we may of course regard that power as "a deluding power."[4] We may regard it as the enemy of its own work, giving life and then destroying it, giving hope and then dashing it, instilling desire, including the fundamental desire to be, and then frustrating it. This, too, is a faith, even if it is faith in the form of a distrust of that "alien and inscrutable power" in whose hands we seem but expendable pawns. To live in this faith, in this distrust, is to be anxious, to close one's fist tight to grasp what little security one can pretend to have in a world ruled by the enemy and by death, to close one's fist tight ready to strike in self-defense.[5] But here death has the last word. We may try for a time to appease this Enemy rather than to resist him, but in the end to die faithfully in this faith, in this distrust, is to die in despairing defiance, in a kind of assertive hopelessness.

Another interpretation of the world in which we live and die, however, is possible; a different account of the power in whose hands we are, both in life and in death, is possible. We can respond to the truth of our absolute dependency by learning to trust that "alien and inscrutable power." We cannot learn this by ourselves. We can only learn it in community. Indeed, we only learn it within particular communities of faith. The doctrines and stories of particular communities report the trustworthiness of the power on which, or on whom, we depend; and they evoke from us faith and trust. Still, the doctrines of the community are, as Calvin insisted, not a matter of the tongue alone but also of living and dying. Christian doctrine, he said, "is not apprehended by the understanding and

4. Niebuhr, *The Responsible Self*, p. 117.
5. Niebuhr, *The Responsible Self*, p. 140.

memory alone, as other disciplines are, but it is received only when it possesses the whole soul, and finds a seat and resting place in the inmost affection of the heart. . . . [I]t must enter our heart and pass into our daily living, and so transform us into itself that it may not be unfruitful for us."[6] Such faith is at once communal and personal, at once "ensouled" and "embodied."

It is obviously not my claim that only Christians have faith or can die faithfully. Neither is it my claim that only Christians can learn to respond to their vulnerability to death by learning to trust the power in whose hands they are as they lie dying. Nor is my claim an apologetic one, as if I could prove the moral or aesthetic superiority of dying well and faithfully within the context of the Christian story. I do not claim a point of view outside of the Christian story that would allow me to compare impartially different ways of dying. It is my claim, however, that Christians have a story that can nurture and sustain both faith and faithfulness in the face of death.

One other clarification is called for. I am not simply claiming that the story of Jesus' death and resurrection is an example or illustration of the human condition, as if we could dispense with Jesus once we achieved some insight into that condition. Jesus is not just an example of faith; the story of Jesus is fundamental to the faith of Christians. When God raised the crucified Jesus from the dead, God vindicated God's own trustworthiness, God's own righteousness, God's own faithfulness. God can be trusted. And when God raised the crucified Jesus from the dead, God vindicated this Jesus, vindicated the faithfulness of Jesus, vindicated him as the agent of God's cause for the world, vindicated him as the truth of God's self-giving love and as the truth of our own humanity. Because he was raised, we look to Jesus as "the pioneer and perfecter of our faith" (Heb. 12:2) and to his faith as the paradigm for our living and our dying.

The faith of Jesus is displayed in trust in God and in loyalty to the cause of God. Jesus trusted God in his dying. Even the dreadful cry of lament was, as we have seen, drawn from Psalm 22, a psalm of confidence. Like the psalmist, Jesus made lament. His faith did not require the commendation of suffering and death. The threat of death, the threat of being sundered from his own flesh, from those he loved, and from God by death, prompted lament. But like the psalmist, under the threat of death he

---

6. John Calvin, *Institutes of the Christian Religion,* ed. John T. McNeill, Library of Christian Classics, vol. 20 (Philadelphia: Westminster, 1960), 3.6.4.

trusted God to deliver him and to triumph over death. Jesus made the evening prayer of the pious Jew his own prayer at his death: "Father, into your hands I commend my spirit." This prayer is drawn from Psalm 31, another psalm of lament marked by confidence in God. Jesus recognized the truth of his own dependence, the truth that he too was finally, as Santayana said, "in the hands of some alien and inscrutable power." Jesus did not respond by attempting to ignore his neediness. He did not respond by denying the awful reality of death. He did not allow himself to be distracted from the tasks of faith and faithfulness. (Those tasks of faith and faithfulness were not reduced to the "spiritual" task of contemplating the bliss of a soul in heaven; they included rather, as we have noted, the quite mundane tasks of caring for one's body and for one's family and friends.) And Jesus did not respond in distrust. He did not lash out in defiance and in self-defense or attempt a last-ditch effort to appease this "alien and inscrutable power." He responded in trust. This power was "Abba" to him, and he trusted the self-giving love of the Father to provide for him. He was dependent upon the Father, but he knew he would find security and refuge in those hands.

Jesus' faith was of one piece with his faithfulness. It was displayed not only in trust but also in faithfulness, in loyalty to the cause of God. He came announcing the good future of God. He made that future felt in his works and in his words, in his life and in his ministry. It was a future in which the poor would be blessed, in which the humiliated would be exalted, in which justice and peace would finally embrace. It was a good future in which God would finally set the world right, in which God's self-giving love would overrule death and sin. It was God's cause, a cause worth living for, a cause worth dying for.

To live well you have to care about life, to be sure, but you also have to care about some things more than you care about survival. And Jesus lived well. He cared about some things more than he cared about his own survival. It is, I think, at least one meaning of his cryptic remark to the disciples: "Those who try to make their life secure will lose it, but those who lose their life will keep it" (Luke 17:33). Without this kind of loyalty to God and to the cause of God, life can shrink to self-absorbed and egocentric anxiety. And suffering and dying can tempt our lives to shrink. Against that egocentric anxiety Jesus spoke early and often. "Do not be anxious," he said (cf., e.g., Matt. 6:25). God can be trusted. God has promised the world's good future, a future in which we have by God's grace a part. To die well, no less than to live well, you have to care about life, but you also have to care about some things more than you care about survival. Self-absorbed anxiety is the enemy of faithfulness unto death. And this egocentric anxiety may include the anxiety about whether our souls will go to heaven when we die. The remedy for that anxiety is not to make a last-ditch effort to appease God with the right words or the right works, as if either the little truth we know well or the little good we do well could provide a ticket to heaven. The remedy is not faith in faith but faith in God. The remedy is to trust the God who created the world and promises to make it new. Then, faithful to God and to the cause of God, we may find words and works that honor God and the cause of God, even while we are dying.

And since faith is the primogenitor of all the virtues, those words and works will display faith at work in hope and love and patience and humility and serenity. Such faith and faithfulness are not displayed in an asceticism that is born of dualism and takes flight from this world to some "other world." It is displayed in gratitude to God for the gifts of God, which include our lives surely, but which may also include a little time for the tasks of reconciliation and forgiveness, justice and generosity, even while we are dying.

Hope

This faith exists as hope, as the confidence that God will be faithful to the cause of God, as the trust that God and the cause of God will triumph over sin and death. The hope of Jesus is paradigmatic for a Christian's hope in the face of death.

Ars Moriendi had it right. Dying can tempt one to despair. Death threatens not just an end to one's existence but the unraveling of meaning, the severing of relationships, the shattering of hopes. Death threatens to have the last word. It threatens to overcome the life and the light by its darkness. Then it is life that seems ephemeral. And hope seems like folly.[7] If it is true, as the old proverb says, that "where there's life, there's hope," then the contrary seems also to be suggested, that in death there is no hope. Then we are right to be fearful of death, to tremble in the face of darkness and hopelessness.

---

7. One is reminded, I suppose, of the schoolboy's definition of faith: "Faith is believin' what you know ain't true" (Robert McAfee Brown, *The Spirit of Protestantism* [New York: Oxford University Press, 1965], p. 69). Hope that has no basis is simply wishful thinking, but the Christian hope is not just whistling in the dark.

What would have to be the case for it to be otherwise? For it to be possible — without illusion, evasion, or fantasy — still to hope in the face of death? "Can these bones live?" someone asks, echoing the question put to Ezekiel. And we are inclined to answer in grief and anger, "Don't be ridiculous! No, these bones cannot live! There is no hope." But when we turn toward God, the God of Ezekiel, the God of Jesus, toward the God who was and ever shall be and *is* God, then we are able to whisper hope. "Can these bones live?" "O Lord God, *you* know!" We turn toward God in the midst of some desolating valley of dry bones, in the midst of death and grief and doubt and tears, and we hear God's last word in Jesus. "Yes," God says, "these bones can live." "Yes," God says, "I make all things new!" And that word echoes to all the corners of our world's sadness, to all the niches of our despair, giving us hope.

God is our hope. And God has given us grounds to hope that death will not have the last word in our world or upon our lives. Christians do not deny the awful reality of death, but they do insist that death will not have the last word, that the last word belongs to God, and that the last word is not death but life, not suffering but *shalom*. In the face of death and its power Christians hope. With faith in God they share the hope of the church and of its creed. The Apostles' Creed, for example, has a nice sense of an ending; it closes with these words of hope: "I believe . . . in the resurrection of the body and the life everlasting."

The grounds for this hope, for this confidence that death will not have the last word, are found in the story Scripture tells, and in the "short story" the creed tells between its initial "credo" and "the resurrection of the body and the life everlasting" at its ending. The grounds for this hope are found in the story — and in the faithfulness — of the triune God.

At the beginning of that story, "God the Father almighty, creator of heaven and earth," made a cosmos by a mighty and creative word. By that same word God created humanity; by God's breath and gift the dust was made "a living being" (Hebrew *nephesh*; Gen. 2:7).[8] From that beginning it was clear that without God there was no hope. From that beginning it was clear that without God human weakness and mortality would make their

---

8. The "living being" (Hebrew *nephesh*) was and remained "flesh" (Hebrew *basar*); that is, whole selves were and are "flesh" in their creatureliness, in their contrast to God and in their dependence upon God, in their weakness and mortality. To be sure, the *nephesh* is *basar*; but the *basar* is *nephesh*, too. The "flesh" is *not* without God. The flesh, too, is from God. Whole selves — embodied selves, mortal and dependent, creative and powerfully gifted — are "flesh," and it is good (but not without God).

inevitable way toward death, and that without God great human powers would demonstrate their weakness, their "flesh," by their inability to preserve the cosmos from tilting back to chaos. From that beginning it was clear that the grounds for hope are not in some "soul" that has its immortality independently of God and that finds liberation in the death of the body. It was clear that the grounds for hope are not located in some romantic account of the cycles of nature, as bringing always the return of life and spring. And it was clear that the grounds for hope are not to be found in the technological mastery over nature. The beginning points us toward the powerful and creative word of God that can call a cosmos out of chaos and give light to the darkness and life to the dust. That is the basis of our hope.

The creation, of course, is not the end of the story. The canonical narrative continues with the story of human sin and of a "curse" that rests upon the whole creation and on all life. Sin brings alienation in its wake — not mortality, it should be said, which was and is a simple sign that we do not have life the way God has life. But with sin death threatens alienation from our own flesh, from our communities, and from God. Human sin might have smashed the cosmos back to chaos, but God would not let evil have the last word. Even under the burden of a "curse," there were grounds for hope, hope that God would be faithful to what was the cause of God from the beginning, that God's power and love would refuse to let sin and death have the last word in the world God made. So, "the Fall" — or the flood — is not the end of the story either. God comes again to covenant and to bless. And the blessing with which God would visit the world is not a rescue from the world but a vocation within it, a vocation to be a blessing (e.g., Gen. 12:1-4), to restrain and to lift the power of the "curse" in the world God made and preserves and loves.

The center of the Christian story — and of the creed — is Jesus of Nazareth. The story is that in Jesus we see "Emmanuel," "God is with us" (Matt. 1:23). He came announcing the good future of God, and he made its power felt in works of healing and in words of blessing. The coming cosmic sovereignty of God was the center of Jesus' proclamation and of his life. It was his hope, and that hope gave shape and meaning to the present. When the dead were raised, the good future of God was revealed. When the sick — those under the power of death — were healed, the good future of God was present. When demons were cast out and the "possessed" were returned to themselves and to their communities, the good future of God was made known and made real. And when the poor were blessed and sinners forgiven, the good future of God made its power felt. That good future remained future, of course, but it was always there on the horizon, ready to dawn. Sometimes the brightness of the horizon threw its light on this world ruled by sin and death, and sometimes it made the darkness seem darker yet. This hope prompted both great joy and lament, joy that God's good future was breaking into the present and lament that it was not yet, still sadly not yet, that future.

This Jesus "suffered under Pontius Pilate, was crucified, dead, and buried." That was a time of darkness, first the darkness at noon and then the greater darkness of the tomb. That was a time when not only Jesus but also hope was dead. But then God raised this Jesus up, "the first fruits of those who have died" (1 Cor. 15:20).[9] The power of God and the love of God reached into death to raise this Jesus up, vindicating both Jesus and Jesus' hope, vindicating both Jesus and God's own faithfulness. God had the last word on that Sunday morning, the first day of the week, the first day of a new creation. This is the reason for the hope that is in us (1 Pet. 3:15). The New Testament fairly thunders with that sense of victory and expectation. Sometimes the best we can do is, like Ezekiel, to whisper hope, but even if it is only a whisper and not a shout of victory, it is possible because on that ordinary Sunday in Jerusalem God said, "Yes, these bones can live."

Because Jesus has been raised, the Spirit, "the first fruits" (Rom. 8:23) and the "guarantee" of God's good future (2 Cor. 1:22; 5:5; Eph. 1:13), has been poured out, and the Spirit is included in the creed and in the grounds for Christian hope. The Spirit was there at the beginning, of course, brooding on the waters of chaos, the breath that made the dust a living creature. And then, when sin brought death and a curse in its wake, the Spirit that gives life was still there to renew and to bless, still brooding on the waters of human tears, pledging that death would not have the last word.

The Spirit was there in the hurt, there when Israel took notice of its pain in Egypt and gave it voice, there when the psalmist took note of his suffering and cried out to God in lament, there when Jesus joined his voice to theirs on the cross — "My God, my God, why?" — there when, as Paul

---

9. It was a curious body, to be sure, but it was recognizable as Jesus' body — as the body of the one who preached and healed and suffered. His wounds were raised with him. It was no mere "spirit" (Luke 24:39); this embodied person was identifiable — had an identity — in ways no mere "spirit" could. "It is I myself," he said (Luke 24:39). "Touch me and see." See above, chapter 11, pp. 207-14.

wrote, the whole creation groaned in travail (Rom. 8:22). All these cried to God in the hope — against hope — that there was someone there to hear their cry.

And the Spirit *was* there, hearing the cry, feeling the hurt, answering the pain with promise. The Spirit was there in the promise then, and when the promise was given token, when Israel was delivered from its bondage, when the psalmist was assured that he would not be abandoned, when Jesus was raised, and when — the promise is still outstanding — the whole creation is made new, and death shall be no more, and neither mourning nor crying nor pain shall be any more (Rev. 21:4).

The Spirit, as Paul says, "helps us in our weakness" (Rom. 8:26). While we "groan inwardly" (8:23), when there are no words, while we wait for "the redemption of our bodies" (8:23), the Spirit gives us words, "Abba! Father!" (8:15), and makes us "heirs," "joint heirs" (8:17), of God's good future. The Spirit is at work where the groaning find words and where God's future makes its power felt: when the sick are healed, when the grieving are comforted, when (like Pentecost and unlike the tower of Babel) people understand each other, and when the threat of death is met with confidence in God and with care for persons as embodied and communal selves.

And the Spirit is at work in the church, in that community where the resurrection is celebrated and where the good future of God is anticipated in practices of friendship and forgiveness, or as the creed says, "the communion of saints, [and] the forgiveness of sins."

Christians hope because they know the faithfulness of the One who made all things, because they know the story of one who was raised from the dead, and because they know a life-giving Spirit. The Christian church owns a story in canon and in creed that begins with the power and love of the Creator, centers in the resurrection of the crucified Jesus, and ends with talk of God's good future — and our own. They cannot but hope.

If these are the grounds for Christian hope, then the virtue of hope must somehow be fitting to this story. And if it is to be fitting to this story, hope may not shrink to the egocentric hope that a solitary individual may experience the bliss of heaven. The scope of Christian hope is nothing less than cosmic. The story begins with the creation of all things, and it reaches finally to "all things" made new.

That was John's vision in a prison on Patmos. Domitian was emperor then. Jerusalem and its temple lay in ruins again. Roman greed and violence still asserted their doomed reign. Death and desolation filled the earth again. John didn't have to be a visionary to see dry bones afoot or the possibility of his own execution. But John did not just hope for release from prison. Under the threat of death he did not just hope that his soul would be transported to heaven. This was no egocentric and otherworldly hope. Neither did John talk nostalgically about turning things back to the way they were in some good old days. He did not hope simply for a slightly revised edition of the same old life. He envisioned God's good future, an embodied and communal future. He was not just talking about a little alteration or two. He was talking about God setting the world right. He was talking about resurrection. And to talk of resurrection is not just to talk about individuals. It is to talk about the arc of history and the future of the cosmos. If God does not defeat sin and death for the universe, then God did not win the victory over sin and death for Jesus, either. And if God did not win the victory by raising Jesus from the dead, then our faith and our hope are vain (1 Cor. 15:13-14). John hoped for the renewal of the creation. He hoped that God would set the world straight. What he saw was "a new heaven and a new earth." He saw a new Jerusalem. And he heard a voice from the throne, "Death shall be no more; mourning and crying and pain will be no more. . . . I am making all things new!"

That is the word that echoes to all the corners of our world's sadness, to all the niches of our own despair. That is the word of blessing that reaches "far as the curse is found." And that is the word that shapes the virtue of hope, also in the face of death. We will die well and faithfully when we care for others, also while we lie dying. The virtue of hope strengthens us in our weakness to resist self-absorption, to resist the temptation to care only for ourselves and our survival. Hope encourages us and inspires us, and like Ezekiel we learn to speak and to live that word a little — haltingly sometimes — but a little, even as we are dying. Sometimes, like Ezekiel, the best we can do is a whisper of hope, "O Lord God, *you* know." But sometimes we can find a word of our own, or some deed, some small act of kindness we can show or some little injustice we can right. Such words and deeds will not, of course, suddenly usher in a new heaven and a new earth. They will not utterly destroy the pain and hurt and sadness around us, but they may at least lessen the weight of pain that someone else carries. They may at least lighten the burden of someone else's grief. They may at least relieve the bitterness of someone else's tears. And they may help some dry bones to move a little, and even — with the Spirit's aid — to dance to the tune of things made new.

The word encourages us, but it is also a burden to us. It is a burden to us not just because there is so much around us that is "old" and broken but also because there is so much in us and of us that is just dry bones. A hope that is fitting to the story is not inconsistent with lament. Our own withering can properly prompt lament. But so can a sense of our failures to live and die faithfully. There is much in us and of us that is fearful and slothful, much in us that is proud and presumptuous, so much, if we are honest, that we feel the condemnation of Revelation 21:8 weighing heavy on us and on our own lives. Revelation 21:8 condemns the "the cowardly, the faithless, the polluted, the murderers, the fornicators, the sorcerers, the idolaters, and all liars" to a second death. We don't need the demons that circled the bedside of Moriens to remind us that the spirit of the murderer, the spirit of the fornicator, the spirit of the liar is a spirit that continually haunts these dry bones we call a life. And the weight of that bends our backs until we fall to our knees and claim the promise of that voice from the throne, "I make all things new — *even you.*"

Christian hope remains cosmic, but it is also inalienably personal. It surely was for the thief on the cross. His request is the hope of Christians: "Lord, remember me when you come into your kingdom." Christians hope for the kingdom of God, and hope to have a part in it. Dying prompts, however, not only a sense of dependence upon that power in whose hands we are but also a sense of remorse and shame. There was much good we might have done that we failed to do. There was some evil that we did that we can no longer rationalize. *Ars Moriendi* may have focused too much on the sins of Moriens in its account of the temptation to despair, but it was on the mark in insisting that the shame and remorse of Moriens must be considered. The life review that frequently accompanies dying will frequently, if it is honest, be accompanied also by a sense of shame and remorse. If we would die well and care well for the dying, that sense may not be ignored or neglected. That shudder of self-recognition that can only approve another's disapproval should not be lightly dismissed, as it often is in a guilt-free culture. We need not coerce this sense of shame, need not insist upon it as though shame is itself the saving act of God. But we should not ignore it when it is present. The sense of shame leaves one feeling unworthy of any small share in God's good future.

Christians do not deny the awful reality of sin any more than they deny the awful reality of death. They do not claim that the little good they have done well or the little truth they know well makes them "worthy" to have a share in God's good future. But they do insist that sin, too, will not have the last word. God will set the world straight. That requires judgment, to be sure, but God brings us — together with the cosmos — safely through the judgment. And on the far side of the judgment of God are God's renewing righteousness and mercy, forgiveness and life.[10] Christians do not find hope by looking at themselves, whether at the quality of their works or at the quality of their faith; they find hope by looking to God, to the power and love of God that can deliver the cosmos from the power of both death and sin, to God who can raise us up from both the dust and from our shame. We die well and faithfully when we look to God who has the power to raise the dead and the grace to forgive sinners. Christian hope points the dying who sense their dependence "on some inscrutable and alien power" toward the faithful hands of God, the God who can be trusted. Jesus was the paradigm for such hope when he commended his life to God. Christian hope points the dying who shudder with a sense of their unworthiness to the self-giving love of God, the God who forgives. Jesus was the paradigm of God's self-giving love on the cross, and his word of forgiveness was God's own word.

This hope, then, is neither egocentric nor otherworldly. It is at once cosmic and personal. The thief was told in effect, "I make all things new . . . even you."

It is not yet that good future, of course, still sadly not yet that future. That is why Christian hope is not inconsistent with lament. Indeed, as C. Clifton Black has said, "[T]he spine of lament is hope: not the vacuous optimism that 'things will get better,' which in the short run is usually a lie, but the deep and irrepressible conviction, in the teeth of present evidence, that God has not severed the umbilical cord that has always bound us to the Lord."[11] The creation and the Christian still "wait" and "watch" and pray for God's good future (Rom. 8:19-23). This hope is not only displayed in hymns that dance to the tune of all things made new; it is also displayed in lament, in sorrowful sighs to God, "How long, O Lord?" It is not just that we are not to mourn as those who have no hope. It is rather that hope mourns. Jesus said it on a hillside in Galilee, "Blessed are those who mourn," and he displayed it on that hill called Golgotha when he made the

---

10. It is what Christians practice in baptism. They are brought into judgment. It is a pleading guilty. See below, pp. 326-28.

11. C. Clifton Black, "The Persistence of the Wounds," in *Lament: Reclaiming Practices in Pulpit, Pew, and Public Square*, ed. Sally Brown and Patrick D. Miller (Louisville: Westminster John Knox, 2005), pp. 48-58, p. 54. See also Ellen T. Charry, "May We Trust God and (Still) Lament? Can We Lament and (Still) Trust God?" in the same volume, pp. 95-108: "Without hope, one cannot lament, for there is no meaningful pattern to life to be disrupted" (p. 96).

human cry of lament his own cry. The mourners are those who have caught a glimpse of God's good future and who weep because it is not yet. They weep that any should weep, they mourn that any mourn, they lament because God's final vanquishing of death and sin is sadly not yet. Hope is displayed in such expressions of sorrow joined to the confidence that at the limits of this life and in the withering of these bodies, God can still be trusted to be faithful. God's good future is sure to be, and we shall — and do already — by God's grace have a share in it.

In Jesus' dying Christians find the paradigm of hope. He did not hope for death, as though death were a good. But neither did he cling to life, as though life were the greatest good. Because he hoped for the good future of God and was committed to the cause of God in the world, he recognized that there were goods more compelling than his own survival. And as he was dying, he hoped — in spite of death — to live by God's power. He displayed that hope in lament. The sadness and the sorrow of death were given voice, even while God was trusted to make things right. As he was dying, he displayed his hope in words of forgiveness and in mundane tasks of care.

Hope that has no basis is a pipe dream. Hope that is attentive only to one's self is egocentric and shriveled. Hope that cannot lament denies the awful reality and the continuing power of death and sin. And hope that does not shape life, even in the dying of it, is mere optimism, airy and nebulous. But the hope of Jesus and of the Christian has a basis in God's power and love. Its scope is cosmic without ceasing to be personal. It is quite capable of lament. And it already shapes our living and our dying. Hope is displayed in works and words that reflect God's future and make it already present and real, even as we lie dying, works and words of forgiveness and comfort, works and words of care for those we leave behind, works and words of love.

Such hope is an alternative to the presumption and the despair that are sometimes on display in a medicalized dying. When death is seen as the great enemy to be defeated by the greater powers of medicine, presumption and despair can surround the bedside of the dying like two malicious little demons that would catch us in their own catch-22. Like Moriens caught between despair for his sins and pride in his virtues, we seem caught between presumption and despair concerning the technology that can surround the dying. Presumption speaks first, insisting that the technology can rescue us from our mortality and deliver us to our flourishing. When that presumption is defeated by the progress of disease, despair speaks, or whispers at least, sometimes first in the hallway or in the elevator, "It's a hopeless case." That despair can prompt deceit, lest the patient "lose hope," but the "hopeless case" in the bed hears the voice of despair as well. In order not to be "hopeless," to resist despair, patient or doctor or family or all of them together invite presumption to revisit the room, promising that the latest tool or a new protocol may yet defeat death. Thus the patient is caught between presumption and despair when technology is the basis of hope.

When, however, death is seen as the enemy already and finally defeated by the greater power of God, then technology can be received and used as a good gift of God, without presumptuous expectations of it. When death is seen as the enemy already and finally defeated by the greater power of God, then — even in the face of technology's limits — one is not without hope. To be dying is not to be "hopeless" — unless the basis of our hope is technology and the object of our hope can be measured by a lab report. One may certainly hope, of course, for a good lab report, but if the basis of our hope is God's faithfulness, and if the object of our hope is God's good future, then we are not "hopeless" even when the lab report is bad.

Love

The third temptation in *Ars Moriendi* was to impatience, and the remedy for impatience was the love of God. Surely *Ars Moriendi* was right to call attention to love as a virtue important to dying well and faithfully. Surely it was right to insist on the priority of the love of God. The first commandment must remain first. Surely it was right to say, as Paul did, that "love is patient." And surely it was right to regard Jesus as the paradigm of love in the face of death.

But *Ars Moriendi* went badly wrong when it insisted that to receive sickness and death with sorrow is a sign of not loving God sufficiently.[12]

---

12. *Ars Moriendi* cited Jerome, but it might also have cited Augustine (or at least his early works). In *Of True Religion* Augustine argues that such sadness and grief are inconsistent with the love of God. They are signs of loving some "material thing" inordinately, of having "abandoned God" (*Of True Religion* 12.23, trans. J. H. S. Burleigh [Chicago: Henry Regnery, 1959], pp. 21-22). In the same work he goes on to say, "If we are ablaze with love for eternity, we shall hate temporal relationships" (46.89, p. 85). The test for the genuineness of our love for God is whether we can let go all else — our own life or the life of another — "without grieving" (46.92, p. 89).

In his *Confessions* he confesses his grief and tears at the death of ones he loved, first at

To love God is not to delight in suffering or death. To love God does not make masochists of us. On the contrary, to love God should prompt a pi-

---

the death of his friend (4.4-7) and then again, in spite of his best efforts to restrain his tears, at the death of his mother Monica (9.12-13). He reports these incidents in order to repent of them. His grief was the sign of too much "worldly affection." He says concerning the death of his friend, "I was unhappy, and so is every soul unhappy that is tied to its love for mortal things" (*The Confessions of St. Augustine* 4.6, trans. Rex Warner [New York: New American Library, 1963], p. 76). That was before his conversion. Later, when his mother was "freed from the body" (9.11, p. 204), Augustine says he "reproached" himself for his sorrow; "I grieved at my grief with a new grief and so was consumed with a double sorrow" (9.12, p. 205).

Such grief at his grief makes sense in the context of Augustine's account of the love of God in *On Christian Doctrine*. There to love God is to desire God, and to desire God is to long for spiritual union with God. That yearning is simply given with the creation. When that union is achieved there is joy, "rest," beatitude. Until that union is achieved, until the human being finds its "rest" in God, it will remain "restless" (*Confessions* 1.1). The root assumption here is provided by Plato's notion of *eros*, that desire of the soul for the truly good, the truly beautiful, the truly immortal. Human happiness finally depends upon possession of an immortal and unchanging Good. Love, *eros*, is the yearning for that Good. The soul, therefore, is inevitably in motion. In that sense every human being loves; every human being is in motion toward something, drawn to it by its attractive power. Moreover, like Plato in his *Symposium*, Augustine insists that the final object of our longing must be immutable and changeless (*On Christian Doctrine* 1.8). For Augustine, however, the contrast between God's perfect and unchanging life and our own unstable state is further complicated by human sin. Created by God, we yearn for fulfillment in true being, in true goodness, beauty, and truth, in God, but in our sin we look for fulfillment elsewhere. So, while every soul is in motion toward something, sin disorders and disorients our yearning souls. Since love is desire and since we become what we desire, the object of love is decisively important. There is always *eros*, always yearning, but there is also always the struggle between two fundamental forms of this yearning, which Augustine calls "charity" and "cupidity." "Charity" is the love of God, and it leads to union with God. "Cupidity" is the love of the world, the love of this life, and it leads to nothingness. In *On Christian Doctrine* Augustine stipulates the meaning of these terms in this way: "I call 'charity' the motion of the soul toward the enjoyment of God for His own sake, and the enjoyment of one's self and of one's neighbor for the sake of God; but 'cupidity' is a motion of the soul toward the enjoyment of one's self, one's neighbor, or any corporal thing for the sake of something other than God" (3.10.16, trans. D. W. Robertson [Indianapolis: Bobbs-Merrill, 1958], p. 88). It is by the object of our love, our *eros*, that we are oriented either toward God or away from God toward nothingness. "Cupidity" is *eros* qualified and ordered by sin; "charity" is *eros* qualified and ordered by God's grace.

Earlier in *On Christian Doctrine* Augustine had famously distinguished between the things to be "enjoyed" and the things to be "used" (1.3-4). We are to enjoy God, that is to say, we are to love God, move toward God, desire communion with God. That is our nature and our destiny. Our hearts are restless until they rest in God (*Confessions* 1.1). All other things, he insists, including our neighbors and ourselves, are to be "used" (*On Christian Doctrine*

ous delight in the good gifts of God. To love God should prompt a love of the world God loves, the bodies God gives, and the "carnal" relations in

1.22.20-21; 1.33.37), that is to say, we are to relate to them in ways that help and sustain our desire for union with God, our movement toward God. To invoke this terminology, the grief and sorrow that Augustine rejected in *Of True Religion* and that he regretted in his *Confessions* are signs that he was guilty of "enjoying" what he should have been "using."

There are problems with this language of "enjoy" and "use," of course, that even Augustine seemed to recognize. The language of "use" invokes the logic of means and ends, and is at risk of reducing the beloved to a means to the lover's own ends, but that hardly seems an appropriate account of love. Augustine seems uncomfortable with this language, first, when he talks of loving the neighbor. At least he recognizes the possibility of someone becoming "angry" when "used" in this way (1.22.21). And again, when he considers God's love for us, the distinction hardly allows him to say that God "enjoys" us, but he is also plainly not comfortable with the language that God simply "uses" us. He insists that God "does not use a thing as we do" (1.32.35). God's "use" of us is finally made "not to His utility but to ours" (1.32.35). God's love serves both God's "good" and our own, for God's "good" is our good.

In the Middle Ages *On Christian Doctrine* was the most popular work of this most influential theologian. There can be no doubt that Augustine was influenced by the Platonists of his time in his account of love. In *On True Religion* he speaks warmly of the Platonists, even suggesting that "with the change of a few words and sentiments, they would become Christians" (4.7, p. 9), and that if Plato himself "were to come to life again," he would become a Christian (3.6). In his *Confessions* he says candidly that he has been greatly influenced by reading certain works of the Platonists (7.9.13). There can also be no doubt that *Ars Moriendi* was influenced by the Platonists of its time — and surely influenced by Augustine's *On Christian Doctrine* — when it rejects sorrow and grief and when it disparages "worldly attachments."

On Augustine's account of grief and its influence on Christian piety, see further Nicholas Wolterstorff, "Suffering Love," in *Philosophy and the Christian Faith*, ed. Thomas V. Morris (Notre Dame, Ind.: University of Notre Dame Press, 1988), pp. 196-217. For a different view of Augustine's account of grief, see Gibert Meilaender, *The Way That Leads There: Augustinian Reflections on the Christian Life* (Grand Rapids: Eerdmans, 2006), pp. 143-60. David Albert Jones, *Approaching the End: A Theological Exploration of Death and Dying* (Oxford: Oxford University Press, 2007), pp. 37-89, argues that, although Augustine begins with a view of death and grief that is close to Ambrose (and to Ambrose's Platonism), his developed thought (as in *The City of God*) departs from it, acknowledging death as an evil, insisting that the union of soul and body is good, and giving place to lament and grief. Joanne E. McWilliam DeWart, "Augustine on the Resurrection," in her *Death and Resurrection* (Wilmington, Del.: Michael Glazier, 1986), pp. 164-89, also argues for such a development in Augustine's account of death and resurrection. For Augustine's later view of the resurrection body, see the final books of *The City of God* (19–22); it is that account that he considered his best in his *Retractions* (1.16). Similarly, it can be argued that Augustine's account of love also develops and changes over time — and notably that he finally rejects the instrumental associations of "use," that he "avoids repeating the classification [of some thing to be 'enjoyed' and other things to be 'used'] but rather reverses it, classifying love-of-neighbor as a form of

which bodies inevitably involve us. And if these are worth loving, then their loss is worth grieving. We have already noted that faith is not inconsistent with lament and that hope sometimes takes the shape of lament, and now we may note that it is love that prompts grief and lament.

Ars Moriendi goes wrong when it, following the tradition of Plato, Plotinus, and Augustine, understands love as fundamentally desire, as *eros*. But love is not reducible to desire. If it were, then love would always mark a lack, a need, and when the desire was fulfilled by union with the beloved, it would no longer exist as love but as rest and joy. Then love could never be a mark of fullness of being. For Plato, for example, it makes no sense to say that God or the gods love. It is true, of course, that love frequently expresses itself as desire when one is separated from one's beloved, the desire for her presence, for example, but in that case desire is born of love, not reducible to it. And it is surely the case that we desire good things for those we love, but then desire expresses a more fundamental attitude, namely, care. Perhaps, then, we should understand love as fundamentally care for another, but care, too, presupposes some need, some lack, now in the beloved, and when that need is met, love does not cease. We desire to be with another because we love that person, and we do what we can to care for another, to meet that person's need, because we love him or her, but the love that desires and cares cannot be simply reduced either to desire or to care.[13]

So what is love? To be sure, "love" is a rich and multifaceted notion, "a many splendored thing." Scripture itself uses "love" in a great variety of ways,[14] and theologians have used the concept in an even greater variety of ways. There have been a number of theological quarrels about "love." I will not attempt to resolve these quarrels in a paragraph or two, but I do want to resist accounts of love that reduce it to desire, to *eros*.[15]

'enjoyment'" (Oliver O'Donovan, "*Usus* and *Fruitio* in Augustine, *De Doctrina Christiana* I," *Journal of Theological Studies*, n.s., 33, pt. 2 [October, 1982]: 361-97, p. 397).

13. See Jules Toner, *The Experience of Love* (Washington, D.C.: Corpus Books, 1968).

14. See Amy Laura Hall, "Complicating the Command: Agape in Scriptural Context," in *The Annual of the Society of Christian Ethics 1999*, pp. 97-114. There is, for example, the compassionate love of the deliverance from slavery in Egypt, the covenant love of Deuteronomy that creates community, and the love of God imaged in Hosea's love for Gomer, a love at once passionate and resolute.

15. Anders Nygren's *Agape and Eros*, trans. Philip S. Watson (Philadelphia: Westminster, 1953; first published in 1930) famously complained about the rendering of Christian love as *eros* and insisted upon a fundamental contrast of *agape* and *eros*. Many have criticized the work, but few have thought it possible or prudent to ignore it.

Nygren regards *agape* as the "fundamental motif" of Christianity and *eros* as the

Love is fundamentally an affective affirmation of the other. Love affirms the beloved for her own sake; it does not "use" the other for the sake of achieving some other desired end. It affirms the beloved not only for herself but also in herself; it is a response to her lovable actuality.[16] One great advantage of such an account of love is that it coheres with the human experience of love, as Jules Toner has quite persuasively shown. But another great advantage is that it is fitting both to God's love and to the love of God and both to the love of God and to the love of the neighbor. If we start with this root notion of love, we can understand that it should sometimes be expressed as desire and sometimes as joy in the presence of the beloved. We can understand that it should be expressed sometimes in

"fundamental motif" of Hellenism. That is to say, Nygren regards *agape* not just as one idea among many within Christianity, but as the central idea, as the *sine qua non* of Christianity, as the notion without which Christianity would lose its coherence and its significance (p. 37). It is the "fundamental motif" of the Christian religion because Christianity conceives of fellowship with God as initiated by God's *agape*, or God's love freely bestowed upon the sinner. Hellenism, on the other hand, according to Nygren, conceived of fellowship with God as initiated by the human desire for God, by the egocentric longing for human fulfillment in the divine, by *eros*. Nygren also draws a sharp contrast between Judaism and Christianity. The "fundamental motif" of Judaism was *nomos*, for fellowship with God in Judaism depended, according to Nygren, on obedience to the law, or merit (pp. 250-51, 67-70). He says, "Agape comes to us as a quite new creation of Christianity. It sets its mark on everything in Christianity. Without it nothing that is Christian would be Christian. Agape is Christianity's own original conception" (p. 48).

Nygren insists that if we are to understand the Christian idea of *agape*, we must begin with God's love for sinners (pp. 61-67). It is Paul's theology of the cross that provides the definitive account of God's *agape* for Nygren. If we would understand *agape*, then, we must start with God's love for sinners made known on the cross. The four main features of *agape* are that it is "unmotivated," "indifferent to value," "creative," and "the initiator of fellowship with God" (pp. 75-81). God's love for the sinner is the basis and prototype for human love of the neighbor (p. 91).

But there are significant problems with Nygren's analysis of *agape*. One problem is obvious as soon as we begin to talk about loving God. That love can hardly be regarded as "unmotivated" or "indifferent to value," or "creative." Nygren himself admits that loving God "lacks all the essential marks of Agape" (p. 125), and he adopts instead the language of faith to talk of one's response to God's love. But it is no less problematic when this notion of *agape* is taken to be paradigmatic for human love of the neighbor. That love, too, is not "unmotivated"; it is hardly "indifferent to value"; and it is as much responsive as creative. Even the love of the enemy is motivated by the recognition that the enemy too is the creature of God and worthy of our love. As the following paragraph makes clear, I have left Nygren's notion of *agape* aside, following instead the account of love in Jules Toner, *The Experience of Love.*

16. Toner, *The Experience of Love*, p. 167.

care for the one in need and sometimes in sorrow that the neighbor's need goes unmet.

H. Richard Niebuhr's account of love is, I think, among the most adequate — and surely among the most eloquent — brief descriptions of love:

> By love we mean at least these attitudes and actions: rejoicing in the presence of the beloved, gratitude, reverence and loyalty toward him.
>
> Love is rejoicing over the existence of the beloved one; it is the desire that he be rather than not be; it is longing for his presence when he is absent; it is happiness in the thought of him; it is profound satisfaction over everything that makes him great and glorious.
>
> Love is gratitude: it is thankfulness for the existence of the beloved; it is the happy acceptance of everything that he gives without the jealous feeling that the self ought to be able to do as much; it is a gratitude that does not seek equality; it is wonder over the other's gift of himself in companionship.
>
> Love is reverence: it keeps its distance even as it draws near; it does not seek to absorb the other in the self or want to be absorbed by it; it rejoices in the otherness of the other; it desires the beloved to be what he is and does not seek to refashion him into a replica of the self or to make him a means to the self's advancement. As reverence, love is and seeks knowledge of the other, not by way of curiosity nor for the sake of gaining power but in rejoicing and in wonder. In all such love there is an element of that "holy fear" which is not a form of flight but rather deep respect for the otherness of the beloved and the profound unwillingness to violate his integrity.
>
> Love is loyalty; it is the willingness to let the self be destroyed rather than that the other cease to be; it is the commitment of the self by self-binding will to make the other great. It is loyalty, too, to the other's cause, to his loyalty.[17]

In that light we may consider again loving God as a virtue important to dying well and faithfully. To love God is at its root an affective affirmation of God. It is the praise of God. It affirms God for God's own sake; it does not simply "use" God for the sake of achieving some other desired end, whether a return to health or "eternal bliss." It is a response to God's

17. H. Richard Niebuhr, *The Purpose of the Church and Its Ministry* (New York: Harper and Row, 1977), p. 35.

lovable actuality. Loving God is to rejoice that God is God. It is gratitude for God's gifts of life and love, for a good night's sleep, for a little relief from pain, for God's companionship even in suffering and dying. It is reverence for God as God, a readiness to let God be God and to rest in God's hands. It is loyalty to God and to the cause of God, making that cause our own cause. It is to hope for and to pray for the good future of God. And because that future is not yet, still sadly not yet, loving God will sometimes prompt lament.

There is a second virtue, the love of the neighbor. There is no loving God that does not also love the neighbor (1 John 4:20; see also 3:17; 4:12). It is not, as Augustine said, that we "enjoy" God and therefore "use" the neighbor. Rather we love God as God and love all else as all else is related to God. Surely the neighbor is related to God, and worthy of our affectionate affirmation as another cherished child of God. We will consider more fully the love of the neighbor as a virtue for dying well and faithfully in a moment, but first consider "all else."

Because we delight in God, we may take pious delight in the bodies God made, in the natural relationships that come with our embodiment, in the friends and companions God gives. To be sure, if we relate to all else as all else is related to God, we will not delight in sin or death. They are not the cause of God; God has won the victory over them. Death still threatens alienation from our flesh and from our communities and from God. But when God won the victory over death, death lost the power to make good on those threats at the end of the story. Because God won the victory over death, we may die in hope for the redemption of our bodies, for the renewal of relationships, and for the blessing of God. And so, as we die, we may take "pious delight" in the pleasures of our flesh, listening to the music we love, looking at old photos we cherish, tasting a favorite beer. Perhaps, of course, sickness will have dulled the senses, but even then we may take delight in a little rest in a familiar bed and in a little relief from pain. As we die, we may take "pious delight" in the pleasures of the companionship of family and friends, remembering pleasant days and recalling shared struggles, admiring the little (or great) accomplishments of a grandchild or sibling or niece or friend, affirming them as a blessing of God. To be sure, sometimes death has made its power felt in the breaking of relationships long before we lie dying, but then as we die, we may seek some reconciliation, forgiving and being forgiven even as we pray for God's forgiveness.

That readiness to be reconciled, to forgive, is part of what the virtue of love of the neighbor requires. It is part of dying well and faithfully. Jesus' word from the cross, "Father, forgive them," was the paradigm of such a love, and we do not die well or faithfully by carrying a grudge to our graves.

Love for the neighbor is also displayed in the desire to be with those we love and caring for those we leave behind. Love is not reducible to either desire or compassion, but the affective affirmation of the other expresses itself both as a desire to be with family and friends if they are absent and as care for their needs. So we take pious delight in the visits and calls of family and friends and do what we can to meet their needs both as we lie dying and when we are dead. Jesus is the paradigm for such a love when he longs for the companionship of the disciples and when, in John's Gospel, he instructs the beloved disciple to care for his mother and his mother to care for John. This care, this compassion, extends not just to family and friends; it extends to others as well. It is expressed in gracious and generous attention to the needs of others even as we are dying. Jesus is the paradigm of such a love when he responds so graciously to the request of the thief dying beside him.

Care for the needs of family and friends and others can take form in instruments as prosaic as a will and instructions for one's care as one is withering and dying. The will can help meet the needs of those we love and can exercise some generosity toward others in need or toward institutions that serve the cause of God. Some conversation or written instructions about one's care at the end of life might release loved ones from any burden of guilt in refusing heroic measures to keep you alive. Not everything that can be done must be done. Everything that needs to be done to win the victory over death has been done; the victory over death is a divine victory, not a technological one. Medical technology is a good gift of God, but there comes a time when it makes Christian sense to seek not to live longer but to live well while one is dying. There is no algorithm here, but there is Christian discernment. (We will come back to discernment and to the matter of preparing advance directives as a Christian practice in a subsequent chapter.)

Love, of course, is intimately related to faith and hope. Paul already regarded these three as a triad (1 Cor. 13:13; 1 Thess. 1:3). Faith and faithfulness exist as love; faith "works" as love (Gal. 5:6). And love is the mark of the new creation, the good future for which we hope.[18] The Spirit is the

18. Compare Gal. 5:6 and 6:15, where after almost identical opening clauses, "in Christ Jesus neither circumcision nor uncircumcision counts for anything," the first text has "the

"first fruits" (Rom. 8:23) and the "guarantee" (2 Cor. 5:5) of that good future, and the "fruit of the Spirit is love, joy, peace, patience, kindness, generosity, faithfulness, gentleness, and self-control." Love is simply set first in that list of virtues. But in 1 Corinthians 13:4-7 the other virtues are the work of love. "Love is patient; love is kind; love is not envious or boastful or arrogant or rude. It does not insist on its own way; it is not irritable or resentful; it does not rejoice in wrongdoing, but rejoices in the truth. It bears all things, believes all things, hopes all things, endures all things." The spiritually gifted in Corinth may boast that their gifts of tongues and prophecy and knowledge mark them as having arrived spiritually, but Paul insists that all these gifts will come to an end. It is love that "never ends" (1 Cor. 13:8), for love is the mark of God's good future. Or, as John says, "We know that we have passed from death to life because we love one another. Whoever does not love abides in death" (1 John 3:14). So, even as we lie dying, love is a sign of the resurrection, a testimony that we have a share in the victory of God over death, a witness that we participate already in God's good future.

Patience

Love is patient. *Ars Moriendi* had that right. It went wrong, however, when it confused Christian patience with Stoic resignation. It went wrong when it, citing Seneca, identified patience with taking death "gladly and wylfully, with reason of his mynde that rewleth hys sensualyte" (*Crafte*, p. 2).

Stoic contentment in the face of death was formed by reason ruling over the passions. Reason required two things, *autarkeia* and *apatheia*. *Autarkeia* is self-sufficiency, independence from anyone or anything other than oneself. The wise man should never become dependent upon anyone else for his happiness or upon anything else than his reason. *Apatheia* is a matter of suppressing the passions, of quitting desire. The wise man avoids suffering by attaining indifference; he learns patience by unlearning sadness.[19] It is no easy matter, of course. Epictetus, the Stoic, suggested that the one who would learn contentment should start by learning not to care

---

only thing that matters is faith working through love," and the second text has "a new creation is everything."

19. This is Martha Nussbaum's account of Stoicism in *The Therapy of Desire: Theory and Practice in Hellenistic Ethics* (Princeton: Princeton University Press, 1994), pp. 388-99.

about little things, a cup that is easily broken, for example. From there he might advance a little to a dog, a horse, a little bit of land, learning not to care if anything should happen to these things. Finally, he may reach a stage where he will not care what happens to his body or his family.[20] Little wonder that Epictetus regards love as a kind of slavery, the enemy of freedom from care, for love cares.[21]

Christian patience, on the other hand, is formed by sharing the passion of Jesus in watchfulness for God's good future. In striking contrast to Stoic contentment, it does not pretend to self-sufficiency; it recognizes and affirms that we depend upon God and upon each other and upon the good earth God made. We are created for community and in relations of mutual depending. We are all born as babies, dependent upon the care of others, and throughout our lives we remain dependent upon others in more ways than we can count, and finally when we are withering and dying, we grow again more obviously dependent upon caregivers.[22]

It is not just the Stoics, of course, who made *autarkeia,* autonomy, and independence the norm. Western culture has outdone the Stoics in its emphasis on independence and autonomy and in its horror of dependency. Ironically, this horror of dependency only adds to our suffering on our way to death. Dependency has become a threat to our identity as self-sufficient agents, and so we suffer it. Our culture makes it difficult to receive care graciously because care reminds us that we are not as independent and self-sufficient as we pretend to be. (And when care is not received graciously, it becomes more difficult to provide graciously.) But Christian patience acknowledges and affirms that we are dependent creatures. It trains us to receive care graciously and gratefully. It trains us to accept both the dependency of others and our own dependency. Then our identity is not threatened when we depend upon others, and we do not suffer our dependency in quite the same way. It need not shame us. It is only threatening when caregivers cannot be trusted.

Christian patience, formed by the passion of Jesus in watchfulness for God's good future, knows this at least, that God can be trusted. God is faithful when we are dependent, as we always are. God is faithful when we are dying, as we all will. "We do not live to ourselves, and we do not die to

20. Epictetus, *Discourses* 4.1.110-112, trans. W. A. Oldfather, 2:283.

21. Epictetus, *Discourses* 4.1.60; 2:265.

22. See Alasdair MacIntyre, *Dependent Rational Animals: Why Human Beings Need the Virtues* (Chicago: Open Court, 1999).

ourselves. If we live, we live to the Lord, and if we die, we die to the Lord; so then, whether we live or whether we die, we are the Lord's" (Rom. 14:7-8). In life and in death we depend on God, and patience is the faithful watching for the faithfulness of God. It is hope in God that makes us patient, not Stoic self-sufficiency.

A second contrast between Christian patience and Stoic resignation is no less striking. Love is no enemy of Christian patience, formed as it is by sharing the passion of Jesus in watchfulness for God's good future. Love is the basis of Christian patience. Epictetus may have been right to insist that, if we did not love, we would not suffer. But those who are formed by the passion of Jesus are less ready to surrender love than to suffer because of it. Christian patience would rather suffer than give up on love. The Stoics would teach us how not to care, how not to love. The passion of Jesus calls us to care deeply and passionately about others, to be ready to endure suffering on their behalf and ready to suffer with those who hurt. It does not make suffering a good. It does not celebrate suffering any more than it celebrates death. But patience is ready to endure and to share suffering for the sake of love. Such patience would seem foolish to the Stoic, and perhaps it would be foolish if it were not joined to the confidence that "love is strong as death" (Song of Sol. 8:6), if it were not joined to watchfulness for God's good future.

These two contrasts imply a third. The Stoics had no place for lament (and little patience with it). They did have a place for suicide, for quitting life. Christian patience, formed by sharing the passion of Christ in watchfulness for God's future, is quite capable of lament. Because Christians have caught a vision of that future, they weep and mourn that it is not yet, still sadly not yet. In God's good future, death will be no more, but it has not yet surrendered its power to threaten. So Christians grieve not as those who have no hope but precisely as those who do. Christian patience, however, makes no place for suicide.[23]

The patience formed by watchfulness does not deny that death and sickness and suffering are real. And it does not pretend that they are not real evils. But it knows that because God took the crucified Jesus from the dead,

---

23. Early Christian theologians were quite explicit and consistent in prohibiting suicide. See Darrel W. Amundsen, *Medicine, Society, and Faith in the Ancient and Modern Worlds* (Baltimore: Johns Hopkins University Press, 1996), pp. 70-126. It is well known that there is no explicit prohibition of suicide in the Bible, but the narrative of Judas's suicide sets suicide in the context of his denial and of his impatience. See Allen Verhey, *Reading the Bible in the Strange World of Medicine* (Grand Rapids: Eerdmans, 2003), pp. 304-44.

God and not death or sickness or suffering will have the last word. It knows that all human resistance to death and sickness, all human affirmation of embodied and communal life, is necessarily in vain if God is not God, if God has not vindicated both God's own faithfulness and Jesus by raising him from the dead. More than that, patience knows that because God *is* God, because God's faithfulness *has* been vindicated, because Jesus *has* been raised, sickness and weakness and withering signal not just the power of death but also our human limits and our dependence finally upon God. And more than that, because God *is* God and Jesus *has* been raised, patience knows that at those limits and in that dependence God may still be trusted.[24]

Christian patience is marked neither by independence nor by indifference. It is characterized, rather, by hope and love. Indeed, the two Greek words that are translated as "patience" in the New Testament, *makrothumia* and *hupomone,* may be distinguished (roughly) by their respective associations with love and hope. So, for example, when Paul says that "love is patient" (1 Cor. 13:4), he uses *makrothumei;* when he says, "Rejoice in hope, be patient in suffering" (Rom. 12:12), he uses *hupomenontes.*

Makrothumia was hardly an important part of the vocabulary of classical Greece. It entered Christian vocabulary through the Septuagint, the Greek translation of the Hebrew scripture. There it was included in the catalogue of God's attributes that runs through the Old Testament like a refrain:

> a God merciful and gracious,
> slow to anger,
> and abounding in steadfast love and faithfulness.
>
> (Exod. 34:6; cf. Num. 14:18; Neh. 9:17; Pss. 86:15;
> 103:8; 145:8; Jer. 15:15; Joel 2:13; Jon. 4:2; Nah. 1:3)

Makrothumia is used by the Septuagint for "slow to anger." (Formed from *makros,* "large" or "long," and *thumos,* "temper," it means quite literally "long-tempered.") God is not short-tempered; he is slow to anger, eager to forgive. It is not apathy or indifference. The legitimacy of wrath against an unfaithful people is acknowledged; the claims that are God's to make are not surrendered, but God delays the display of wrath to give the people an opportunity for repentance. God's patience is God's refusal to give up on God's children; it is God's refusal to give up on the desire to bless them (even the Ninevites, Jon. 4:2); it is God's decision to accept suffering rather than to surrender love.

24. Karl Barth, *Church Dogmatics* III/4 (Edinburgh: T. & T. Clark, 1961), pp. 372-73.

Jesus was a son of his Father in his *makrothumia,* in his being "slow to anger" and "long-tempered." Such patience is surely on display when Jesus is on the way to the cross and when he hangs there. He does not seek revenge; he does not return evil for evil; he does not return insult for insult (1 Pet. 2:23). That way of suffering and dying is "an example" (1 Pet. 2:21). Christ's patience is the paradigm for human patience. And those who would follow him, even as they are dying, should also be characterized by a love that is "slow to anger." Again, it is not mere passivity or feigned indifference. It is the refusal to give up on those one cares for and on those upon whose care one depends. In dying there are plenty of opportunities for short-tempered anger, anger at the nurse with too many patients, anger at the spouse who seems angry with you for dying, anger at the children who cannot come the moment they are called, anger at friends who say foolish things. And pain and suffering can tempt us to impatience, but as God has been patient with us, so we should be patient with one another. It is a part of not giving up on them. It is a part of loving them. It is a part of dying well and faithfully. It is part of what it means "to lead a life [and die a death] worthy of the calling to which you have been called, . . . with patience, bearing with one another in love" (Eph. 4:1-2).

Hupomone, on the other hand, the second word for patience in the New Testament, was a familiar word in classical Greek. It was used by Plato, for example, in *Theaetetus* for the courage to hear out an argument rather than running away (177b). Biblical usage is consistent with this emphasis on courage, but in Scripture courage is founded on hope. The faithful can endure hardship courageously because they trust God to be faithful and because they hope for the good future of God. Revelation, for example, calls the churches of Asia Minor to "patient endurance" (1:9; 2:2; 2:19; 3:10; etc.) in the confidence and hope that God has won and will win the victory over sin and death, over the bestiality of empire, and over all that corrupts and destroys God's creation. And when in Romans 8 Paul declares that "the sufferings of this present time are not worth comparing with the glory about to be revealed to us," he declares as well that "the creation waits [for it] with eager longing" and that we "groan" for it while we wait for the redemption of our bodies (vv. 18, 19, 23). "But if we hope for what we do not see, we wait for it with patience [*hupomones*]" (Rom. 8:25). That is to say, we wait for it courageously. This is not apathy or fatalism; this is the courage to live and to die well and faithfully in watchfulness for God's good future. This is the virtue of patience.

The story of Jesus' passion is paradigmatic for a Christian's dying with patience. It is a story of courage, courage formed by the hope that God will be faithful to God's own cause, courage nurtured by the hope for God's good future in the face of the threats of death. It is a story of love, a love that was gracious both to those for whom he cared and to those who would care for him, a love that was slow to anger and quick to forgive, a love that refused to give up on love or on the people he loved. In this story — from Gethsemane to Golgotha — lament had a place and suffering was given voice. The patience of Jesus was not indifference. It was not mere resignation. It did not celebrate death or suffering, but it was ready to endure both patiently in the confidence that the last word belonged to God.

Humility

We may learn not only faithfulness, hope, and love from the death of Jesus, not only patience; we may also learn humility. In *Ars Moriendi* the temptation of pride came to Moriens as he lay dying. The demons, having failed in their efforts to tempt Moriens to give up on faithfulness and on hope and on love, commended him for his virtues. It was a diabolically clever attempt to tempt Moriens to self-righteousness, to suppose that he had no need of God's grace in the judgment. Poor Moriens seemed caught between despair for his sins and pride for his virtues. The wise message of the angel commended the virtue of humility, advising Moriens not to focus on either his sins or his virtue but on the grace of God.

There is considerable wisdom there. Surely the *Ars Moriendi* was right to warn against self-righteousness. It echoed Jesus' warning in the parable of the Pharisee and the tax collector (Luke 18:9-14). The Pharisee in the parable is proud, of course, but he is also thankful; indeed, he evidently makes a habit of giving thanks. "Thank God," he says, "that I am not like other people: thieves, rogues, adulterers, . . . and this tax collector." But this is not the way to be thankful. And Luke makes it clear just why this is not the way to be thankful. In introducing the parable, he says Jesus told this parable against the habits of some who regarded themselves as righteous and who regarded others with contempt. The Pharisee's thankfulness divided the world into two parts, the righteous and the sinners, and it counted the Pharisee among the righteous and others among the sinners. The Pharisee's thankfulness was corrupted by self-righteousness and by contempt for others. This is a thankfulness that divides, that nurtures self-righteousness and contempt. This is a bad thankfulness.

The same wisdom is wonderfully narrated in Flannery O'Connor's story "Revelation."[25] In that story the self-righteous Mrs. Turpin sits in a doctor's waiting room and counts her blessings that she is not like the others in the room. "'If it's one thing I am,' Mrs. Turpin said with feeling, 'it's grateful. When I think of all I could have been besides myself . . . , I just feel like shouting, "Thank you, Jesus, for making everything the way it is!"'" (pp. 205-6). She was thankful that she was not "white trash," or a "nigger," or "ugly," or . . . Like the Pharisee, she was in the habit of giving thanks, and like the Pharisee's, her thankfulness was a thankfulness that divided, that nurtured self-righteousness and contempt for others. It was a bad thankfulness. But Mrs. Turpin was about to have a revelation. It came in the form of a disturbed and disturbing college student who also sat in that waiting room. The young woman first threw a textbook *(Human Development)* at Mrs. Turpin, then attacked her physically, and finally whispered to her, "Go back to hell where you came from, you old wart hog" (p. 207). It was outrageous behavior, but it was also, Mrs. Turpin worried, a revelation. It nearly drove her to despair. Finally, out in the field behind her farm, she cried out to God to confirm or to deny that the accusation was a revelation. "'Go on,' she yelled, 'call me a hog! Call me a hog again. From hell. Call me a wart hog from hell. . . .' A garbled echo returned to her" (p. 216). She stood there for a moment "absorbing some abysmal life-giving knowledge" (p. 217) until her self-righteousness was broken, and she looked up and saw a purple streak in the sky. "A visionary light settled in her eyes. She saw the streak as a vast swinging bridge extending upward from the earth through a field of living fire. Upon it a vast horde of souls were rumbling toward heaven" (p. 218). On that bridge to heaven there were hordes of the people she had thought unlikely to be on their way to heaven, and toward the end of the procession she saw also respectable people like herself with their self-righteousness burned away. And then she heard in the choruses of the crickets "the voices of the souls climbing upward into the starry field and singing hallelujah" (p. 218). If there is hope for Mrs. Turpin, then there is hope for Moriens and for all of us. Perhaps we can learn humility and a thankfulness that does not divide.

In contrast to the Pharisee and to Mrs. Turpin in the doctor's office, the tax collector throws himself upon the mercy of God, relying not on himself or on his own righteousness but on God's grace, like Mrs. Turpin

25. Flannery O'Connor, "Revelation," in *Everything That Rises Must Converge* (New York: Farrar, Straus and Giroux, 1976), pp. 191-218. Page references to this short story are provided in parentheses.

in the field. The tax collector is humble, and it is the tax collector who is justified. The concluding aphorism, found frequently among the teachings of Jesus, serves to underscore the point: "all who exalt themselves will be humbled, but all who humble themselves will be exalted" (Luke 18:14).[26]

The tax collector, too, of course, should be thankful. But suppose he returns to the temple to give thanks and says, "Thank God that I am not like other people, proud people, people like that Pharisee." Suppose, that is, that he is proud of his humility, that he boasts about it. Then his gratitude, no less than the Pharisee's, will be a thankfulness that divides, that nurtures self-righteousness and contempt of others. It will be a bad thankfulness.

We do the parable no injustice if we take its lesson to be "justification by grace through faith," but injustice is done both to the parable and to that doctrine if we take them to refer to a purely individualistic and introspective reality. It is a social reality. The Pharisee's lack of humility before God entails the contempt of others. The publican's humility establishes solidarity with others, at least until it is subtly perverted by pride. Humility is not just a characteristic of our proper posture before God; it is also always a characteristic of our proper relations with others. There is no place for arrogance in the community of God's people, no place for dividing the world into the righteous and sinners, no place for the contempt of others.

Therefore, insofar as the *Ars Moriendi* focuses exclusively on the dyad of Moriens and God, it misleads us even concerning humility. We should observe, by the way, that this little effort of ours to consider how to die well and faithfully may also be tempted to the wrong kind of thankfulness. If we say, "Thank God that we are not like other people, like the Stoics and the Platonists and the devotees of the Baconian project who do not know how to die well or faithfully," then we have not yet learned humility. If we boast about our little knowledge or have contempt for those who die poorly, then we have not yet learned humility. We stand in solidarity, on the one hand, with all who are dying, and on the other, with Jesus whom God has already raised from the dead.

Ars Moriendi is surely right, I think, to insist that pride gets in the way of dying well. The work may be faulted, as we said, for focusing too exclusively on the dyad of Moriens and God, and it may also limit its account of pride too much to the self-righteousness that pretends to have no need

---

26. Cf. Matt. 23:12; Luke 14:11; cf. also Matt. 20:16; Mark 10:31; Luke 13:30; Mark 9:35; Matt. 20:27.

of God's grace in the judgment. Pride is not just the pretense of self-righteousness; it is also any pretense to self-sufficiency. Pride pretends to have no need of either the grace of God or the grace of another human being. It refuses to acknowledge neediness. That is why it is no good at gratitude, or at least no good at good gratitude.

When my mother used to tell me, "Pride goes before a fall," she was simply quoting a still more ancient sage (cf. Prov. 16:18). And of course, she and the more ancient sage were right. Life sometimes has a way of bringing down those who exalt themselves, but if life doesn't do it, dying surely will. Death is, after all, the great leveler. And dying inevitably reminds us of our neediness.

The temptation of pride is a common one in our culture, given its emphasis on autonomy and independence. Like my mother's son, our culture is not particularly good at acknowledging neediness — or at gratitude. The temptation of pride comes long before the deathbed, of course, but when we are dying, the habit of pride makes dying well difficult. Pride can keep us from receiving care graciously. It can make those in need of care ashamed of "being a burden" and resentful of those compassionate caregivers whose very care reminds us of just how needy we are.

Such pride is folly, of course. None of us is as autonomous and independent as we like to claim. I have been a burden to those I love — and to those who love me — for quite a while now. I started as a baby, as all of us do, and I remain dependent upon others, as all of us also do, whether we acknowledge it or not. The utter helplessness while being sick from the chemotherapy for my amyloidosis was just a vivid reminder of it. But to acknowledge it — to acknowledge gratefully our dependence upon God and upon other human beings — is a mark of wisdom and a key both to living well and to dying well. Both living well and dying well require help from others. Both living well and dying well take community. It is not good to die alone.

But leave the temptation of pride aside for a moment. Let's just admit that even if we acknowledge our dependence upon God and upon others, dying can sometimes be, well, humiliating. Perhaps if we were to find a remedy for our pride, we could more easily accept the loss of some measures of our independence. But even if we acknowledge our neediness, the events that sometimes accompany dying can be humiliating. You do not have to be very proud to find the loss of control over your bowels to be a little humiliating. You do not have to be outrageously arrogant to be humiliated by throwing up on your wife's lap. Such things seem to assault not just our pride but our dignity. They are unwelcome messengers of the alienation from our own flesh that death threatens. And we need not celebrate such humiliation any more than we celebrate death. Sometimes, thankfully, the good care of a palliative care doctor or a hospice nurse can alleviate the symptoms that humiliate, but it cannot eliminate the humiliation. We will need humility to deal with that.

When we feel like dirt because of such humiliation, it may be at least a little helpful to remember that we are all, after all, dirt, that we are dust and to dust we shall return, that "human," "humility," and "humus" all have the same root. Then it is also worth remembering that God took that dirt, that dust, breathed into it, and made human beings living creatures. God can do it again. And above all, it is to be remembered that Jesus was not just humble but was humiliated on his way to death. People insulted him, mocked him, spat on him. Roman crucifixion was quite deliberately humiliating to the victim. Jesus died in solidarity with the humiliated, with those who are beaten down and broken, whether by the bestiality of empire or by the bestiality of disease. But God raised this Jesus up. God, as God had promised, made the last first, exalted the humiliated.[27] The final resurrection is of one piece with that resurrection of Jesus, even if it is separated in time. Solidarity with the humiliated and exalted Christ can help us to bear the humiliation that sometimes accompanies dying.

Greek moralists did not think highly of humility; at least they did not think highly of the quality *tapeinos* named. They used the term *tapeinos* disparagingly.[28] The Christian church, however, with the help of its Jewish heritage, changed the status of this word in the Greek vocabulary. The transformation can be found within the New Testament itself. When Paul quotes the accusation of his Corinthian opponents that Paul is "humble [*tapeinos*] when face to face . . . but bold" when he is away, it is hard to escape the sense that "humble" is meant disparagingly (2 Cor. 10:1; cf. 10:10). When Paul, however, appeals to the "meekness and gentleness of Christ," he vindicates his own humility and convicts his opponents; "it is not those who commend themselves that are approved, but those whom the Lord commends" (2 Cor. 10:1; 10:18). Again, *tapeinophrosune* is used in Colossians to name both an attitude that is condemned (Col. 2:18,

27. Most of the Hebrew and Greek terms translated "humble" can also be translated as "humiliated." The context will usually suggest one rendering rather than another, but frequently either is appropriate.

28. Epictetus, for example, in *Discourses* 3.2.14, sets *tapeinos* first among the set of qualities he finds censurable in another philosopher.

23) and an attitude that is commended (3:12; cf. Eph. 4:2). The attitude that is condemned is "self-abasement" (Col. 2:18) and "humility" (2:23). The "humility" that is condemned is associated with "severe treatment of the body" (2:23), is consistent with an ascetic dualism, and seems to have provided the basis for dividing the church into the spiritually elite and the ordinary Christians. Such "humility" is at bottom religious pride, and the writer of Colossians refuses to commend it. Still, the same term returns in the list of virtues with which all Christians are to clothe themselves: "compassion, kindness, humility [*tapeinophrosune*], meekness, and patience" (3:12). Humility must be formed by the pattern of Christ's life and death if it is to count as a genuine virtue for Christian living and dying. It is not formed by indifference to the body — whether feigned or genuine — and it is not displayed in "severe treatment of the body." It is not formed by indifference to the community, and it is surely not displayed in a spiritual elitism.

The change in vocabulary is related, of course, to a transformation of values. The announcement of God's good future promised a great reversal. Jesus had told of it. The poor would be blessed. The last would be first. The hungry would be fed. The humiliated would be exalted. But even before Jesus was born, his mother Mary saw it and sang of it in her Magnificat (Luke 1:46-55). The humble Mary submits to the reign of God, already celebrates God's good future. Humility is submissiveness, to be sure, but not submissiveness to the reign of sin and death, not submissiveness to the fates or to the rule of Mother Nature *(que sera sera)*, but submissiveness to (indeed, delight in) the coming reign of God.

We began this section by acknowledging that *Ars Moriendi* was right in condemning self-righteousness and right in observing that pride is the enemy of dying well and faithfully. Along the way we have tried to supplement and sometimes correct the account of humility in *Ars Moriendi*. But let's close this section by observing that *Ars Moriendi* was also right in this: that attention to God and to the grace of God can nurture humility. Attentive to God, we can acknowledge our neediness and no longer fear it. Attentive to the grace of God, we need not pretend that it is our little righteousness that makes us worthy of God's care (or anyone else's); we can learn to receive care graciously. Attentive to God and to the power that exalted the crucified and humiliated Jesus, we can even cope with the humiliation of dying. Attentive to God, we need not anxiously hoard the little resources we think we have against our vulnerability to suffering and death; we can be a little less anxious, a little more carefree.

Letting Go/Serenity/Generosity

That freedom from the anxiety that prompts us to hoard the little resources we think we have against our vulnerability to suffering and death brings us, finally, back to the temptation of avarice, the final temptation of Moriens, and to the virtue we hardly know how to name. *Ars Moriendi* is surely right to call attention to our anxious and tightfisted refusal to "let go" — the refusal to "let go" of possessions, of our family members, of our friends, of life itself, and, we may add, of the hope that medical technology may yet deliver us from our finitude and to our flourishing. Such tightfistedness, such avarice, displays something closer to idolatry than to affection and gratitude. It surely makes dying well more difficult. Let go of them, of course, we finally must. Death will take them from us. That is the threat of death. To die is to be dispossessed, to be sundered from the things and the people we love.

Nevertheless, the remedy *Ars Moriendi* proposed for this temptation is deeply flawed. The antidote to this anxious tightfisted grasping is not to be found in Stoic indifference or in a Platonic vision of a disembodied and "spiritual" otherworld to which our souls will be transported. The remedy is not to deride or neglect the things and the people that God made good. On the cross Jesus still showed his concern for his mother. The problem is not that we love what God also loves, and the solution is not to love them less — or to "use" them but not "enjoy" them. The problem is to let go of our anxious tightfisted grasping.

There are, of course, quite different proposals for an antidote to the anxiety that prompts the refusal to "let go." Some would medicalize the anxiety. There must be, we suppose, an antidote to anxiety in some pill. But this, too, is flawed. To medicalize our human condition in the face of death is to refuse the meaning of our suffering. When antebellum doctors described as a disease the rage and grief of slaves torn from their homeland and from their families, the culture was helped to ignore the meaning of their suffering. By medicalizing the condition of slaves, the culture could refuse to attend to the meaning of their suffering. And by medicalizing the anxiety that attends those who are dying, we are enabled to refuse to attend to the meaning of their (and our) suffering. To be sure, it is sometimes necessary and appropriate to offer palliatives, but "it is drastically wrong to offer or to accept a palliative as if it were a cure."[29]

---

29. Marilynne Robinson, *The Death of Adam: Essays on Modern Thought* (Boston: Houghton Mifflin, 1998), p. 82.

Looking to Jesus, however, we may discover an antidote for this anxiety. He commanded us, after all, not to be anxious (e.g., Matt. 6:31; Luke 12:22). Of course, a command not to be anxious might well only increase anxiety. But this command comes clothed with the gospel of God's good future. We need not be anxious because God is faithful; God's good future is sure to be. Jesus, moreover, not only commanded freedom from anxiety; he displayed it on the cross. Once more his death is a paradigm for a Christian's dying. Without commending death, he was able to face it without fear because he was confident of the grace of God. Because he did not commend death, he could and did lament. His freedom from anxiety was not a matter of indifference to life or to his family and friends. The freedom from anxiety that he commanded and displayed was not freedom from sadness in the face of death; it did not mute the voice of the sufferer. Lament moves always from the honest expression of sorrow and sadness toward the certainty of a hearing, and it finally expresses the confidence that God is faithful. So, it is in the context of lament that both Jesus and the psalmist say, "Into your hands I commend my spirit" (Luke 23:46; cf. Ps. 31:5). Jesus and the psalmist — and we — can let ourselves go into the hands of God, knowing God can be trusted. God raised this Jesus from the dead, and by that apocalyptic deed assures us that God can be trusted and that God's good future is sure to be. Therefore, even at the limits of our lives, we need not be anxious, for we may know that God's love is stronger than death. We may let go also of those we love, confident of God's care. Dying well and faithfully will mean commending also them into the hands of a God who can be trusted. Then we can be calm in the chaos of dying. Then we can "let go." Perhaps the name for this virtue is serenity.[30]

30. Martin Luther's famous hymn expresses this confidence, this serenity, quite eloquently.

> A mighty fortress is our God,
> a bulwark never failing;
> our helper he, amid the flood
> of mortal ills prevailing.
> For still our ancient foe
> does seek to work us woe;
> his craft and power are great,
> and armed with cruel hate;
> on earth is not his equal.
>
> Did we in our own strength confide,
> our striving would be losing,

Jesus' command not to be anxious did not, however, prohibit concern for others. Paul, for example, can commend Timothy for his concern, his anxiety, for the Philippians (Phil. 2:20; Paul uses the same word, *merimnao*, that Jesus used). He can call on members of the church at Corinth to exercise some "care for one another," some concern, some anxiety, for the welfare of other members of the body (1 Cor. 12:25; again the same word is used). Responsible care for others is evidently not forbidden. What seems forbidden is both the egocentric anxiety that only worries about one's own welfare and the pride that supposes we can establish our own identity and security. Such egocentric anxiety and pride mark the wealthy farmer of Jesus' parable in Luke 12:15-21 as a rich "fool." He delights in the abundance of his harvest and thinks that building bigger barns will guarantee his security (v. 18). He thinks (and speaks) only of himself. He neglects gratitude both to God and to the laborers in his field, and he neglects the obligation to share the harvest with the poor. Such folly is one more occasion for Jesus to urge his hearers to be not anxious (v. 22), for God can

---

were not the right Man on our side,
the Man of God's own choosing.
You ask who that may be?
Christ Jesus, it is he;
Lord Sabaoth his name,
from age to age the same,
and he must win the battle.

And though the world, with devils filled,
should threaten to undo us,
we will not fear, for God has willed
his truth to triumph through us.
The prince of darkness grim,
we tremble not for him;
his rage we can endure,
for lo! his doom is sure;
one little word shall fell him.

The Word above all earthly powers —
no thanks to them — abideth;
the Spirit and the gifts are ours
through him who with us sideth.
Let goods and kindred go,
this mortal life also;
the body they may kill;
God's truth abideth still;
his kingdom is forever.

be trusted. Perhaps the name for this virtue capable of "letting go" is generosity. And again the paradigm is the self-giving love of the cross. We are not Jesus, and our deaths do not have the same cosmic significance that his does. Nevertheless, when our dying is marked, not by indifference to those we leave behind, and not just by serenity and calm, but also and especially by generosity, by gratitude to God for the gifts of God, by gratitude to others for the ways in which they have enriched our lives, and by sharing what we have with those in need, then it may provide a definitive disclosure of our Christian identity.

Surely our anxiety and pride are related to our avarice, to the anxious tightfistedness that is unwilling to let go of the things we think will establish our independence and our security against need. Death will leave us empty-handed, but on the way to death we will die well and faithfully if we learn to open our hands, to open them humbly and thankfully toward the blessing of God and to open them gratefully and generously toward others in love. In both cases we open them toward the good future of God.

That is the answer to our anxiety — the good future of God, the kingdom of God, the renewal and redemption of this world and these bodies. The antidote for our tightfisted avarice is to be found in God's power and promise to give life to the dust, to raise the dead. God's good future is sure to be. It is God's grace and power that secure our identity and our hope. Then we can hear the command "Be not anxious" as a blessing. Then we can be carefree, serene, even in the face of death. Then we may let ourselves go into the care of God, into the hands of God, confident of God's power and grace. That confidence, with its attendant freedom from anxiety, is displayed in words and gestures of gratitude to both God and to those who have been gifts of God to our lives. It is displayed in generous expressions of affection and in the generous distribution of our possessions. It is the remedy for our avarice and wisdom for living well and dying well.

The same point can be made another way. Looking to Jesus, we may discover that the antidote for this anxiety and pride is finally prayer. When in the midst of suffering our way toward death, we learn from Jesus to cry "Abba! Father!" we may learn as well "that we are children of God, and if children, then heirs, heirs of God and joint heirs with Christ" (Rom. 8:15-17). As Paul said, "Do not worry about anything, but in everything by prayer and supplication with thanksgiving let your requests be made known to God" (Phil. 4:6). Prayer is an important practice if we are to find an antidote for anxiety and if we are to learn to die well and faithfully.

Taking another cue from the *Ars Moriendi,* we will consider this practice more thoroughly in a subsequent chapter. Here it is enough simply to note its significance as an antidote to anxiety.

Courage

All these virtues — faithfulness, hope, a love that is patient, humility, and serenity — finally support another virtue, namely, courage in the face of death. Without commending death, we may nevertheless learn from the death of Jesus the courage we need in the face of death. His faithfulness was displayed in his steady and heroic fidelity to God and to the cause of God, even when it was clear that it would end in his death. He knew that there are some goods more important than survival, some duties more compelling than the preservation of one's own life. His confidence that God would display God's own faithfulness and finally establish the good future that he had announced nurtured and sustained his courage. His self-giving love was the very image of the Father's love, and the model for those who would follow him. That love was patient, not indifferent. He acknowledged his dependence upon a God who could be trusted. Like the God he trusted, he was slow to anger and quick to forgive. Without celebrating suffering, he was ready to suffer with others who suffered, ready to share the human cry of lament. Without celebrating death, he courageously endured even dying for the sake of God's cause, the neighbor's good, and his own integrity. That love was humble. Though he was master and lord, yet he was among us as one who served. He trusted the God who could make the last first, who promised to exalt the humble. His humility enabled him to endure with courage even the humiliation of the cross. His confidence in God allowed him, in the midst of lament, still to let himself go into the hands of God. Perhaps that "letting go" was the greatest display of his courage.

We are not Jesus. Our deaths do not have the cosmic significance that his did. Still, the *Ars Moriendi* had it right: by remembering Jesus and his dying, we may find a paradigm for dying well and faithfully.

We find and follow that paradigm, however, only in the light of the resurrection. When God raised Jesus from the dead, God vindicated both Jesus' faithfulness and God's own faithfulness. When God raised Jesus from the dead, God won the victory over death. This is no commendation of death. The *Ars Moriendi* went badly wrong when it made death a good. We live and die with the confidence that death will not have the last word. God's victory over death has robbed death of its sting, of its terrors. The resurrection assures us that we will not finally be alienated from our flesh or from the community, and that nothing can separate us from the love of God. It is that assurance that nurtures our own courage in the face of death. It nurtures the faithful readiness to acknowledge that at the end of life and at the limits of human powers God can still be trusted. Precisely because death will not have the last word, we need not always resist it. And because the triumph over death is finally not a technological victory, but a divine victory, we will resist not only the commendation of death but also the medicalization of dying.

PART FOUR

The Practices of Christian Community and the Practices of Dying Well and Caring Well for the Dying

The Lord of the church is not ruler of a surface kingdom. His dominion is nothing if it does not go at lest six feet deep. The church affirms the one Lord who went down into the grave, fought a battle with the power of death, and by his own death brought death to an end. For this reason, the church must be unafraid to speak of death.

William F. May, "The Sacral Power
of Death in Contemporary Experience"[1]

Dying well in America is hard work. And American Christianity has not helped much. Those were the problems we identified already in part 1. We attended there to the medicalization of death in the middle of the twentieth century. While we celebrated the advances in medicine and its new powers to intervene against disease and premature death, we joined the chorus of voices that complained about a "medicalized death." The commanding image of death in a "medicalized" dying is that death is an enemy to be defeated by the greater powers of science and medicine. A "medicalized" dying has fundamentally one focus: avoiding death by means of medical technology. So dying usually happens in a hospital, in a

---

1. William F. May, "The Sacral Power of Death in Contemporary Experience," in *On Moral Medicine: Theological Perspectives in Medical Ethics,* ed. Stephen E. Lammers and Allen Verhey, 2nd ed. (Grand Rapids: Eerdmans, 1998), p. 201.

sterile environment, in the company of technology, and under the control of those who know how to use it. We did not quarrel with the notion that death is an enemy. It threatens, after all, the sundering of persons from their own flesh, from their communities, and from God. But we did challenge the confidence that medicine is finally stronger than death. It does not and cannot finally deliver us from our mortality. And ironically, the result of the new technologies and our confidence in them has sometimes been a premature alienation of the dying from their own bodies, a premature sundering of the dying from their communities, and a forgetfulness of God — in a hospital and for the sake of our survival. The medicalization of death has made dying well difficult.

We noted in that first part some of the complaints about medicalization and the proposals to correct it. Standard bioethics, for example, complained about "depersonalization" and proposed "patient autonomy" as a way to allow dying patients to wrestle control over their dying away from the doctors. However, because patient autonomy allows the question of who should decide to monopolize our attention, it fails to nurture either a conversation about what should be decided or an alternative moral imagination. It is easy to blame physicians when people do not die well, but it is not their responsibility to teach people how to die well. The problem is not their skill but our imagination. The death awareness movement also complained about medicalized dying. It promised that, if we would stop our silence and denial and learn to regard death as "natural," we could avoid a medicalized death. To regard death as "natural" does suggest, of course, an alternative imagination. When we considered it carefully, however, we found the mantra that "death is natural" to be deeply flawed. The hospice movement provided, we said, the most powerful voice in the chorus of complaints and the most hopeful alternative to a medicalized death. Even in the hospice movement, however, we noted some reasons to worry a little.

The first part of the book concluded with a complaint about the silence of the churches about medicalized dying and their surrender of death to medicine. It called on the churches to resist the medicalization of death not by relying on the bioethics movement or the death awareness movement but by faithfully and creatively retrieving their own resources.

Among those resources may be counted the tradition of *Ars Moriendi*. In part 2 we focused on the fifteenth-century beginnings of that tradition and especially on the little self-help book from that century called *Ars Moriendi*. Its instructions about how to die well — and the wood-block prints that accompanied them — formed the imagination of the Christian community for centuries.

Ars Moriendi, like most other early works in the genre, began with a commendation of death. It moved quickly to an account of the deathbed temptations of Moriens, temptations of faithlessness, despair, impatience, pride, and avarice, and of the virtues necessary to meet those temptations, faith, hope, the patience of love, humility, and the ascetic surrender of worldly attachments. After the account of the temptations and the virtues, there was (although much-abridged in *Ars Moriendi*) a little catechism for the dying, an instruction to the dying that they should look to the cross and find in Christ a paradigm for their own dying, and finally, advice and prayers for trusted friends to use when Moriens grew too weary for "self-help."

We noted the considerable wisdom of *Ars Moriendi*. There is here no silence or denial of death. There is a recognition that Moriens has decisions to make, and the doctors cannot make them for him. His integrity, if not his autonomy, is of crucial concern. It calls Moriens to faith and faithfulness in the face of death. It encourages Moriens to practice the virtues of dying well. And most noteworthy of all, I think, it urges Moriens to "thynke on" the story of Jesus' death as a paradigm for a Christian's dying.

But we also noted some problems. And the problems began at the very beginning, with the commendation of death. The work echoed Plato more clearly than Christian Scripture. And that dualism between body and soul at the beginning ran like a virus through the whole, corrupting even its account of the virtues and its attention to Christ as the paradigm for a Christian's dying. Its account of hope, for example, became the longing of an individual soul for heavenly bliss. Its account of patience left no place for lament. Its call to humility was attentive to our sins but not to our finitude. And its call for an ascetic detachment from "carnal" attachments disparaged relationships with family and friends. Although Christ is the paradigm, it was curiously inattentive to the place of lament in Christ's dying, to his simple thirst, and to his concern for his mother and friend.

In part 3 we began the attempt to imagine a contemporary *ars moriendi*. We took a cue from the instruction of *Ars Moriendi* to remember Jesus. By the story of Jesus our imagination can be re-formed. We began with the story of his resurrection and with a celebration of embodied and communal life, not with a commendation of death. Then we attended to the stories of Jesus' dying — and especially to the words from the cross — as instructive for a Christian's faithful dying. If we are to follow Christ, then the single focus of our living (and of our dying) may not be to avoid death. The story of Jesus' death provides an important corrective both to the tradition of *Ars Moriendi* and to our own medicalized dying. Finally we turned to the virtues for dying well in *Ars Moriendi,* now formed and re-formed by the story of Jesus.

In this fourth and last part we turn our attention to the Christian community and to the practices of Christian community that can nurture and sustain practices of dying well and caring well for the dying. Here, too, we take our cue from *Ars Moriendi.*[2]

It is not good to die alone. *Ars Moriendi* knew as much. And *Crafte and Knowledge For To Dye Well* said as much in its fifth chapter. There it called upon the friends and caregivers of Moriens to help him die well and faithfully.[3] It complained about deceptive assurances of recovery, about "false cherying and comfortyng and feyned behotyng of bodyly hele" (p. 14). It insisted instead that friends and caregivers tell the sick honestly of their condition, that they encourage the dying to make peace with God and order their affairs, making a will and testament. It urged that friends and caregivers do what they can to help Moriens engage in those practices that could help one to die well and faithfully, and among those practices it counted confession and sacrament and, above all, prayer. And it suggested that the whole community, "all a cyte" (p. 16), should come to the aid of the sick and dying.

Taking this cue from the *Ars Moriendi* tradition, we return to the complaint about the silence and denial of the churches and attempt to remedy it a little. We will attend to certain practices of the church that are

2. The significance of this cue was underscored by a student, Jillaine VanEssen, who responded to my talk about the virtues for dying well with some suspicion. "For pity's sake," she said. "They're dying! Cut them some slack! Dying is hard enough without requiring the exercise of all these virtues." I admitted that dying well and faithfully is no easy matter, but then neither is living well and faithfully. Still, it was only when I acknowledged that it is al-most impossibly hard if you have to do it alone, only when I insisted that the community must care well for the dying if the dying are to die well, that I won back her trust.

3. *Crafte and Knowledge For To Dye Well* (hereafter *Crafte*), in *The English* Ars Moriendi, ed. David William Atkinson, Renaissance and Baroque Studies and Texts, vol. 5 (New York: Peter Lang, 1992), chapter 5. Page references to this work will be placed in the text. We complained earlier about one feature that marred this chapter of *Crafte,* the in-struction to focus solely on the "spirituell helthe" of Moriens (p. 15) and to help him to ig-nore his "carnal" relationships, including his "carnal friendys," his wife and children. Our complaint against the dualism of the *Ars Moriendi* tradition, clearly on display in such ad-vice, has been something of a refrain, and we need not reiterate it here.

themselves formed by the story of Jesus and that bear the promise of re-forming communities that are capable of supporting practices of dying well and faithfully and of caring well and faithfully for the dying.

The churches and their practices can form our imagination. They can help to form certain habits while we are healthy that, when we are dying, will help us to die well and faithfully. As *Crafte* observed, one should learn the art of dying well "whyles he ys in hele [while one is in good health]" (p. 16). If the churches can imagine and display a contemporary *ars moriendi*, then their members might learn both to die well and to care well for the dying. Perhaps then the culture's imagination may also be free to consider an alternative to "medicalized" dying.

Because community is so important, we will begin with the simple practice of gathering. We will continue with the practices of reading Scripture, prayer, and the sacraments of baptism and Eucharist. Those practices, central to the life of the church, form and inform others, and we will attend to the practices of mourning and comforting, the practice of funerals, and the practice of remembering saints. Then we will recommend that Christian communities engage in a practice of catechesis concerning death and dying. That practice could include the writing of advance directives for health care, now set in the context of the Christian community and its memory of Jesus. It should include moral discourse and communal discernment concerning the ways people die and care for the dying. We will attend also to the Christian practice of caring for the dying, a practice without which dying well and faithfully is very hard work indeed, and a practice that may finally be the best testimony to Christian confidence in the God who has triumphed over death.

CHAPTER FOURTEEN

Gathering on the Lord's Day

[T]he gathering of the ekklesia *for worship is itself a response to God's prior action. The Christian liturgy assumes that God, by virtue of who God is and what God has done, is worthy of praise, adoration and thanksgiving. Such an assumption has important ethical implications to the extent that the liturgy forms those gathered with a particular orientation or posture toward God, the world, and other people that flows from and is consonant with the* ekkesia's *practice of worship.*

Phillip Kenneson, "Gathering:
Worship, Imagination, and Formation"[1]

The Practice of Gathering

Christian churches gather regularly. That itself is a significant practice, signaling and forming relationships of friendship, gesturing and nurturing a common life. It is not so much that Christians gather as that they are gathered. They come together in response to the call of God. The greeting at the

---

1. Phillip Kenneson, "Gathering: Worship, Imagination, and Formation," in *The Blackwell Companion to Christian Ethics,* ed. Stanley Hauerwas and Sam Wells (Malden, Mass.: Blackwell, 2004), p. 63.

beginning of their worship is God's greeting. And it announces the fact that this gathering is not based on anything other than God's grace and call. They do not come together on the basis of their status in society or their race, their wealth or their health, but simply on the basis of God's grace and call.[2]

That greeting, like any greeting, calls for a response. God's grace and greeting alone make us able to respond, but they also make us responsible. The answering includes the praise of God in the worship service, to be sure, but that praise spills over into lives and a common life "to the praise of [God's] glory" (Eph. 1:12, 14). The answering, the response to God's gift of grace, includes learning to trust God's grace and learning loyalty to God's cause. Here we learn faith. Lives and a common life "to the praise of God's glory" include learning to see ourselves as "members of one another" (Eph. 4:25), learning to see the other as another loved by God, learning to greet one another in the name of the one who greeted us. It means learning to practice hospitality to those who would be strangers but for the grace and call of God. It means learning to rejoice with those who rejoice and to weep with those who weep. It means learning that sickness, withering, and dying cannot separate us from the love of God and need not alienate us — or another — from the community. It means learning to care and to be cared for. Here we learn love.

By the greeting and grace of God we are gathered as a community. That greeting already forms identity and community. It initiates us into worship and into a community, into an alternative culture. Here we learn to trust God at the center of our lives and at the end of them. Here we learn to set our living and our dying, and our care for the dying, in the context of this greeting, as a response to the God of grace who can be trusted. Here we learn that, as God had the initiating word, so God will have the last word, and that it, too, will be a word of blessing. Here we learn hope.

The Practice of Reading Scripture Together

When the church is gathered, one thing they do is read Scripture together. It is in many ways a strange practice. And Scripture itself is in many ways a

---

2. It must be shamefully acknowledged, of course, that many congregations reflect the divisions of social status, wealth, and race, but the grace and call of the one God of all the world and of all people still gather many diverse members into one body and shall judge its divisions.

strange book. But in this practice of reading Scripture, the church remembers the story of God's grace. It remembers the story of creation and covenant, of promise and hope, of judgment and renewal, of Christ and of God's good future. It remembers the story not as an archivist might. It does not read Scripture in search of some objective account of "what really happened." It remembers the story as the story of its own life, as the story that gives the church its identity and makes it a community. Without memory, there is no identity. That is the tragedy of amnesia. And without common memory, there is no community.

The church sets Scripture apart, calls it "Holy Scripture," and sets apart a time and a place to read it. By reading it the church remembers its story, and then sets all the stories of their lives alongside it to be tested and made new by it. It sets the stories of our sexual lives, our economic lives, our political lives, our dying and our caring for the dying alongside Scripture to be challenged, qualified, and sanctified by it. It is not a rule book. It does not give us a timeless code. But it does give us the story we love to tell and long to live. To live the remembered story requires both fidelity and creativity. It will require both discipline and discernment. There is no recipe for discernment, but reading Scripture together the church and its members can begin to see whether certain acts and practices fit the story or not, whether certain deeds and dispositions are worthy of the gospel or not. By reading Scripture the church remembers the story that is constitutive of its identity and determinative for its discernment.

I hope this practice of the church has been on display in this book. In regarding Scripture as somehow normative for our dying well and faithfully, I have simply taken a cue provided by *Ars Moriendi* (and, of course, by the larger Christian tradition as well). By rereading Scripture and by remembering Jesus, I have tried to test both the medicalized death of the mid–twentieth century and the *Ars Moriendi* of the fifteenth century. I have tried to set the stories of our dying alongside the remembered story in the hope that they may be re-formed by it.

The practice of reading Scripture as somehow normative for discernment belongs to the church, of course, not to one minor theologian within the church. My work is not intended to be a substitute for the church's reading of Scripture, nor to be a substitute for the communal work of discernment of ways of dying and caring that are fitting to the story. The intention is much more modest, to contribute to the community's task.[3]

3. The significance of the practice of reading Scripture as determinative for discern-

The Practice of Prayer

When the church is gathered by God's grace and call, it also prays.[4] In the gathered church we learn to pray. A wise and wonderful teacher once told me that in the practices of reading Scripture and prayer, we not only commune with God but also find new strength — new virtue — for our daily lives. I won't tell you whether that teacher was a theology professor or my mother, but she was right. And *Ars Moriendi*, of course, insisted that with prayer we may nurture the strength, the courage, the virtues for dying well. We need to heed that advice, and not just on a Sunday in church. We need to take that advice with us to the hospital, to the nursing home, to the hospice, to all the places we endure and care in the face of sickness and suffering, pain and death. These practices may provide strength — and virtue — for our dying and for our caring for the dying. To emphasize this practice in the formation of virtues for dying well and faithfully is simply to take yet another cue from *Ars Moriendi*.

Earlier in this book, while complaining about the silence and surrender of the church, we told the story Robert Coles told of a Catholic friend of his, a physician become a patient who knew his cancer would not likely be beaten back, a Christian who knew that the final triumph belongs to the risen Christ.[5] He wanted and needed someone with whom to talk of God, someone with whom to talk to God. What he got instead was a visit from a chaplain who neglected the practices of piety for the sake of the "religionless" and generic language of psychology. He seemed more familiar with Kübler-Ross than with Scripture. He dwelt on the stages of dying as if they were "Stations of the Cross." Coles's friend got angry with the chaplain, calling him a "psychobabbling fool." And Robert Coles, the emi-

---

ment stands at the center of my earlier works, *Remembering Jesus: Christian Community, Scripture, and the Moral Life* (Grand Rapids: Eerdmans, 2002) and *Reading the Bible in the Strange World of Medicine* (Grand Rapids: Eerdmans, 2003). For a fuller account of this practice and its significance, the interested reader may consult either of these works. The significance of the practice for decisions at the end of life is treated especially in *Remembering Jesus*, pp. 79-154. The practice is brought to bear on the question of physician-assisted suicide in *Reading the Bible*, pp. 304-44.

4. This section on the practice of prayer draws upon my essay "The Practice of Prayer and Care for the Dying," in *Living Well and Dying Faithfully: Christian Perspectives on End-of-Life Care*, ed. John Swinton and Richard Payne (Grand Rapids: Eerdmans, 2009), pp. 86-106.

5. Robert Coles, "Psychiatric Stations of the Cross," in *Harvard Diary: Reflection on the Sacred and the Profane* (New York: Crossroad, 1990), pp. 10-12.

nent Harvard psychiatrist, agreed. What his friend needed, he said, was some "good hard praying."

There has been a good deal of attention lately to the question of whether prayer is effective therapeutically.[6] That is not the question here. Indeed, when prayer is rendered a technology in the service of medicine, when it is authorized or judged in terms of its therapeutic effectiveness, as an alternative or supplementary medical technology, then prayer has been corrupted. Then it is no longer a practice of piety but a practice of medicine, attentive not to God but to something other than God, something for which God and prayer may (or may not) be useful. And then the practice of prayer can hardly be expected to re-form our dying or our care for the dying. Our question is not whether prayer is medically useful; our question is whether the practice of prayer can guide and govern our dying and our care for the dying, whether we can set medicine in the practice of prayer, not prayer in the practice of medicine.

We may nevertheless take courage for the task from the simple fact that prayer is as commonplace in hospitals as bedpans, indeed as commonplace in hospitals as it is in churches. Think of that: as noisily secular as modern medicine is, this practice of piety is commonplace. When people hurt and suffer, when they face death, we are not surprised to find them under the care of a physician and in a hospital — and we are not surprised to find them praying.[7] To be sure, sometimes such prayers seem to regard God as a divine last resort, a heavenly pharmacopoeia. But the simple fact that prayer is commonplace suggests that it is not unreasonable — and may be important — to ask how a faithful practice of prayer can and does and should guide and challenge the ways we endure pain and suffering and dying and the ways we attend to the sick and dying. (At the very least, ethicists like me should find it curious that large numbers of patients — and large numbers of doctors and nurses, too — keep calling on God for guidance rather than on the "experts" in medical ethics.)

Suppose that the chaplain, chastened by the angry rebuke of Coles's friend, resolves to visit Coles's friend one more time, this time to pray — and suppose we go with him in an effort to learn perhaps how the practice of prayer might govern and guide our dying and our care for the dying.

6. See the discussion (and critique) of the social scientific studies of the healing power of prayer in Daniel Sulmasy, *The Rebirth of the Clinic: An Introduction to Spirituality in Health Care* (Washington, D.C.: Georgetown University Press, 2006), pp. 147-60.

7. Perhaps that is why some seem intent on co-opting prayer, rendering it serviceable to the therapeutic ends of medicine.

Why Prayer Is Important

"We have heard that you want to pray," we say. "But before we begin, may we ask why prayer is so important to you?" His reply, I imagine, would go something like this: "It is important because I am a Christian and because I long to live the Christian life, even in the dying of it, and prayer is part of the Christian life. Indeed, it is, as John Calvin said, the most important part, 'the chief exercise of faith.'[8] Moreover, it is a part of the whole Christian life that cannot be left out without the whole ceasing to be the Christian life. The Christian life is a life of prayer. It is, as Karl Barth said, a life of 'humble and resolute, frightened and joyful invocation of the gracious God in gratitude, praise, and above all petition.'"[9]

Well, perhaps his response would not go exactly like that. Not many people quote Calvin and Barth in their hospital rooms, and fewer Catholics. Perhaps his reply would rather go something like this: "Prayer is important to me because it is a practice of piety. As you know, chaplain, Alasdair MacIntyre defined a practice as a 'form of socially established cooperative human activity through which goods internal to that form of activity are realized in the course of trying to achieve those standards of excellence which are appropriate to, and partially definitive of, that form of activity with the result that human powers to achieve excellence and human conceptions of the ends and goods involved are systematically extended.'"[10]

Well, OK, probably not. But even if he has not memorized an important and difficult passage from MacIntyre's *After Virtue*, even if he has never read a philosopher or a theologian, he may still make a reply to which John Calvin, Karl Barth, and Alasdair MacIntyre would nod their heads and say, "Yes, that's what I meant."

He is a Christian. He has learned to pray in the Christian community. And in learning to pray, he has learned as well the good that is intrinsic to prayer. He has learned, that is, to attend to God, to look to God. And he has learned it not just intellectually, not just as an idea. In learning to pray, he has learned a human activity that engages his body as well as his

8. John Calvin, *Institutes of the Christian Religion*, ed. John T. McNeill, trans. Ford Lewis Battles (Philadelphia: Westminster, 1960), 3.20.1.

9. Karl Barth, *The Christian Life:* Church Dogmatics *IV/4, Lecture Fragments*, trans. Geoffrey Bromiley (Grand Rapids: Eerdmans, 1981), p. 43.

10. Alasdair MacIntyre, *After Virtue: A Study in Moral Theory* (Notre Dame, Ind.: University of Notre Dame Press, 1981), p. 175.

mind, his affections and passions and loyalty as well as his rationality, and that focuses his whole self on God.

To attend to God is not easy to learn — or painless. And given our inveterate attention to ourselves and to our own needs and wants, we frequently corrupt prayer. We corrupt prayer whenever we turn it into a means to accomplish some other good than the good of prayer, whenever we make of it an instrument to achieve wealth or happiness or life or health or moral improvement.

In learning to pray, Coles's friend has learned to look to God and, after the blinding vision, to begin to look at all else in a new light. In prayer he does not attend to something beyond God, which God — or prayer — might be used in order to reach; he attends to God.[11] That is the good intrinsic to prayer, the good "internal to that form of activity."

In learning to pray, he has learned as well certain standards of excellence[12] that belong to prayer and its attention to God, that are "appropriate to" prayer and "partially definitive" of prayer. He has learned *reverence,* the readiness to attend to God as God and to attend to all else in his life as related to God. He has learned *humility,* the readiness to acknowledge that we are not gods, but the creatures of God, cherished by God, but finite and mortal and, yes, sinful creatures in need finally of God's grace and God's future. He has learned *gratitude,* a disposition of thankfulness for the opportunities within the limits of our finiteness and mortality to delight in God and in the gifts of God. Attentive to God, he has learned *care;* attentive to God, he grows attentive to the neighbor as related to God. He has learned to care even for those who are least, to care especially for those who hurt and cry out to high heaven in anguish. Looking to God, he has learned *hope,* a disposition of confidence and courage that comes not from trusting oneself and the little truth one knows well or the little good one does well, but from trusting the grace and power of God.

These standards of excellence form virtues not only for prayer but also for daily life. The prayer-formed person — in the whole of her being and in all of her doing — will be reverent, humble, grateful, caring, and

11. On prayer as attention see especially Iris Murdoch, "On 'God' and 'Good,'" in *Revisions: Changing Perspectives in Moral Philosophy,* ed. Stanley Hauerwas and Alasdair MacIntyre (Notre Dame, Ind.: University of Notre Dame Press, 1983), pp. 68-91.

12. Consider John Calvin's attention to the "rules" of prayer in *Institutes* 3.20.4-16. Calvin's "rules" are reverence, a sincere sense of want (i.e., to pray earnestly), humility, and confident hope.

hopeful.[13] One does not pray in order to achieve those virtues. They are not formed when we use prayer as a technique. But they are formed in simple attentiveness to God, and they spill over into new virtues for daily life — and for dying and caring for the dying.

"That's why prayer is so important to me," Coles's friend might conclude. "That's why I called it the 'chief exercise of faith,'" Calvin might say. "That's why I said the Christian life was 'invocation,'" Barth might say. "That's what I meant by a 'practice,'" MacIntyre might add. And if I may add my own word here, that's how we can begin to see the links between this practice of piety and the practice of medicine, between our praying and our dying and our caring for the dying. We can try to envision the prayer-formed patient and the prayer-formed physician and the prayer-formed community that supports and sustains them both.

Invocation and Adoration

We are ready at last to offer prayer with Coles's friend. "And how should we begin?" we ask, and he replies, "With invocation, of course, for prayer is to call upon God and to adore God as the one on whom we depend."[14]

To call upon God is to recall who God is and what God has done. It requires remembrance,[15] for we invoke not just any old god, not some nameless god of philosophical theism, not some idolatrous object of someone's "ultimate concern," but the God remembered in religious community and in other practices of piety, especially the practice of reading

13. See Donald Saliers, "Liturgy and Ethics: Some New Beginnings," *Journal of Religious Ethics* 7 (Fall 1979): 173-89: because prayer is a "characterizing activity," the standards of excellence that belong to prayer are formed in those who practice prayer.

14. I take as my guide for the components of prayer, or the forms of attention to God, the acronym ACTS: adoration, confession, thanksgiving, and supplication. I learned it in Sunday school many years ago and learned to appreciate it in the congregational prayers of Rev. Ren Broekhuizen. William F. May, "Images That Shape the Public Obligations of the Minister," *Bulletin of the Park Ridge Center* 4, no. 1 (January 1989): 20-37, considers the same set of components. Notably (and regrettably) absent from both lists is lament. In a thoughtful recent little book on prayer, however, by Martha Moore-Keish, *Christian Prayer for Today* (Louisville: Westminster John Knox, 2009), lament is included as a mode of prayer along with adoration, confession, thanksgiving, and supplication; she calls it "a five-finger exercise" (p. 60).

15. On prayer as an act of remembrance, see Nicholas Wolterstorff, "Justice and Worship: The Tragedy of Liturgy in Protestantism," in his *Until Justice and Peace Embrace* (Grand Rapids: Eerdmans, 1983), pp. 146-61, especially 152, 154-56. Donald Saliers, "Liturgy and Ethics," p. 178, also emphasizes that "the shape and substance of prayer is *anamnetic*."

Scripture. Invocation is remembrance, and remembrance is not just recollection but the way identity and community are constituted. So we invoke the God made known in mighty works and great promises, and as we do we are oriented to that God and to all things in relation to that God.

We invoke God as *creator;* and as we do we learn to make neither life nor choice an idol; for nothing God made is god. That is a good and simple gift to medical ethics, when talk of "the sanctity of life" would sometimes require our friend to make every effort to preserve his life and when "respect for autonomy" would prohibit every moral question besides "Who should decide?"

We invoke God as creator; and as we do, we learn as well not to turn our back to life or to choice; for all that God made is good. That, too, is a good and simple gift to medical ethics, when a "compassionate" doctor would kill or when another would exercise some arbitrary power to keep Coles's friend alive.

We invoke God as creator; and as we do, we learn to refuse to reduce the embodied selves God made either to mere organisms or merely to their capacities for agency. And resistance to both forms of reductionism is a gift to medical ethics both at the beginnings and at the endings of life, and in all the care between as well.

Then we invoke God as the *provider.* We do so in remembrance that God has heard the cries of those who hurt, that God has cared. We do so in remembrance of one who suffered and died, and we attend to that cross as the place the truth about our world was nailed. The truth about our world is the horrible reality of suffering and death. The truth about our world is the power of evil in the story of the cross and in the myriad sad stories others tell with and of their bodies. The truth about our world is dripping with blood and hanging on a cross, but the same cross that points to the reality and power of evil also points to the real presence of God and to the constant care of God.

So, in invocation and remembrance we learn again that in spite of sickness, in spite of cancer, in spite of death's apparent triumph, God's care is the world's constant companion and our friend's constant companion. Invocation and remembrance do not deny the sad truth about our world or about our friend; they do not provide any magic charm against death or sickness; they do not provide a tidy theodicy to "justify" God and the ways of God.[16]

16. See Stanley Hauerwas, *Naming the Silences: God, Medicine, and the Problem of Suffering* (Grand Rapids: Eerdmans, 1983).

But by attention to this God we may learn that God is present in spite of sickness and death, that God cares, that God suffers with those who hurt, even in places no medicine can touch.

Then our friend — and every patient — may cry out, "God, why?" and still be assured that he is not abandoned by God. And the rest of us — including the physicians among us — may be formed by such a prayer and by such a providence to embody care even when medicine cannot cure, to be present to the sick even when our powers to heal have failed, to resist the temptation to abandon the patient who reminds us of our weakness — and the great weakness of our great medical powers.

Such prayer is not an alternative to medicine, "not a supplement to the insufficiency of our medical knowledge"[17] and skill; rather, it forms and sustains as a standard of excellence in both medical practice and communal life simple presence to the sick — and a simple refusal to abandon them to their hurt. Such invocation and such a prayer-formed medicine will not always triumph over disease or death, but it will always gesture care in the midst of them and in spite of them.

We will return to these themes of lament and care before we leave the practice of prayer, but for now note that we invoke God also as *redeemer* and as healer. We make such invocation, too, of course, in remembrance of Jesus and, indeed, in the name of Jesus, hoping for the good future Jesus announced and made real and present by his works of healing and his words of blessing, the good future God made sure by raising him from the dead.

As we invoke this God, as we attend to the redeemer and healer in prayer, we orient ourselves and our lives and our medicine — along with our prayers — to God's promises and claims. So a prayerful people and a prayer-formed medicine will celebrate and toast life, not death, but they will be enabled to endure even dying with hope. A prayerful people and a prayer-formed medicine will delight in human flourishing, including the human flourishing we call health. They will not welcome the dwindling of human strength to be human, including the loss of strength called sickness, but they will be enabled to endure also that in the confidence that God's grace is sufficient (cf. 2 Cor. 12:9).

A prayer-formed community will not despise medicine, as if to turn to medicine were to turn against God and God's grace. Medicine is a good

17. Stanley Hauerwas, *Suffering Presence* (Notre Dame, Ind.: University of Notre Dame Press, 1986), p. 81.

gift of God the creator, a gracious provision of God the provider, and a reflection and servant of God the redeemer. To condemn medicine because God is the healer would be like condemning government because God is the ruler, or condemning families because God is "Abba."

Of course, if medicine presumes for itself the role of faithful savior or ultimate healer, then its arrogance may be and must be condemned. One cannot invoke the one true God and take a presumptuous medicine too seriously (or a presumptuous state or a presumptuous parent). Perhaps Coles's friend, like other good and honest doctors, is less tempted to this sort of idolatrous and extravagant expectation of medicine than many other patients who sometimes enter the hospital speaking some version of the line from Auden: "We who must die demand a miracle."[18] But when we invoke God as redeemer, we are freed from the vanity and illusion of wielding human power to defeat mortality or to eliminate the human vulnerability to suffering. An honest prayer could "let the air out of inflationary"[19] medical promises and restore a modest medicine to its rightful place alongside other measures that protect and promote life and health, like good nutrition, public sanitation, a clean environment, and the like.

One thing more here: a prayer-formed people, celebrating life and health as the good gifts and wonderful promises of God, will acknowledge in remembrance of Jesus that a life oriented to the kingdom may be shorter and harder, for there are goods more important than our own survival, and there are duties more compelling than our ease.

Confession

Having made invocation, we pause to ask whether we should continue. Coles's friend says, "Yes," and we ask, "How?" "With prayers of confession, of course," he says, "for those who have invoked God can make no pretense to be worthy of God's care and presence. Those oriented to God are reoriented to all else; it is called, I think, *metanoia,* a turning, repentance."

It seems obvious to us that we have no major-league sinner here, but we humor him. "What would you confess?" we ask. "Are you a smoker?"

---

18. W. H. Auden, *For the Time Being,* in W. H. Auden, *Collected Poems,* ed. Edward Mendelson (London: Faber and Faber, 2007), p. 253.

19. See May, "Images," p. 25, concerning prayers of invocation and adoration and their effect on political rhetoric.

"That, too," he says. "But I see a reflection of my life in my doctor, and I don't like it. I have been where she is, angry at the patient who refuses another round of therapy, angry at her powerlessness to save him, eager to use her authority as a physician to convince him to try again, and eager to avoid him when he refuses to try again or dies before she can try again. It is no great callousness I confess; it is the failure to acknowledge the fallibility and limits of medical care.[20]

"And now I find myself where my patients have been; and I don't like it much better, angry at the doctor who cannot deliver a miracle, judging her much too quickly and severely, angrier still that she would try to tell me how to live while I am dying, and eager to render her still more powerless and optionless. It is no great callousness I confess here either; it is the failure to acknowledge the fallibility and limits of my own autonomy."

Confession is good for the soul, of course, but it also serves discernment. It helps us see the fallibility of both medicine and patients. It helps us recognize the evil we sometimes do in resisting evil, the suffering we sometimes inflict in the effort to banish suffering and those who remind us of it.[21]

A prayer of confession, this form of attention to God, may help the dying to turn from despising the doctor because the doctor is a reminder of his sickness and mortality. And it may help the doctor to turn both from the disposition to abandon the patient because the patient is a reminder of her powerlessness to save him and from any readiness to eliminate suffering by eliminating the sufferer.

A prayer of confession may form the possibility of a continuing conversation. When assertion of authority by a physician would ordinarily have put a stop to an argument and reduced the patient to manipulable nature, a prayer of confession may enable the conversation to continue.[22] And when the assertion of autonomy by a patient would ordinarily have put a stop to a discussion and reduced the physician to an animated tool, a prayer of confession may enable the conversation to continue. We may at

20. See Douglas Anderson, "The Physician Experience: Witnessing Numinous Reality," *Second Opinion* 13 (March 1990): 111-22, especially 117-22, which focus on confession, the freedom it gives from being "blinded by the utopian images arising from uncritical overestimations of technology's power" (pp. 121-22) and the freedom it gives for presence to those who hurt or grieve.

21. See further Hauerwas, *Suffering Presence.*

22. See further Allen Verhey, "Christian Community and Identity: What Difference Do They Make to Patients and Physicians Finally?" *Linacre Quarterly* 52 (May 1985): 149-69.

least talk together longer and listen to each other better if in confession we turn from the pretense of being either final judge or final savior, for we are formed by prayers of confession to be critical without condescension and helpful without conceit. And that is a good and simple gift to medical practice and to medical ethics.

"Moreover," our friend continues, "when we make prayers of confession, we are prompted to be forgiving ourselves. As we stand praying for forgiveness, we are to forgive others (Mark 11:25-26). The practice of prayer in the form of confession supports and sustains another practice of Christian community, the practice of forgiveness. The grace of God upon which we depend can be quite demanding, requiring that we forgive those who have hurt us (e.g., Matt. 18:23-35) and that we ask forgiveness also of those whom we have hurt (e.g., Matt. 5:23-24). Prayers of confession nurture the humility necessary for reconciliation with those we will leave behind." He does not ask for forgiveness in order to become more forgiving, but he does become more forgiving — and for the tasks of dying well and faithfully he must.

Thanksgiving

"There are prayers of thanksgiving to be made as well," our friend says, and he begins to mention gifts great and small. And not the least among the gifts for which he gives thanks are opportunities to fulfill some tasks, great and small. He thanks God for a little time to be reconciled with an enemy and for enough relief from pain for the tasks of fun with the family. He gives thanks for the opportunity and the task of being a witness, a "martyr," he says, to demonstrate even in his dying that some things are more important than mere survival, and that many things are more to be feared than death. There is a gift here to medicine and to medical ethics in the simple and joyful acknowledgment that the sick and dying are still living, that they may not be reduced to the passivity of their sick role. Moreover, their choices may not be regarded simply in term of the arbitrary self-assertiveness of their autonomy. The sick and dying have tasks and opportunities that must be considered both by themselves and by their caregivers.

Among those tasks and opportunities is the simple and joyful one of saying thanks to those who have enriched his life and to those who have challenged him, to those upon whose care he has depended and to those who allowed him to care for them. "In prayers of thanksgiving to God," he says, "I am reminded to be grateful also to those who have been gifts of God. There are so many, I wish I had started long ago. I wish there was more time for the tasks of gratitude."

Lament

Then our friend mentions one more gift for which he is thankful. He gives thanks to God, he says, that he does not always have to give thanks to God. He is grateful, he says, that he does not always have to be grateful. The psalms of lament have been a gift, he says, and he follows them by attending to God sometimes in the form of *lament*,[23] crying out to God and against God in anger and in anguish.

The first gift, he says, was simply noticing that they are there, included in that songbook of the Second Temple and in the story of the cross. In ancient Israel the practices of faith allowed for the expression not only of praise and joy but also of grief and doubt and fear and anger. They not only acknowledged the reality of such emotions, they also gave them social sanction. The community of faith gave the suffering a voice, and lament gave the voice of the sufferer form and direction. In contemporary liturgical practices, however, one seldom finds lament. We make little room for the cry of anguish in our prayer books. Even our funeral liturgies rush to talk about the life and the light that death and darkness cannot overcome. Little wonder, I suppose; lament is hardly "good news." Little wonder, but still a pity, for we neglect the cry of anguish to our harm and to the harm of our communities.

When we leave aside the language of lament, we obscure the hurtful realities of human experience and drive both suffering and response to suffering outside the practice of our faith. We marginalize, then, not only suffering but also sufferers. When we make so little room in liturgy for lament, then in their hurt and their anger and their sense of absurdity, sufferers think they sit alone in the congregation. They must struggle to lift themselves by their bootstraps to the heights of some triumphant liturgy. When we neglect lament, we alienate the suffering from worship and from community precisely when they need both the most. Lament had a place in ancient liturgies. Where is it in ours?

If we retrieve lament, we may again give the suffering voice and pre-

---

23. On lament see the works cited above on p. 227 n. 16.

serve for them a place in the community. Those who suffer might realize that they may cry out to God in anger and in anguish and that, when they do, they are not alienated from the community. If we retrieve lament, the rest of us gain some leverage against our triumphalism — both against our spiritual triumphalism that supposes that righteousness and faith provide a charm against sickness and sadness and that prayer works like magic to end our suffering and to ensure our flourishing, and also against our medical triumphalism that supposes that some new piece of medical wizardry will finally rescue us from the human condition with its vulnerability to death and suffering. If we retrieve lament, we may also renew our capacity for genuine compassion, for we may learn again to give the suffering a voice, to preserve for them a place in community, to be present to those who suffer.

In lament suffering finds a voice looking heavenward. By its attention to God it may be contrasted to a dirge. In a dirge, notably in David's dirge at the death of Saul and Jonathan in 2 Samuel 1:19-27, God is not addressed or even mentioned. The dead are eulogized, but the decisive feature of this and every dirge, as we have noted before, is the contrast between past glories and present misery. The greatness of Saul and Jonathan is remembered, but the refrain and conclusion of David's dirge call attention to the great contrast of the present, "How the mighty have fallen!" Once Saul and Jonathan were "swifter than eagles, . . . stronger than lions," but *now* "how the mighty have fallen!" The "tragic reversal" of the dirge moves from glory to shame, from strength to powerlessness. It is suffering finding a voice, to be sure, but in lament, in this form of attention to God, there is a reversal of the reversal. Looking heavenward, lament moves from distress toward wholeness, from powerlessness to the certainty of a hearing, from anger toward confidence in God's justice, from guilt toward the assurance of God's forgiveness. The distress and powerlessness and anger and guilt are still there, still finding voice, but the very form of the lament moves sufferers toward their share in Israel's faith that a saving reversal — and not the tragic reversal — is the pattern of their existence. Attention to God allows the pattern to change, but it does not disallow the sorrow. Looking heavenward in lament helps the sufferer both to find words that express the pain and to find hope for a saving reversal, to find words and works that nurture the reconstruction of a faithful identity, a faithful direction.

There is no pretense here, no denial, no withdrawal to some otherworldly consolation. Lament calls faith and worship to deal with life as it comes to us. To look to God is not to look away. Moreover, the psalms of lament show clearly that biblical faith — as it faces life fully and honestly — is without embarrassment communal. The ones who suffer have to do with God, and God has to do with them. The ones who suffer have to do with the community, and the community has to do with them. The ones who lament know that they need not fake it or be polite in the presence of God and of God's people,[24] and they know that they need not face the hurt alone. They may also know that God does not neglect their cry, that Christ weeps in their tears. They may believe the reversal of the reversal. But even if they cannot get so far, even if they do not share just now the faith of the church, even if they have no certainty of a hearing (like the author of Psalm 88, the saddest of the laments),[25] still they may know that the community accepts their cry as their own cry, that the community believes for them even in their doubt, that the community keeps faith with them — and *for* them — even in their lack of faith just now.

Petition

There is little time left when we turn finally from lament to *petition,* and we apologize a little, but our friend will have no apologies. "Prayer is not magic," he says. "It is not a way to put God at my disposal. It is the way to put myself at God's disposal. It is not a technique to get what I want,[26] either a fortune or fourteen more healthy years. It is not a spiritual technique to be pulled out as a last resort when medical technologies have failed. Prayer is not a means, not even a 'means to make God present.'[27] It attends to God; and as it does, it discovers in memory and hope that God *is* present. To treat prayer as a means to some other good than the good that

24. To be sure, the lament gave both form and limits to the venting of emotions. Indeed, if there were no forms and limits for the expression of rage and sorrow, then perhaps politeness would be reasonably preferred. The forms and limits not only make the venting of emotions communally manageable, however; they also help, as we have seen, to give direction to the sufferer, to help encompass the hurt within a faithful identity.

25. See Allen Verhey, "Meditation: Is the Last Word 'Darkness'?" in *Medical Ethics: Looking Back, Looking Forward,* ed. Allen Verhey (Grand Rapids: Eerdmans, 1996), pp. 142-50.

26. Henry Stob, "Prayer and Providence," in his *Theological Reflections* (Grand Rapids: Eerdmans, 1981), p. 91: "[At] the bottom, and in its purest state, prayer is not a way to get things out of God, but rather to receive what he freely offers — fellowship with himself. At the heart of prayer is *communion.*"

27. Against Hauerwas, *Suffering Presence,* p. 81.

315

belongs to prayer makes prayer a superstition and trivializes God into some 'great scalpel in the sky.'"[28]

"May we not then make petition together?" we ask, a little shocked. "Of course we can," he says. "But carefully, for here it is easy to attend to ourselves rather than to God, and to our wishes rather than to God's cause."

So we form our petitions on the model of the one to whom we attend. We pray — and pray boldly — that God's name and power may be hallowed, that God's kingdom may come, that God's good future will be established "speedily and soon"[29] — in this man's own lifetime. And because that good future is *already* established, we pray — and pray boldly — as the Lord taught us, for a taste of that future, for a taste of it in such ordinary things as everyday bread and everyday forgiveness, in such ordinary things as tonight's rest and tomorrow's life, in such mundane stuff as the workings of mortal flesh, and in the healing of our embodied and communal selves. But because that good future is *not yet* — still sadly not yet — we may continue to make lament and to pray no less boldly for the presence of the one who suffers with us, the one who made the human cry of lament his own cry, the one who hurts in our pain. We pray no less boldly for that than for the power of the one who promises in God's good future to raise up and heal us: "the redemption of our bodies" (Rom. 8:23).

Praying for a Miracle

"Shall we pray for a miracle?" we ask. And then, a bit surprised that our friend hesitates, evidently a bit unsure of how to respond, we ask, "But don't you believe in miracles?"

He seems a little irritated, as though we had failed to pay attention to what he had been saying. "Of course I believe in miracles," he says. "The good news is a miracle. The Word made flesh, made vulnerable to suffering

28. Interior quotation from William F. May, *The Physician's Covenant* (Philadelphia: Westminster, 1983), p. 60.

29. The Lord's Prayer was modeled after the Kaddish, which was (and — in an expanded form — still is) used in synagogue services. Joachim Jeremias, *The Prayers of Jesus*, Studies in Biblical Theology, 2nd ser., 8 (London: SCM, 1967), p. 98, offers this reconstruction of the oldest form of this prayer: "Exalted and hallowed be his great name in the world which he created according to his will. May he let his kingdom rule in your lifetime and in your days and in the lifetime of the whole house of Israel, speedily and soon."

and death like all flesh, that's a miracle. The love of God that makes the human cry of lament God's own cry, that's a miracle. The love of God that is stronger than death, that's a miracle. In Auden's *For the Time Being,* that's the miracle needed and demanded by those who must die. That's the miracle I needed and need. The gospel is hilariously good news — even and especially as I approach my death.

"Of course I believe in miracles," he says. "But by the grace of God's miraculous love I am made God's servant, not God, mine. Prayer is not some magic that puts God at my disposal. It is not some technology of last resort to be pulled out when nature and conventional technologies have failed. Prayer is simple attention to God in adoration, confession, and gratitude. Isn't that what I have been saying?"

"Yes," we say, "you said that. But you also said that it was petition. And when faithful people pray, they often ask God for good things. And when they encounter threats to their well-being or to the well-being of those they love, they frequently cry out to God for help. Yesterday a child was brought to the emergency room, bleeding and broken, after being hit by a car, and when his mother arrived shortly after the ambulance, she just repeated again and again, 'Oh, God, please let him be all right!' Was that simply presumptuous? And when the author of this little narrative in which we are characters was himself near death, his good and faithful wife told God, 'I want this old fart to live, and you should too.' Was that simply presumptuous?"

Our friend smiles a little at the last story. "That last one might be a little presumptuous, I suppose, but no more presumptuous than many of the psalms of lament. But you misunderstand my reticence to ask for a miracle. It is altogether appropriate for faithful people to ask God to bless them with good things. God promises a good future, and that good future is full of good things. It is fitting that faithful people cry out to God in their suffering. They are sheep who know something of a good shepherd, and it is fitting and proper that sheep bleat when they are hurting. I have cried out to God myself a good deal lately."

"So what's the problem with praying for a miracle, then?" we ask.

Our friend pauses for a moment or two before answering. Finally, he says, "Well, first of all, I worry that praying for a miracle can be a form of the denial of death, as if when the technology does not deliver us from our mortality a prayer still might. Perhaps you remember the story of Baby Rena. She was an eighteen-month-old child, dying from AIDS and heart disease. She had spent six weeks in the intensive care unit of Children's

Hospital in Washington, D.C. She was on a respirator and in so much pain that she had to be constantly sedated. The simplest procedures, like weighing her, prompted tears of pain and so much anguish that her blood pressure shot up. The doctor thought that further efforts to keep her alive were 'futile' and could only prolong her suffering on her way to her death. He thought that caring for Baby Rena should focus now on medication to ease her pain rather than on the technology to keep her alive. When he suggested removing Baby Rena from the respirator, however, her foster parents rejected his suggestion. They were praying for a miracle, they said, and refused to consent to the removal of Baby Rena from the respirator.[30] I leave aside the obvious point that if God is going to do a miracle, God does not depend on the respirator. The more compelling point, I think, is how closely this praying for a miracle parallels the denial of death in medicalized dying. It is the same refusal to acknowledge the limits of our finitude, the same refusal to acknowledge our mortality and the mortality of those we love. It is the same tightfisted and avaricious hanging on to biological life, and it gestures the same anxiety that death may have the last word. It is sad but not unfaithful to let a beloved child die when it is suffering its way to its death. It may be 'pious' but still unfaithful to presume that the triumph over death is in our hands — if not in some physician's hands, then in our hands when they are folded in prayer.

"But there is a second point related to that first one. I worry that praying for a miracle may divert me from the task at hand, from the task, that is, of dying well and faithfully. Like the 'false cheering' that *Ars Moriendi* warned against, like the deception that attended medicalized dying, praying for a miracle may divert me from the tasks of forgiveness and reconciliation, saying good-by to those I love, and attending to the care of those I will leave behind. In stunning contrast to the story of Baby Rena, when Dayna and Eric Olson-Getty learned that the baby they were expecting and already cherishing had a fatal birth defect (acrania, so the skull never forms), they decided not to pray for a miracle.[31] They had friends who reported that they were praying for a miracle, but the Olson-Gettys did not join them. From the story Dayna Olson-Getty told it was clear that they already loved this child, whom they named Ethan; it was

30. The story was told by Benjamin Weiser, "A Question of Letting Go," *Washington Post*, July 14, 1991, p. 1, and retold by Vigen Guroian, *Life's Living toward Dying* (Grand Rapids: Eerdmans, 1996), pp. 67-75.

31. The story was told by Dayna Olson-Getty, "Life Expectancy: On Not Praying for a Miracle," *Christian Century*, September 22, 2009, pp. 11-12.

clear that they were people of deep faith and faithfulness; and it was clear that they were committed to care for this child, however 'achingly short' their time with him would be. While still waiting for the birth (and death) of Ethan, Dayna wrote, 'But I am not praying for a miracle. I am not capable of praying for healing while simultaneously preparing for Ethan's death. I have to choose one or the other — the two possibilities are simply too much for me to hold together. Eric and I have only this one opportunity, now, in these days of waiting to parent Ethan well. We don't want to waste this precious opportunity by denying the reality that his life will be very short or by failing to acknowledge that what he needs most from us is our preparation to care for him in his dying.' They prepared a plan with their hospice team to be sure Ethan would be 'protected from pain and surrounded by love.' They made other preparations for his short life, for his funeral service, and for his burial. It was a story of faith and hope and love, a story of patience and humility and letting go, a story of courage to face the death of a dearly desired child in the comfort (the *com-fortis*, the strengthening) of the faithful love of God. Dayna did not call attention to the virtues they had displayed, but she did report this: 'I have not been praying for the miracle of his healing, but I have been taking great comfort in the miracle that is already assured — the miracle that Ethan's life will not end with his death.' That's it exactly, you see. She and Eric believed in the miracle of the resurrection, in the miracle that God's love is stronger than death, and because they did, they did not use 'praying for a miracle' as a way to deny death or allow 'praying for a miracle' to divert them from the task of dealing well and faithfully with Ethan's dying.

"These are stories about parents dealing with their children dying, but I recognize in myself the temptations to deny death and to allow myself to be diverted from the tasks of dealing well and faithfully with my own dying. Those are my worries about 'praying for a miracle.'

"And there is one more worry. I worry that 'praying for a miracle' always seems to mean praying for a miraculous cure. It fails to recognize the other ways in which the good future of God comes upon us as we are dying. That is, after all, what the miracles of Jesus were about. 'The miracles of Jesus were all "miracles of the kingdom," evidence that God's sovereignty was breaking in, with a new effectiveness, upon the confusions of a rebellious world.'[32] That is at least what Jesus said: 'But if it is by the finger

32. G. B. Caird, cited in C. F. D. Moule, *Man and Nature in the New Testament* (London: Athlone Press, 1964), p. 17.

of God that I cast out the demons, then the kingdom of God has come to you' (Luke 11:20). That good future comes upon us and is effective among us also in a faith that is not anxious, in a hope that gives courage, and in a love that forgives and is patient. It comes upon us in the Spirit whose fruit is 'love, joy, peace, patience, kindness, generosity, faithfulness, gentleness, and self-control' (Gal. 5:22-23). So, yes, I invite you to pray for a miracle. Pray that the good future of God will be displayed even in my dying, that the Spirit, the promise and guarantee of that future, will bear some fruit even in the confusions of my rebellious heart.

"I know that in God's good future by God's grace I have a part. I know that death will not have the last word. So pray, if you like, that I shall live, but please recognize that such a prayer may be answered on the far side of my death."

We pray then for the presence and the power of the Spirit as he is dying. We do not — and I think we may not — pray for death. Death is not the cause of God. In the good future of God death will be no more. Attending to God rather than to ourselves, to God's cause rather than to our own wishes, we are unlikely to bring a petition for death to our lips. Until that good future comes, however, there will sometimes be good reasons to cease praying for a patient's survival. Attending to God in confident hope of God's final triumph frees us from desperately holding on to this life, frees us to let go of it, leaving it in the hands of the one who can be trusted.[33]

Perhaps only a prayer-formed person will see clearly that there is an important moral difference not only between praying for someone's death

---

33. Incidentally, these questions of what we may pray for are interesting and illuminating moral questions. They are found in the Talmud and in the early theologians of the church, but they are not found in the recent literature on medical ethics. Consider, for example, the wonderful story and subsequent debates about the behavior of Rabbi Judah's maid in the Babylonian Talmud, tractate *Ketubbot* 104A. The maid saw Rabbi Judah's unrelieved suffering and, in fact, "prayed that it should be God's will that the immortal [angels who wanted his death] should win over the mortal [humans, who did not]." When the rabbi's gathered colleagues continued to pray for his survival, she dropped a jar from the roof. When it crashed onto the ground, the rabbis stopped praying, and Rabbi Judah died. On this story and the debate see Baruch A. Brody, "An Historical Introduction to Jewish Casuistry on Suicide and Euthanasia," in *Suicide and Euthanasia: Historical and Contemporary Themes,* ed. Baruch A. Brody, Philosophy and Medicine 35 (Dordrecht: Kluwer Academic, 1989), pp. 39-75, at pp. 63-64. I suppose medical ethics does not really need any additional interesting questions right now, but it is poorer for its failure to attend to prayer. It is poorer for its failure to attend by prayer to God.

and ceasing to pray for someone's survival but also between suicide and letting go our desperate hold on life. At least it seems increasingly difficult to make that distinction in moral "Esperanto," whether the language chosen is one of utility or autonomy.[34]

Doctors and nurses make intercession, too, of course — as well as patients. They make petition for those for whom they care, and over whom they exercise responsibility. Conscientious caregivers, especially the ones who take themselves too seriously and regard themselves messianically, will be tempted to make prayer a means again, a supplementary technology, to insure the effectiveness of their own work. But such a prayer is no less corrupted into superstition because the petitioner is a medical practitioner, and "God" is no less trivialized as the "great scalpel in the sky" because the bloody hands of a surgeon are lifted up in such a prayer.

Prayer and Compassion

There is a petition chiseled on an urban cathedral, "Christ, look upon us in this city. And keep our sympathy and pity fresh and our faces heavenward lest we grow hard."[35] It is a petition that might well form a church in the city, but it might also form the vocation of doctors and nurses, of chaplains and ministers, and of all who, by being "members one of another," are called to care for the sick and the dying.

"Lest we grow hard," the chiseled inscription says. It can happen, as even the softest heart knows. Why is it that we grow hard? Why is it that compassion withers and hearts harden? And how might simple attention to God in prayer help? How might prayer strengthen and enliven and direct compassion?

There is, first, sometimes something about those who suffer that makes our hearts shiver and shrivel and makes our eyes look away. And sometimes the thing about those who suffer that makes our eyes look away is simply and precisely their suffering. How can "looking heavenward" help? Let it be said again, first of all, that "looking heavenward" is not finally to look away. Looking heavenward, we call upon one who hears the cries of those who hurt and one who calls people to something like the

34. See below, p. 366 n. 33.
35. Bernard O. Brown, "The Problem of Compassion," *Criterion*, Winter 1990, pp. 24-26.

same uncalculating compassion. Looking heavenward, we name a risen Lord and remember that his wounds were raised with him. Looking heavenward, we see enthroned the one who says, "Inasmuch as you have not been kind or considerate or even moderately helpful to one of the least of these, you were not kind or considerate or helpful to me" (cf. Matt. 25:45). Looking heavenward directs our eyes back to those who suffer, and we see their weakness and vulnerability, their hurt and pain, their loneliness, in a new way — as the very image of the Lord we serve.

Then, still looking heavenward, we may intercede for the suffering, and intercession, too, cultivates compassion when we grow hard. When we pray, "Please be with that fool," we cultivate a readiness to be with him ourselves. And if, looking heavenward, we can identify why it is important for God to be present to this person or that, we will have made some progress toward compassion and found some direction for it. For example, "Please be with her because she is tired of being probed and poked and prodded and has forgotten the power and pleasure of a genuinely human touch." Or, "Please be with him because he is accustomed to commanding his world of subordinates and now the humblest subordinate, his own body, seems to be in revolt." Or even, "Please be with him because . . . well, because you are the sort of God who loves even fools like me and him."

Sometimes, however, what makes our hearts grow hard is not something in "them" but something in us. Fear, for example, is fertile soil for hard hearts. Compassion for a person with AIDS still takes some courage. If fear is the soil, pride is the seed of hard hearts. Not many of us are enormous egotists — not like the character who turns to his dinner companion and says, "But look, I've been talking about myself long enough. What do you think of me?" — but all of us know how self-absorbed we can be and how difficult it is to be really attentive to another's suffering. Compassion takes not just courage but humility. And guilt can make compassion wither, too. If some preoccupation or carelessness of ours gets in the way of compassion in a first encounter with the one who suffers, it is often very tempting not to notice the person's suffering in subsequent encounters.

But how can "looking heavenward" help? Looking heavenward, we are reminded that we rely on a grace that we should not be reticent to share. Looking heavenward, we find ourselves in the presence of one who is present to our weakness and our horror no less than to the weakness and horror of the sick and dying. Looking heavenward, we may even discover that, if our embodied self is identified with Christ, our integrity is threatened not so much by hurt as by the failure humbly to share the suffering of another. Looking heavenward, we may learn courage and humility. And when we are feeling guilty, we may, looking heavenward, form a prayer of confession; and forming a prayer of repentance, we may also form the self, freeing the self from being fated by that first careless and self-absorbed encounter. We may learn of turnings and new beginnings in repentance. It is not magic, of course, but to look heavenward can help reconstruct a compassionate self in spite of fear, pride, and guilt.

Another reason compassion sometimes withers is this: suffering is always individual; it differentiates — and it alienates. Compassion, on the other hand, is always communal; it shares and it unites. Jesus said, "It is more blessed to give than to receive" (Acts 20:35), but he might have added that it's a lot easier, too. To receive care is to be reminded of one's suffering, and in a culture that values independence as much as this one does, it can add to one's suffering. To experience the kind, good works of a friend (or a nurse) is sometimes to experience the hard division of the human race (and a hospital) into two groups: the relatively self-sufficient benefactors and the needy beneficiaries — and to be reminded of the side of that divide that one inhabits. To receive care graciously is hard work, and where it is not received graciously, compassion becomes hard work, too.

And how can "looking heavenward" help? Prayers of thanksgiving help provide a different picture and different relations, a world — and a hospital — in which each is a recipient of gifts, in which human giving is set, as Bill May says, in the context of primordial receiving.[36] Looking heavenward, sufferers may be reminded that dependency and indebtedness do not alienate them from the human condition or from the other dependent and indebted humans who care for them. Prayers of thanksgiving can commend and form in doctors and nurses and all of us simple works of mercy, not as a self-important conceit of philanthropy but as little deeds of kindness, which are no less a response to gift than the prayers of thanksgiving themselves.

Finally, compassion withers when we expect too much from it or from ourselves. When compassion simply arms itself with artifice and not with wisdom, it can self-deceptively lose sight of the limits of technology. In the context of the extravagant modern expectation that technology will deliver us from our mortality and from our human vulnerability to suffering, it may be little wonder that we suffer "compassion fatigue," for we expect so much, so limitlessly much from ourselves and our tools. And in the

36. May, "Images," p. 28.

context of the failure of such expectations, compassion withers. Indeed, caregivers who make it their identity and purpose to eliminate mortality or suffering will experience the death or suffering of one for whom they care as a threat to their identity; they will suffer.

And how can "looking heavenward" help? Looking heavenward can remind us of our limits. Doctors and nurses and parents and friends who look heavenward and make petition for the sick and suffering may of course be tempted to corrupt and trivialize prayer by making it into a means, a supplementary technology, an old and desperate artifice, to ensure the effectiveness of their own work. On the other hand, looking heavenward, attending to God in the form of a petition for the one who suffers, may form an altered (and an "altared") sense of compassion.

In petition doctors and nurses and all of us hand the one under our care over to the hands of God. Looking heavenward, we are reminded that we need not anxiously substitute for an absent God; we learn again that we are not Messiah and that we need not accept that intolerable burden. But there is a Messiah, and the Messiah can be trusted. When we hear again the always stunning "Inasmuch . . . ," we are reminded that, if anyone is to be counted Messiah in our encounters, the one who suffers is. Looking heavenward, we will provide the best care we can, but we can let go the anxious control we had conscientiously assumed. We can take ourselves a little less seriously. We can freely acknowledge the limits of our tools and our own limits. We can learn again a more carefree care.

One final word. We said before that a prayer-formed people will not despise medicine. It may also be said that a prayer-formed people will not despise medical ethics either. Only let them pray now and then. Prayer is not magic for decisions either, of course. It is not a technique to get what I want, even when what I want is an answer or a solution to a dilemma rather than a fortune or fourteen more healthy years. It is not a technology to be pulled out as a last resort when medical ethics has failed to tell us clearly what we ought to do. It does not rescue us from moral ambiguity. Part of what we know to be God's cause may still conflict with another part of what we know to be God's cause. You will still have to work hard, attending to cases, sorting out principles, identifying the various goods at stake, listening carefully to different accounts of the situation. Prayer does not rescue you from all that, but it does permit you to do all that in ways that are attentive to God and attentive, as well, to the relations of all that to God.

"In prayer," Coles's friend might say, "we not only commune with

God but find new strength — new virtue — for daily life and for dying and caring for the dying. A wise teacher once told me that."

The Practice of the Sacraments

When the church is gathered, it also makes a practice of the sacraments of baptism and Eucharist.[37] The story of Jesus' death and resurrection is at the heart of these sacraments, and in both sacraments the churches remember that story. It is not, of course, simply a matter of recalling some facts. There are facts to be reported again and again, of course, but they are not the sorts of facts that one can regard with an objective indifference. They are remembered not just that we might be better informed, but that we might be formed. The story is remembered as our story, the story that gives us our identity and nurtures it, the story that makes us a community, the story that orients us in our living and our dying toward God's good future. By these practices the church keeps company with the one who died and was raised. The sacraments could and should nurture and sustain other practices of keeping company with others who are suffering and dying.

These practices, however, have too often been allowed to shrink in significance. When infant baptism becomes an occasion for parents publicly to name a child and for a congregation to admire another adorable infant, then the practice has been distorted and shrunken. When the Eucharist becomes an introspective occasion, a private matter in the midst of a crowd, then this practice too has been distorted and shrunken. A renewal of the sacraments and renewed attention to these practices might form Christians and Christian communities capable of taking back death, more able to die well and faithfully and more willing to care well and faithfully for the dying.

---

37. My reflections on the sacraments of baptism and the Eucharist are indebted on the one hand to the quite remarkable ecumenical consensus represented in *Baptism, Eucharist, and Ministry*, Faith and Order Paper No. 111 (1982), and on the other to the work of Markus Barth, *Rediscovering the Lord's Supper* (Atlanta: John Knox, 1988), which criticized that document as too sacerdotal and hierarchical and as failing to witness to the unity of all humanity in Christ. I would also recommend a thoughtful book by a pastor, Leonard J. VanderZee, *Christ, Baptism, and the Lord's Supper: Recovering the Sacrament for Evangelical Worship* (Downers Grove, Ill.: IVP, 2004).

Baptism

When the church performs a baptism, it is God who acts to sign and seal our participation in the death and resurrection of Christ and in the body of Christ, the church. In Romans 6 Paul reminds the Roman Christians of what they already know, that "all of us who have been baptized into Christ Jesus were baptized into his death" (Rom. 6:3). Baptism is the sign of our solidarity with the crucified Christ. We are crucified with him, "buried with him by baptism." But it is also a sign of our solidarity with the risen Christ. "For if we have been united with him in a death like his, we will certainly be united with him in a resurrection like his" (6:5). That future tense acknowledges the separation in time between Christ's resurrection and our own, but Paul insists nevertheless that our future resurrection is of one piece with Christ's resurrection. In baptism our lives are already marked by that remembered past, already oriented toward that future. Already we are to "walk in newness of life" (6:4). Already we are "one new humanity" (Eph. 2:15; cf. Gal. 3:27-28). We remain mortal, but death and sin no longer rule our lives. The powers of death and sin may still assert their doomed reign, and while they do, our baptism is given to us not only as a blessing but also as a calling. Baptism forms in us and calls from us the very virtues that are important to dying well.

It is a calling, surely, to faithfulness. Baptism calls us to trust in the faithfulness of God, the faithfulness shown in raising Jesus from the dead. Baptism calls us to our own faithfulness, to integrity with the identity we have been given by grace. By signing and sealing our participation in the resurrection of Christ, in God's good future, by making us "heirs according to the promise" (Gal. 3:29), baptism calls us to hope. It calls us not to a private and egocentric hope for an otherworldly bliss; it calls us to hope for God's future, for God's renewal of the cosmos, for God's redemption of humanity, and for a common share in it. By signing and sealing our participation in the body of Christ, the church, baptism calls us to love one another in this community. It calls us to hospitality, to forgiveness and reconciliation, to words and deeds of affectionate affirmation. By signing and sealing these promises while death and sin still assert their doomed rule, baptism calls us to patience, to a love that is slow to anger and quick to forgive. It calls us, while we wait and watch and pray for God's good future, to mourn that it is not yet, still sadly not yet, that future. It calls us to be ready to suffer a little for the sake of it, to be ready to weep with those who weep, to have compassion. It calls us not to celebrate death or suffering but to be ready to endure either faithfully in the confidence that God will have the last word. By signing and sealing our common dependence upon the grace of God, it calls us to humility. It calls us to renounce not only the devil but also our proud assertions of independence. It calls us not only to care but also to receive gratefully the care of others, the constant care of God above all but also the care of others on whom we depend. And by signing and sealing the simple fact that we are finally in God's hands, baptism calls us to trust those hands, to let ourselves go into their care. That is our comfort, and that comfort is the courage that baptism finally forms in us and calls from us.

Let it be admitted that churches and those of us who are members of them (and so members one of another) do not live in ways worthy of the calling of our baptism. Let it be admitted that churches shamefully deny it and contradict it when they fail to live up to the unity of a new humanity that baptism signals. Let it be admitted that we shamefully deny the identity we have been given by baptism whenever we are unfaithful, or despairing, or unloving and unforgiving, whenever we are impatient or proud, whenever we fail to trust the security of God's promise. Still, we may and should look not to ourselves but to the grace of God in our baptism. It still signs our solidarity with Christ in his cross and resurrection, still gives us membership in the church and in "one new humanity," still calls us toward God's good future.

Our dying can be a time for the renewal of our baptism. Sharing in Christ's death, we may hope to be raised with him. Living while we are dying in ways that lean on God's grace and lean toward God's future, we may find strength for the virtues. Then our dying may be a definitive expression of our baptismal identity, a dying worthy of our baptism, a dying with Christ. We will still die, of course, but not as though death will have the last word. We will still mourn, but not as those who have no hope.

In the context of baptism and its memory of Jesus' death, there can be no denial of death or of its awful reality, but in the context of baptism and our solidarity with Christ there need be no fear of death, no anxiety that it can finally make good on its threats. The love of God is stronger than death. God has won the victory over death and sin.

We should not end our consideration of baptism, however, without underscoring that in baptism we enter not only into the death and resurrection of Christ but also (and consequently) into the body of Christ, the church. To share in the common life of that community is no small part of the new life given to us and required of us. Baptism, by the power of the

Spirit, initiates us into "the communion of the saints" and calls us to practice it. To care for the dying can also be a time for the renewal of our baptism and for the practice of that communion. If we share by God's grace in the death of Christ, then we are called to share also in the grief and lament of another's dying. Our solidarity with Christ in his solidarity with human flesh in its very vulnerability to death and suffering is practiced when we are present to the "saints," the members of the communion, who are dying. As we have said, baptism forms in us and calls from us the very virtues that are important to dying well, but the same virtues, faithfulness, hope, love, patience, humility, and serenity, are also virtues important to caring well for the dying.

Eucharist

When the church celebrates Eucharist, it is God who invites us to the table. It, no less than baptism, has the memory of Jesus' death at the center of it. And it, no less than baptism, celebrates the resurrection of that crucified Jesus and looks forward to his appearance at the end of time and to the resurrection to come. It is, as Avery Dulles said, "the sacrament of death swallowed up in Christ's victory."[38] Indeed, it is a foretaste of the eschatological banquet, a foretaste of God's good future. Like baptism, Eucharist is a communal event, not a private affair between an individual and God. But if by baptism the grace of God once and for all time gives us an identity, by regular Eucharist the grace of God again and again nurtures it. If by baptism God once and for all initiates people into the community and into a new humanity, by the Eucharist God again and again refreshes and renews the community. By them both the grace and call of God orient us in our living and in our dying to participation in Christ's death and his resurrection.

Meals were an important part of Jesus' ministry. His delight in them made it clear that he was no ascetic. When he ate with sinners, he displayed his readiness to be a friend to sinners (e.g., Mark 2:15-17 and parallels; Matt. 11:19; Luke 7:34; 15:1-2). When he fed the crowds, he displayed his compassion and his hospitality (Mark 6:30-44 and parallels; Mark 8:1-10 and parallels; John 6:3-15). And on the eve of his death, when he shared a

---

38. Avery Dulles, "The Eucharist, Source and Summit of Ecclesial Life," *Magnificat*, October 2005, p. 6; cited in the thoughtful little book by Daneen Georgy Warner, *Life, Death, and Christian Hope* (Mahwah, N.J.: Paulist, 2009), p. 19.

meal with the disciples, Jesus "took a loaf of bread, and when he had given thanks, be broke it and said, 'This is my body that is for you. Do this in remembrance of me.' In the same way he took the cup also, after supper, saying, 'This cup is the new covenant in my blood. Do this, as often as you drink it, in remembrance of me'" (1 Cor. 11:23-25). When he appeared to the disciples on the way to Emmaus, it was at the meal, when he "took bread, blessed and broke it, and gave it to them," that the disciples recognized this stranger as the risen Christ (Luke 24:30). Again in Jerusalem (Luke 24:35-49) and again at the sea (John 21:1-14), the risen Christ appeared to the disciples and ate with them. And again and again the church has been invited to give thanks at this meal of remembrance and hope, and again and again the risen Lord is somehow present.

Much quarreling has arisen about what exactly those "words of institution" (1 Cor. 11:24-25; cf. also Mark 14:22-23 and parallels) mean, so much that the Eucharist has come to signal the shameful splintering of the churches as much as the unity of the church. I will not pretend to offer a theological resolution to the quarrels, but only to observe that we are invited to this supper neither because we are exceptionally righteous nor because we can give a theologically learned account of exactly what happens to the bread and wine. We are invited to this supper because God is gracious. And however we explain it, the common affirmation of the churches is that the crucified and risen Lord is somehow present in spite of his absence.[39] Again and again the risen Lord has been present. He is the host to our gathering for this meal, and once again we take, eat, remember, and believe.

It is "the sacrament of death swallowed up in Christ's victory," and it is the risen Lord who is present, but the Eucharist will not let us forget or ignore his real death or the not-yet character of our world and of our lives. We celebrate Christ's victory, but we remember his death. In the Eucharist, as Paul says, we "proclaim the Lord's death until he comes" (1 Cor. 11:26). He died in solidarity with sinners, and he still welcomes sinners to his table. He died in solidarity with those who make the human cry of lament,

---

39. I do not mean to demean the significance of these quarrels about the way Christ is present in the Eucharist by some easy appeal to mystery. My own tradition (Calvinist) has quite rightly (in my view) rejected accounts of the Eucharist that suggest that the once-for-all sacrifice of Christ on the cross is repeated (a view it associated with certain Roman Catholic views of transubstantiation) and accounts of it that suggested the "remembrance" was a matter of mere mental recollection (a view it associated with Zwingli and certain Radical Reformation figures). It insisted (again correctly, in my view) that the Spirit brings about Christ's presence in the community.

and he still feels the wounds of those who suffer. He died in solidarity with those who do not count for much as the world counts, and he still grants a place of honor to the weak and sick and dying and to all those whom it is too much our impulse to neglect and shun.

Paul insists that to share this cup and this bread is to share in Christ's death, to share in his blood and in his body. It is, he said, "a sharing," a *koinonia,* a communion "in the blood of Christ"; it is "a sharing," a *koinonia,* a communion "in the body of Christ" (1 Cor. 10:16). And by that "sharing" we are constituted "one body" (10:17). We are made a community, members of the same body. How then can we drink this cup or eat this bread and refuse to share in the suffering of another? How can we share this death and abandon the dying among us to the solitary and lonely death medicalization threatens?

Paul insists that the Eucharist may not be rendered a private transaction between Christ and the believer. That is evidently what the Corinthians attempted — and what Paul condemns as eating the bread and drinking the cup "in an unworthy manner" (11:27). There were shameful divisions in the Corinthian church (11:18; cf. 1:1-12), but most shameful of all was their treatment of the poor (11:21-22). There is no worthy remembering the risen Lord without remembering and being his body, his solidarity with all who die, his solidarity with any who suffer, his solidarity with those whom the Corinthian elite — or any elite, whether they regard themselves as such because they are healthy or wealthy or "autonomous" and in control — regard as not counting for very much. When the dying are regarded as not counting for very much, when the church neglects them or abandons them to the medical experts, then we do not practice "the communion." Then we eat the bread and drink the cup "in an unworthy manner."

"Until [Christ] comes" (11:26), until the dead are raised and death is "swallowed up in victory" (15:54), Eucharist calls the church to solidarity with the dying, the grieving, the suffering, the poor. To be sure, the Eucharist is a token of God's good future, a foretaste of the eschatological banquet.[40] After all, the risen Christ is present at this meal. But until he comes in glory, the Eucharist and the remembrance of Jesus call the community to compassion. And among the works of compassion, caring for the dying has a privileged place simply by the remembrance of the death of Jesus.

40. Incidentally, my image of that banquet is a great table, with plenty of delightful food and drink, but at this table our elbows do not bend, so the only way any of us can eat is by feeding each other, caring for each other.

The community will not celebrate the death of any; indeed, it will grieve any dis-membering of its body and mourn the reminders that it is not yet the good future in which death will be no more. But in the context of such a community and its care, in the context of "the communion of the saints," those who suffer and die may know that they do not suffer and die alone but "with Christ" and within a caring community.

We have noted the eucharistic presence of the risen Lord, the reminders of his death and of the not-yet character of our existence "until he comes." We have noted that Eucharist is communion, that there is no worthy partaking that does not practice solidarity with the suffering and dying. One other observation is important here. The eating of bread and the drinking of the cup signal and celebrate human embodiment and the goodness of the creation. We give thanks in Eucharist for the grains and the human hands that make bread and the vines and the human work that give wine. The point is relevant, of course, to the nurture of an ecological ethic in the church, but it also nurtures a watchfulness against the dualism that dismisses the delights and the groaning of both the creation and embodied selves. We do not partake worthily if we make the supper or our salvation a disembodied bliss of the soul in some world other than the world God gives and loves.

The ancient tradition of bringing the sacrament to the sick and dying, so important also for the tradition of *Ars Moriendi* (but within that tradition, I fear, focused on the disembodied bliss of an individual soul), should continue to be a practice of the community's care for them. Even here — especially here — the Eucharist is not a private act. The community comes with it, gesturing that the sick and dying are still members of the community. The bread and cup are a sharing in the death of the risen Lord, and because of this bread and cup a sharing in the suffering and dying of this member of the body. The body is there. It laments the suffering of the sick and dying, mourns the threat of his or her death, but insists that by God's grace, this member of the body will not finally be separated from God or from them, that his or her flesh will be renewed with the whole creation that serves God and waits for God. Moreover, the sick and dying are given voice, if only to say "Thanks be to God" or "Amen."[41] Perhaps they will express lament, joined to hope. Perhaps they will join their voices to

---

41. M. Therese Lysaught makes this point elegantly with respect to the practice of anointing in the Roman Catholic Church. See Lysaught, "Patient Suffering and the Anointing of the Sick," in *On Moral Medicine*, pp. 356-64, especially p. 362.

the voice of the community expressing the ancient faith. Or, perhaps they cannot get that far on that day. Still the community keeps faith with them — and sometimes for them — offering a taste of a future they can hardly swallow but which is sure to be.

These practices, gathering for worship, reading Scripture, praying, and celebrating the sacraments of baptism and Eucharist, are the central practices of the Christian community and central also to the formation of the virtues for dying well and faithfully and for caring well and faithfully for the dying. But other practices might also be considered, and to them we turn in the next chapter.

CHAPTER FIFTEEN

Some Practices Old and New

The indispensability of shouting out the good news of Easter at a funeral gets highlighted when we realize that there are actually two preachers at every funeral. Death — capital-D Death — loves to preach and never misses a funeral. Death's sermon is powerful and always the same: "Damn you! Damn all of you! I win every time. I destroy all loving relationships. I shatter all community. I dash all hope. . . . I always win!" . . . It is the great privilege of the funeral preacher to shake a fist in the face of Death, to proclaim again [the Easter triumph of God]."

Tom Long, *Accompany Them with Singing — the Christian Funeral*[1]

In addition to the central practices of Christian community — gathering, reading Scripture, praying, and participating in the sacraments — many other Christian practices form our imagination about death and our behavior in the face of it. Some of these are ancient practices, like mourning and comforting, like the practice of funerals. Some were surely important to *Ars Moriendi*, like the practices of remembering the saints and catechesis. And some of them, like creating advance directives, are new, hardly yet

---

1. Thomas G. Long, *Accompany Them with Singing — the Christian Funeral* (Louisville: Westminster John Knox, 2009), p. 188.

warranting the name Christian practice. But old or new, these practices need always to be assessed in the light of the gospel narrative. When they are, they can support and sustain both dying well and caring well for the dying. Consider, first, practices of mourning and comforting.

The Practices of Mourning and Comforting

The denial of death in the mid–twentieth century was accompanied by the denial of mourning. As death was hidden away, made as invisible as we could make it, so was grief hidden away. The visible signs of mourning, the black crepe, the armbands, the "widow's weeds," were all stored away in attics. It was not, of course, that people no longer grieved, but there was not — and there was not to be (after the funeral, at any rate) — any public display of it. Grief was made a private issue.

Perhaps the culture was simply tired of the death and grief that had accompanied war. It wanted to forget it, to move on to something else, something a little more pleasant. Did anyone ever die on *Ozzie and Harriet*? Perhaps the culture was simply tired of the burdens of the Victorian practices of mourning; Scarlett O'Hara was already tired of them in *Gone with the Wind*.[2] But for whatever reason, the culture had evidently adopted a new rule, the rule that, as Ella Wheeler Wilcox put it, "Laugh and the world laughs with you. Weep and you weep alone."[3] Culture required, at least in public, a "happy face."

And so, too often, did the churches. We filled our sanctuaries with choruses of praise, happy songs, but paid too little attention to the ways in which death and sorrow intrude upon our lives and upon our common life. Praise belongs to worship, of course, but so does an honest and communal recognition that it is not yet God's good future. We silenced the cries of abandonment and sadness. Perhaps we did it because sadness does not market well in the consumer culture of American religion. Can you imagine the billboard "Join us on Sunday morning for a little lament"?

But perhaps we let the practices of mourning slip away because we

---

2. Nancy Duff, "Recovering Lamentation as a Practice in the Church," in *Lament: Reclaiming Practices in Pulpit, Pew, and Public Square*, ed. Sally Brown and Patrick D. Miller (Louisville: Westminster John Knox, 2005), p. 6, citing Susan Lyons, "The After Life: Mourning Rituals of the Civil War Era" (from a temporary Web site posting). Scarlett O'Hara, of course, scandalized the community by dancing in her "widow's weeds."

3. Ella Wheeler Wilcox, "Solitude," cited by Duff, "Recovering Lamentation," p. 5.

could no longer tolerate the Platonic platitudes that were provided as consolation. Frankly, the practices of consolation themselves did not help much when, in ways shaped by the *Ars Moriendi*, Christians would chide the one who mourned, "Why are you sad? Your child is better off dead." No one (I hope) said it exactly like that, but the consolation was often heard exactly like that. Little wonder, then, that people tried to "put on a happy face" when they came to church. And little wonder, then, that they stayed away from worship and from community exactly when they needed both the most.

A recovery of mourning practices could nurture a recovery of an honest acknowledgment of the awful reality of death and a compassionate communal response to both the dying and the grieving.[4] It might even

---

4. I do not have prescriptions for what these practices might be, only that there should be such. They and the little rituals associated with them are important not only to sanction grief but also to contain it. When they are lost, it is difficult to recover them and harder to invent new ones. Of course, mourning is always particular, and the practices and rituals should remain flexible. Their performance, moreover, should never be allowed to become perfunctory. They are no substitute for the community's care.

There is much to be learned, I think, from Jewish practices of mourning, starting with *shiva* for a few days (traditionally seven) following burial, and continuing with *shloshim* for the first month, but not ending until the end of the first year at *yahrtzeit.* Following burial those who mourn gather in the home of the deceased or a relative for *shiva.* They turn from honoring the dead in burial to attend to their loss. Visitors come to sit, often silently, with those who grieve. The obligation to visit the *shiva* house falls not just on close friends but on the entire community. On the Sabbath, *shiva* is not observed; instead, those who mourn are encouraged to go to synagogue. The Kaddish prayer is recited three times a day in the home. At the end of *shiva,* those who mourn go outside, frequently to take a walk, and reenter a world poorer for their loss. They enter a period of *shloshim.* They reestablish some of the old routines. Some of the signs of mourning are removed (for example, the mirrors would be uncovered), but not all of them. Even as they reenter the world, they remain apart (for example, the mourners will avoid public celebrations). On the thirtieth day after burial *shloshim* ends, but the rituals of mourning do not. For a year the children of the deceased go to synagogue daily to recite the Kaddish. At *yahrtzeit,* the anniversary of the death, when the mourner goes to synagogue to recite the Kaddish, there is an announcement of the name of the deceased, and at home a candle is lit for twenty-four hours. For a much fuller account of these practices and others in response to death, see Mark A. Popovsky, *Jewish Ritual, Reality, and Response at the End of Life* (Durham, N.C.: Duke Institute on Care at the End of Life, 2007).

Christians can learn from these Jewish mourning practices to provide a communally sanctioned time and space for mourning, for more intense mourning initially and for a more extended recognition of the loss endured. They can learn as well that at such times and in such spaces the community has the opportunity and the obligation to care for and to comfort the mourners.

help us to honor that curious word of Jesus, "Blessed are those who mourn, for they will be comforted" (Matt. 5:4). Jesus said it on a hillside in Galilee, and those who heard it probably asked, "What did he say? Did he really say that, 'Blessed are those who mourn'? What an odd thing to say." Perhaps it is so familiar now that we simply pass over it quickly, no longer shocked, no longer curious, not pausing to wonder over this odd comment. But think of it. "Blessed are those who mourn." Or, as Luke put it, "Blessed are you who weep now" (Luke 6:21). Or, to paraphrase, happy are those with eyes so full of tears they can hardly see. It is a strange thing to say. How shall we make sense of it?

It helps to begin, I think, by setting this odd remark in the context of the Beatitudes and by setting the Beatitudes in the context of Jesus' proclamation of the kingdom of God, his announcement of the good future of God. "The kingdom of God has come near," he said (Mark 1:15; Matt. 4:17). It will be a new day. On that day the humiliated will be exalted. On that day the last will be made first. On that day the dead will be raised. Then the cause of God will be unchallenged by sin or death or greed or hate. Jesus announces the good future of God in the Beatitudes, and he points to the places that good future already makes its power felt.

That is why, for example, Jesus blesses and applauds those who hunger and thirst for justice (Matt. 5:6).[5] On that day God will set the world right, and already that justice is a mark and a token of God's good future. Justice is the food and drink of God's reign, and those who have heard the good news of that future — and long for it — will delight in any little foretaste of God's setting the world right; they will hunger for justice. That is why Jesus blesses and praises the merciful (5:7). In their mercy we catch a glimpse and a promise of the future reign of a merciful God. In their mercy God's good future already makes its power felt. And that is why Jesus blesses and commends the peacemakers (5:9). In the peace they make we may see a token of the *shalom* God promises. What then of this blessing on those who mourn? Who are the mourners?

The mourners are those who have heard the good news of God's good future and weep because it is not yet, still sadly not yet. Their eyes have caught a glimpse of God's future, and their eyes fill with tears because they see it challenged and contradicted in the present. Their spirits ache

---

5. On translating *dikaiosune* as "justice" rather than "righteousness," see Nicholas Wolterstorff, *Justice: Rights and Wrongs* (Princeton: Princeton University Press, 2008), pp. 110-13.

for the coming of the kingdom Jesus announced, the future he made present in his words of blessing and his works of healing. It is because they hope that they mourn. They are eager for joy, ready to celebrate merrily the outrageously good news of such a future, ready to dance. They are hungry for justice, thirsty for peace, longing for the rule of mercy. They are eager to delight in the sight of the blind, to rejoice when the sick are healed, to celebrate when the dead are raised. But the poor are oppressed still. Wars and enmity continue. There is little mercy to be seen. Some are beaten down and crushed by their suffering still. Some who were blind are blind still. Some who were dying are dying still, suffering their way to a lingering death. And the dead stay dead. And the mourners cry out, "How long, O Lord?"

Who are the mourners? The mourners are visionaries who ache with the wounds of the world's sadness. They are, as Nick Wolterstorff said, "aching visionaries."[6] We should not restrict this beatitude to those who grieve at the death of a loved one. But neither should we exclude them from this beatitude! Those who have heard and seen something of God's good future in Jesus do not grieve as those who have no hope (1 Thess. 4:13), but their hope does not keep them from grieving. Indeed, it is precisely their hope for that day that prompts their tears and the cry, "How long, O Lord?"

And Jesus blesses them! He applauds them and celebrates them, for the good future of God also makes itself felt in them, makes itself known in their very sadness now. The compassion of God is disclosed in their tears. In their suffering the suffering of God is revealed.

The promise to them is that the new day for which they ache will dawn. The dead will be raised. The mourners "will be comforted" (Matt. 5:4). God's good future is sure to be, and *that* future, that comfort, already makes its power felt in the assurance to aching visionaries that God is with them. They mourn still, for it is still not yet God's unchallenged reign, but already they know that those who suffer are not alone, that those who mourn are not abandoned, that God is with them.

This blessing on those who mourn does not call us to be somber and humorless; it does not call us to become gloomy and joyless. The future of God does not make its power felt in those ways. On the contrary, it calls us to be eager for joy, ready to celebrate the hilariously glad tidings we are

---

6. Nicholas Wolterstorff, *Lament for a Son* (Grand Rapids: Eerdmans, 1987), p. 86. My account of "Blessed are those who mourn" is much indebted to Wolterstorff.

charged to announce and to perform. But while we wait and watch for that day, while it is still not yet that future, we may — and we must — mourn. It is not yet God's good future. We perform the gospel sometimes by lament, by mourning.

The text permits us — and calls us — sometimes to hurt a little. We've got to care enough to feel our eyes well with tears when another suffers or dies. We've got to so hunger and thirst for God's good future that we weep when yet another person is a victim of this world's sadness. The ancient Stoics celebrated and applauded the one who could stand above the passions and the emotions. They had no room for passion or for pathos. They would not get too upset with evil or delight too much in the good, neither mourn nor dance. But Jesus was no Stoic, and he did not invite his apprentices to become such. He invited people to dance — playing a merry tune of God's grace and future. And he blessed those who mourn. This blessing does not call us to be Stoics. It will not permit Stoic indifference to the wounds of another. It calls us to passion — and to compassion. Aching visionaries see the suffering of another, and they cry out with it, "How long?" Because their horizon is God's good future, and because the scope of their hope is cosmic, they share with the whole creation in its groaning (Rom. 8:22). And because God's good future is as embodied and communal as God's good creation, when a loved one dies, we may mourn. We have Christ's permission and blessing to ache at the loss. And God aches, too. The Spirit joins us in our suffering "with sighs too deep for words" (Rom. 8:26).

So far we have emphasized the authorization to mourn. And if Christ authorizes it, then the church should support it with communally sanctioned practices of mourning. But the text also calls us to be a community that provides some little foretaste of God's future by comforting the mourners. It is God's future that is finally consoling, but while we wait and watch for it, Christians are called to provide some little taste of it. The mourners "will be comforted," and somehow that future too must be made present and real in the life of the churches. Practices of mourning call for practices of comforting.

Here too, however, and perhaps here especially, we must remember that we are not Messiah. We must guard against triumphalism, whether technological or spiritual. The victory over death is finally not a technological triumph, even if we are grateful for the ways medicine can prevent premature death. And the victory over sadness is finally not a technological or a pharmacological triumph either. But it is not just technological triumphalism against which we must guard. There is also a spiritual enthusiasm that proposes that faith and prayer work like magic against death and sadness. It is no comfort to be told one needs to pray a little more or a little harder to avoid death or to vanquish sadness. It is no comfort to be told one needs to have a stronger faith.

Ars Moriendi's strategy of comfort was to commend death as an escape from our bodies into an eternal and disembodied bliss. I have resisted that strategy because it does not fit the story of Jesus, the very story *Ars Moriendi* regarded as normative. Those who mourn, I think, will not be comforted by a commendation of death. Oh, they might be comforted by the presence of well-meaning friends or pastors who talk this way. But it is their presence and their compassion that are comforting, not the celebration of death. And they might take some consolation in the release by death from the indignities and pain that may have been involved in a lingering dying. But while they may be glad that their loved one need not suffer any longer in dying, they know that death is still awful. They know the painful reality of being sundered from one who was loved.

However, those who mourn may not be comforted by talk of the resurrection either. There may be no comfort or comforting if Jesus had not been raised, but the hope of a resurrection like his does not easily fill right now the hole that is left in our lives by the death of one we love. Nicholas Wolterstorff is my witness. In his reflections on the death of his son Eric, he said:

> Elements of the gospel which I had always thought would console did not. They did something else, something important, but not that. It did not console me to be reminded of the hope of resurrection. If I had forgotten that hope, then it would indeed have brought light into my life to be reminded of it. But I did not think of death as a bottomless pit. I did not grieve as one who has no hope. Yet Eric is gone, *here* and *now* he is gone; *now* I cannot talk with him, *now* I cannot see him, *now* I cannot hug him, *now* I cannot hear of his plans for the future. *That* is my sorrow. A friend said, "Remember, he's in good hands." I was deeply moved. But that reality does not put Eric back in my hands now. That's my grief. For that grief, what consolation can there be other than having him back?[7]

---

7. Wolterstorff, *Lament for a Son*, p. 31. Thomas Long, *Accompany Them with Singing*, p. 192, cites William Sloane Coffin as a witness to the same point. In a sermon shortly after the death of his son, Alex, Coffin said, "While the words of the Bible are true, grief renders

Mourners may, like Rachel and the mothers of Bethlehem (Matt. 2:18), refuse to be consoled. Their comfort is, after all, eschatological, and that future is still not yet, more undeniably than ever, not now. Still, even now, the church is called to comfort.

To comfort is not to deny the reality or the sadness of death. It does not require the mourner to disown the grief. To disown the grief would be to disown the love, and then death would triumph. To comfort is, first of all, simply presence, simply being there, listening, not attempting to console immediately but simply sharing the lament. That is the comfort of the cross; Jesus made the human cry of lament his own cry. That is the comfort Job's friends initially offered when they came to "console and comfort" (Job 2:11).[8] They sat in the ashes alongside Job in his grief. For seven days and seven nights there were no words, "for they saw that his suffering was very great" (2:13).

Job's grief was like that of many who mourn. He was struck dumb by his loss. There were no words because there was no sense to be made of it. The structure of his world had been shattered. The meaning of his life had unraveled. His identity as a cherished child of God had been assaulted. It was the presence of his friends, silently ready to share the pain, that broke the desolating isolation of suffering and allowed Job to try to find words to express the pain and to begin to reconstruct a structure, a meaning, and an identity in the midst of it.

When Job did find words, they were words from the edge of hell, furious and despairing words (Job 3). To comfort still required presence, silently listening, of Job's friends, but in response to Job's words they could not stay silent. To comfort required of them, then, some response as well, some words of their own. The problem was not that Job's friends finally spoke. He needed them to speak then, to respond. It was by Job's respond-

---

them unreal. . . . That's why immediately after such a tragedy people must come to your rescue, people who only want to hold your hand, not to quote anybody or even say anything, people who simply bring food and flowers — the basics of beauty and life — people who sign letters simply, 'Your heartbroken sister.'" Long responds instructively, "[This] does not mean that preachers should be silent about the promises of the gospel. It means, rather, that when those promises of victory and joy are directed to those in the pain of grief, they should have the tone of words being held in trust for them until they can claim them for themselves, rather than obligations of the present moment."

8. On Job and his "comforters," see further Allen Verhey, *Reading the Bible in the Strange World of Medicine* (Grand Rapids: Eerdmans, 2003), pp. 114-22, upon which the next few paragraphs draw.

ing to their response that Job was able to discover a better and less bitter voice, a better and less bitter self. They must speak or leave him at this edge of hell, this edge of a place where God is not, or does not care.

The problem was not that they spoke, but what they said. And the problem with what they said was not that they had no answers for Job, but that they thought they had them all. They claimed to know too much and to know it too clearly. They thought they needed to be the defense attorneys for God, but they ended up as prosecutors of Job. Their words defending God and hope and humility painfully accused Job in his suffering and ironically made God out to be a nitpicker and a tyrant.

Still, in spite of them, Job did grow in his answering them.[9] Exasperated with his friends, Job turned toward — and against — God, against — but toward — God. And his voice grew sometimes less assertive in its hopelessness, sometimes less hopeless in its assertiveness. He would not claim to have all the answers against these friends, these comforters, these accusers, but he would not let go either of his own righteousness or of God's. And that holding on without all the answers moved him a little from the edge of hell. That turning toward God — even if only for the sake of confronting God, even if only for the sake of accusing God — turned him away from that place where God was not.

So far, we have observed that the practices of comforting include sometimes silent and compassionate presence and sometimes an expression of the faith of the community. In memory of Jesus and of Job, Christian communities should authorize a mourning that may cry out to God — and against God — from the edge of hell. But to authorize such practices in memory of Jesus and of Job is to be committed as a community to practices of comforting. When meanings unravel, when relationships are sundered, when chaos seems Lord, when God seems absent, we must be there. It is not that we need to anxiously substitute for an absent God. It is rather that we know the gospel that God does not neglect such a cry. It is

---

9. I confess I take great comfort in the fact that, in spite of the folly of these friends (Job 42:8) and the foolishness of their responses to Job, because of them Job is nevertheless helped toward the renewal of his life. I suspect that many of us, including many pastors, have said foolish things to those who mourn. Among my foolish responses I would avoid those who mourned, not because I did not care, but because I did not know what to say. Nick Wolterstorff made a helpful suggestion. Just be there, and when you don't know what to say, say, "I don't know what to say." And I have sometimes said, "I know how you feel." I didn't, and I couldn't. Suffering and grief are always particular. But perhaps my friends knew at least that I cared.

not that we need to have all the answers. It is rather that we share both the suffering of the one who mourns and the confidence of the community that we live and die and suffer, although in darkness, yet not into darkness, but into a life and a light that is finally unconquerable.

There is yet one other aspect of comforting. It is to help with the work of imagining how the next chapter of one's life might be written. The culture wants us simply to put grief behind us, to "get over it." It wants us simply not to think about it anymore. It wants us to disown our grief.[10] But that is not the way a Christian imagination or Christian comfort works. Christ was raised, and he calls us back to life, but it is not and cannot be simply a return to the same old life we had before. The old life is gone; part of it has died. The death of a loved one marks forever one's life in terms of a "before" and an "after." But a Christian imagination is not simply nostalgia. Nostalgia is folly because it wants what is impossible. So does grief, of course. But a Christian imagination and Christian comfort are captured by the fact that Christ's wounds were raised with him. That he was raised is the world's decisive "before" and "after." But he did not disown his wounds. They mark his risen life. And Christian comfort does not call us to disown our grief. It is, after all, because we loved the one who is dead that we are thrown into grief, and that love is not something we should or need regret. If that love was good, then we may and should own our grief as something that is also good and right. It is the failure to grieve that would be unworthy of a wife who loved her husband, a father who loved his children, a friend who loved a friend. In the return to life we do not simply "get over" that love and its suffering. They mark us still — not because we try desperately to live in the past but because we move toward a future in which that love is gratefully remembered and honored. They mark us still when we are able to move toward a future in which we may grow a little more compassionate ourselves, ready to sit with others on that mourner's bench. It is a long bench, but there we sit, "arms linked in undeluded friendship, all of us, brief links, ourselves in the eternal pity."[11]

---

10. The point about "disowning" grief is indebted to a lecture Nicholas Wolterstorff gave at First Presbyterian Church in Durham, N.C., entitled "Living with Grief."

11. These are the last words of the wonderful novel by Peter De Vries, *The Blood of the Lamb* (New York: Popular Library, 1961), p. 237. It is the story of Don Wanderhope and a series of deaths, climaxing in the death of his daughter Carol. (De Vries himself lost a daughter to leukemia.) Just before these closing lines Don Wanderhope observes, "There may be gifts beyond the reach of solace, but none worthy of the name that does not set free the springs of sympathy."

The one whose wounds were raised with him does not call us to disown the grief, but he does call us back to life in his name.

It won't be easy to obey that call. After a time of simple presence and listening, after a time of sharing in the mourner's remembering and lamenting, comforters may help with the mourner's work of imagining how the mourner's story, changed as it is and must be, may nevertheless be continued in ways that are faithful to God, faithful to the remembered loved one, and faithful to the mourner. They can help one who sits at the edge of hell to take some small steps in returning to life. The help may be as mundane as bringing a meal to mourners early in their grief and a little later inviting them to dinner in your home. It may take the simple shape of a little help with the house or a little help in learning to deal with a family's finances. There will still be times of silent presence, of course, still times of listening and sharing tears, as the wounds open up again. Still, comforters can help mourners to imagine how a life may be lived in the absence of a loved one. They can help mourners to envision the next chapter of their life as also good. They can help mourners to return to life, owning their wounds and sharing the wounds of others. And, of course, they can pray. They can pray for and with those who mourn. In prayer they are attentive to God and to God's promise to bless those who mourn.

It is that promise, that vision of God's future, that puts comforters to work. They are themselves mourners in a way. They have caught a vision of God's future in the blessing upon the mourners. They weep that any should look for comfort and find none. And they ache for the fulfillment of God's promise. The vision is no pipe dream. Pipe dreams are airy and nebulous and of no effect. But these aching visionaries see something real and solid, something as sure as the promise of God. It is the ache for it that gives comforters an agenda. It is not yet, still not yet, the good future of God in which mourners find comfort. And because they long for it, because they pray for it, comforters also work for it. Faith and hope and compassion move them to do something to help the one who hurts. Of course, even prayer and work — even hard praying and hard working — do not usher in the new heaven and the new earth. It is still God who will wipe away every tear, still God who will bring a future in which "death shall be no more," in which "mourning and crying and pain will be no more." Comforters may, indeed must, undertake their work, therefore, without the crushing burden of messianic pretensions, without extravagant expectations of being able to find the words that will put sadness to flight. They

343

may undertake their work of sharing the suffering and tears of another in the confidence that God's good future is sure to be.

In the meanwhile, blessed are those who mourn. Blessed are those aching visionaries who see something of God's good future and who weep because it is not yet. Blessed are those aching visionaries who see the mourners uncomforted because the church has abandoned lament and silenced the voice of sufferers. Blessed are those aching visionaries who work to give some small token of the promise that the mourners will be comforted. Blessed are those whose passion for God's good future moves them to compassion. They not only sometimes help to comfort those who mourn; they help to keep the rest of us a little more open to the hurts and the wounds of our neighbors.

The Practice of Funerals

We should not leave the practices of mourning and comforting without some brief attention to funerals. It is commonplace to complain about them, and many of the complaints are justifiable. I am old enough to remember Jessica Mitford's *American Way of Death*[12] and its complaint that funerals in America were extravagantly expensive efforts to deny death. The complaint was justified, but the reaction leaned not toward simplicity but toward getting rid of funerals altogether.[13] In place of a funeral some proposed a "private" gathering of some family and friends before burial in "an old pine box." There is nothing wrong with an old pine box, but there is something quite wrong with getting rid of the funeral or of turning it into a "private" affair. Some social scientists complained then that proposals to get rid of the funeral ignored the importance of the funeral as a "rite

---

12. Jessica Mitford, *The American Way of Death* (New York: Simon and Schuster, 1963).

13. The Calvinists at the Westminster Assembly similarly reacted to the extravagance — and especially the extravagant eulogies — at Anglican funerals of the time. They thought it wise to avoid funerals altogether. "When any person departeth this life, let the dead body, upon the day of burial, be decently attended from the house to the place appointed for publick burial, and there immediately interred, without any ceremony." After the burial, they might meet to hear the Word preached, but the one preaching should not provide a eulogy but put the congregation "in remembrance of their duty." The quotations are from the *Directory for the Publick Worship of God* (1644), cited by Thomas G. Long, "O Sing to Me of Heaven: Preaching at Funerals," *Journal for Preachers* 29, no. 3 (Easter 2006): 22.

of passage," as a way to mark separation and to make a transition. The complaint was justified, and the emphasis on the "therapeutic value" of the funeral was welcomed. It was welcomed, at least, until it was recognized that "the triumph of the therapeutic"[14] risked reducing all of life, including the funeral, to the narcissistic fulfillment of an individual's felt needs and desires without subjecting those needs and desires to moral scrutiny. The felt need might be to deny the death or to display one's grief or simply to get both the funeral and the grief over with. It was time for those churches that had surrendered funerals to the funeral director to take them back. And many denominations did liturgical work — good liturgical work — on the funeral service in the last third of the twentieth century.

The new liturgies both acknowledge the reality of grief and proclaim the hope of resurrection. They do so in the context of the community's worship of God. The practices of gathering, of reading Scripture, of prayer are all there. Many of them quite deliberately remind the gathered of the baptism of the deceased, their participation in the death and resurrection of Christ. Many of them strongly suggest the appropriateness of the Eucharist. Most of them voice a certain wariness about sentimental eulogies. There has evidently been a retrieval of the theological affirmations of the goodness of creation — including the goodness of our finitude — and of the resurrection. Liturgically, at least, there is no commendation of death of the sort one found in the *Ars Moriendi* tradition. It will come as no surprise to the reader patient enough to get this far, that I welcome these new liturgies and hope that they form our practices of dying well and caring well for the dying.

So, what's to complain about? One might complain, of course, that too often the funeral serves as the only communally sanctioned practice of mourning and comforting rather than being the evocation of continuing practices of mourning and comforting. Leave that aside for now. One can still find reasons to complain about some funerals because more things than just the liturgical rubrics shape the funeral service. In spite of the liturgical rubrics, some services still seem captured by the extravagance about which Mitford complained, or by the privatization of death and the funeral about which the social scientists complained, or by the therapeutic narcissism about which Philip Rieff complained. Churches should explain

14. Philip Rieff, *The Triumph of the Therapeutic: Uses of Faith after Freud* (Chicago: University of Chicago Press, 1987).

why they do what they do at funerals long before a few days prior to burial. The failure to provide such explanation is a failure to confront the silence and denial that still surround death, even in churches, even in those places where we remember a story that has a death in the center of it, even in those places where we claim to share in a death in the sacraments. Conversation about funerals, and about one's own funeral, needs to be pushed upstream if it is to form also our practices of dying well and caring well for the dying.

One might complain about the euphemisms that sometimes still get used in funeral homilies and eulogies in an effort to hide death when we should be honest about it. And the homilies themselves sometimes, in spite of the theological assumptions of the liturgies that surround them, adopt the strategy of the *Ars Moriendi,* denying both death and grief by commending death, while they call the mourners to repentance "before it is too late." ("Do not mourn for little Annie. She is not in that coffin. She is in heaven with Jesus." "Death is nothing but the gate to a better world" or "just a birth into eternal bliss." "John is not really dead, and if you listen hard, you can hear him speak to you today, urging you to repent.")

About the liturgical rubrics themselves, one may have legitimate concerns. Many of the liturgies discourage eulogies; some prohibit them. Understandably so, given the frequency with which such remarks engage in the denial of death or in sentimental flattery. When my good friend and colleague R. Dirk Jellema, who taught creative writing at Hope College for years, died, I was asked to preach at his memorial service. I had begun to put some words together in the genre of a eulogy when I faintly remembered an essay he had published in the *Reformed Journal* some years before. It was what that journal called an "As We See It" column, a short opinion piece. The one I had faintly remembered was entitled "Oh, Bury Me Not . . ." It was mostly an objection to expensive caskets, fancy vaults, and the like, but it had a line or two for anyone who dared to speak at a memorial service. Dirk had always had little patience with flattery and especially — as the article made clear — with eulogistic flattery. Such remarks "in the name of memory and for the sake of old Aunt Tillie" too frequently involved "obsequies we couldn't bring ourselves to perform in their presence — for the likely reason that they would have been embarrassed by it all, or corrective of our eulogies, or both."[15] Dirk's words did not make my task easier, but they did, I think, make my words better. Even

15. R. Dirk Jellema, "Oh, Bury Me Not . . . ," *Reformed Journal,* September 1978.

so, while my remarks acknowledged the awful reality of Dirk's death and announced (so I hope) the gospel, they also fell within the definition of a eulogy (literally, a "good word"). It seemed — and seems — to me that a funeral should always be personalized to some extent. We are responding, after all, not to an abstraction, not to death in general, but to the death of a specific person. Those who grieve mourn the death of this particular person. And the funeral as a practice of mourning requires attention to the memory of that person. So, warnings against the tendencies of eulogies to deny death and to engage in the "obsequies" Dirk detested are surely in order, but let there be a "good word" said of the dead.

More significant, I think, is the failure of some of the liturgies to give sufficient attention to grief. As we have said, most of the new liturgies try both to acknowledge the reality of grief and to proclaim the hope of resurrection. But sometimes it seems the liturgy rushes past the grief to celebrate the resurrection. Then, without sufficient attention to the awful reality of death, even the preaching of the resurrection can sound like a denial of death. I am sure this sometimes seems to be the case because funerals are always a response to the death of a specific person. One does not mourn the death of an aged mother who had been afflicted with Alzheimer's for years in the same way one mourns the sudden death of a child. For one thing, the mourning has gone on for a while about the gradual loss of the mother. Even in such a case, however, I have sometimes thought we rushed to Easter without sufficient time in the pain of Good Friday or the silence of Holy Saturday. It is, to be sure, partly a matter of discerning a proper balance, and the proper balance may not be quite the same for all who gather to worship God in response to the death of this particular person. But neither is a proper balance discerned by an inflexible devotion to the liturgical rubrics. In general, and especially in particular cases, funerals should provide more intentionally a time and space for lament.[16]

16. See further Scott Miller, "Reclaiming the Role of Lament in the Funeral Rite," *Call to Worship* 38, no. 3 (2004-5): 34-48. The failure to give sufficient attention to lament mars even Tom Long's recent book on the Christian funeral, *Accompany Them with Singing — the Christian Funeral.* It is in many ways an excellent book. It takes "the gospel narrative" of Jesus' life, death, and resurrection to provide the standard by which Christians should test and adapt the funeral practices of the surrounding culture (p. 16), and I say, "Amen." In the light of that narrative he stresses the theological significance of the body. The resurrection of Jesus and of the Christian is set in contrast to Platonic notions of the immortality of the soul, which inevitably involve the denial of death and the disparagement of the body. The resurrection of the crucified Jesus, on the other hand, acknowledges both the reality of death and

It is still the grace of God that gathers us, of course, and that grace must be announced first of all, but the response we feel might not be praise. The response we feel might well be lament. And a funeral could use sentences of lament to give it voice. There is no shortage of appropriate words in the Psalms. There is, of course, Psalm 22:1-2, and Psalm 77:1-3, and many more. And there could be more silence in worship and especially at funerals, instead of rushing to fill the silence of death with our words or to cover the sounds of weeping with our pretense that we always have something to say. The opening prayers of many of the new liturgies acknowledge the reality of death and grief, but they seldom take words the mourners might recognize as their own; they seldom take the form of a lament. To share a death and to share the grief do not allow us to pretend we know exactly how the mourners feel. We do not. Grief is, as we said, particular. But in a conversation with family and friends and in the story of the one who shared our death a pastor might find authorization to express their grief and the community's sharing of it. If we cannot find a place for lament in the funeral, we are not likely to find it elsewhere in the common life and worship of the community. And if we cannot find it anywhere, then those who suffer and grieve will continue to feel like strangers in the land, aliens and alienated. But if we can honestly make lament in the funeral, then perhaps those gathered will not think it strange in other contexts to attend to God in the form of lament and to expect the community — and God — to hear the cries of those who hurt. Then perhaps in dying as well as in death we will not celebrate death but sadly and honestly acknowledge our limits and the limits of medicine, relying finally on the

---

the goodness of bodies, and again I say, "Amen." Consistently Long affirms the importance of care for the body, including dead bodies, and consistently he criticizes funerals in which the body is ignored or shunned. Long takes the baptismal drama of baptism, our being buried with Christ in a death like his in the hope of being raised to newness of life with him, as the pattern for the dramatic action of the funeral as well. The church brings us to our burial in the hope and expectation of the resurrection, and again, "Amen." But then Long urges us to follow the advice of the fourth-century *Apostolic Constitutions* to "accompany them with singing" (hence the title) on the way to the burial (p. 70), and he contrasts these "cheerful" songs to the "dirges and sad songs" of the Roman funeral. Here, however, I hesitate and resist. The advice of the *Apostolic Constitutions* — and Tom Long's advice — seems to leave too little a place for lament. Surely, Christians need not grieve as those who have no hope, but the gospel narrative does not exclude lament. It includes Holy Saturday, and bringing the body to burial may bring to our remembrance that day of anguish and sadness as readily as the day of God's triumph over death. Lament has a place in the story — and in a Christian funeral.

faithfulness of God. Moreover, there is no real celebration of Easter without acknowledging the anguish of Holy Saturday and the sad reality of death. Only if we make a place for lament, for articulating in worship and in community the awful reality of death and grief in sad cries to God, will we be able truly to celebrate the community's faith in a God who has the hilarious power to raise the dead.

Let this, however, always be the last word at a funeral: that God has won and will win the victory over death. There must be a place for lament — in general and especially in particular cases, a larger place than we frequently allow. But as the lament psalms move toward the certainty of a hearing, toward hope, toward sharing in the faith of the community, so too may and must a Christian funeral. Perhaps the mourners cannot get that far on that day. (The psalmist who wrote Psalm 88 could not get that far either.) Then let the community still keep faith with those who mourn by keeping faith for them. But if the mourners can, if with tears running down their faces they can join the community to affirm the faith, if they can stand and say, "I believe in God the Father Almighty, Creator of heaven and earth . . . and in the resurrection of the body and the life everlasting," then they will have made one giant step toward the renewal of life. If they can at the end stand with the congregation to sing one of the great hymns of faith, to sing, for example, "A Mighty Fortress Is Our God," it will itself be a small token of resurrection.

Death will be there, of course, and its power will be obvious enough. Death needs no words to tell those gathered, "I have won again. I win every time. I make a mockery of every body. I destroy every loving relationship. I dash every hope. You, too, all of you, are mine!"[17] But against that shouting silence of Death, the Christian funeral has the opportunity and the responsibility to say, "The Lord is risen! The last word belongs to God." We need not — and we should not — claim to know more than we do. But remembering Jesus, we do know something about what God intends for God's creation and for us — and we know God's faithfulness. At the limits of our lives and at the ends of the lives of those we love, the faithfulness of God can give us courage.

The funeral should not be the only communally sanctioned practice for mourning and comforting. The community that practices funerals faithfully will be called to other practices that make a space and a time for

---

17. Paraphrasing Tom Long's account of death's "sermon" that we set at the beginning of this chapter.

mourning and comforting. It might keep vigil with the mourners before the funeral, and after the funeral it will surely not abandon the mourners to their grief as if they should have "gotten over it" in that one hour of worship.

The Practice of Remembering Saints

Ars Moriendi had the benefit of a treasure trove of memories of the martyrs and the saints who had died. We noted their appearance more than once in the wood-block prints. We share that treasure, of course, but we, at least we Protestants, have forgotten to tell the stories. We need to rediscover both the treasure and the practice of telling the stories. But we will also need to test those stories by the story of Jesus' death.

The martyrs understood the story of Jesus well enough to know that their own survival and ease should not be the law of their being. But some of them seemed to forget what one also should understand if one understands the story of Jesus, that life and its flourishing are good gifts of God the creator. The martyrs were willing to endure death and suffering for the sake of God's cause and their own integrity. Sometimes, however, they seemed to seek death as though death were itself a good.

There was in the early church unanimous agreement that one should be ready to die if the only alternative was to deny Christ. There was, however, considerable dispute about whether one may (or should) flee persecution and about whether one may (or should) seek martyrdom. Clement of Alexandria, for example, condemned certain Gnostics for their glib indifference about apostasy; they claimed that what you say with your tongue is irrelevant in God's judgment, for God looks upon the heart. But Clement also condemned those who sought martyrdom, provoked it, and volunteered for it: "[T]hose who have rushed on death," he said, display in their eagerness to die "hatred to the Creator."[18] Clement reminded his readers that Christ had told his disciples to flee when they are persecuted (Matt. 10:23),[19] and Clement himself fled from Alexandria to escape persecution. Others, however, denounced flight as itself a denial of Christ and as a display of cowardice.[20] The choice between fleeing and accepting death

18. Clement of Alexandria, *Stromateis* 4.4, in *Ante-Nicene Fathers* (Grand Rapids: Eerdmans, 1951), 2:412, cited by Darrel W. Amundsen, *Medicine, Society, and Faith in the Ancient and Medieval Worlds* (Baltimore: Johns Hopkins University Press, 1996), p. 78.

19. *Stromateis* 4.10, in *Ante-Nicene Fathers*, 2:423.

20. See Amundsen, *Medicine, Society, and Faith*, p. 79.

at the hands of the persecutors was, doubtless, sometimes a difficult one, requiring consideration of the effect of one's choice upon the community. But either choice was a better alternative than either apostasy or seeking martyrdom.

There were some, to be sure, who sought martyrdom. Ignatius quite famously sought his own death as a martyr. In contrast, Polycarp sought to avoid his death.[21] He followed the advice of his friends who urged him to withdraw from the city in an effort to avoid arrest, but when he was arrested and certain to be martyred he endured it with courage and serenity without desiring death. Tested by the story of Jesus' dying, the story of the martyrdom of Polycarp seems to me the more faithful, one still worth telling and celebrating in Christian community. It bears witness *(martus)* to the fact that, while life is not the greatest good, it is good. It bears witness to the fact that, while death is not the greatest evil, it is still evil. It bears that witness by choosing neither death nor suffering but by being willing to endure either for the sake of God's cause and one's own integrity. It bears that witness not by holding on desperately to life, and not by seeking to die, but by living and dying faithfully. The comfort of the martyrs was that they were not their own but belonged to God, the giver of life, from whom not even death could separate them. And their comfort was their courage.

We need to remember and to tell, however, not only the stories of the ancient martyrs like Polycarp but also the stories of those who, in more mundane and commonplace ways, still bear witness *(martus)* in their dying to the same comfort and the same courage. They display that courage and that comfort not only by refusing assisted suicide but also by refusing treatments that may prolong their days but only by rendering those days (or months) less apt for their tasks of reconciliation with an enemy or fellowship with a friend or just plain fun with the family. They display that courage and that comfort by choosing neither death nor a medicalized dying and by living well and faithfully even as they are dying. It is the story of Jesus that liberates them from the tyrannies of survival and ease.

When the persecution of Christians ended, asceticism became a substitute for martyrdom — and sometimes a poor substitute. The ascetic became the new spiritual hero, and the stories of the ascetics were told and retold, also as stories of dying well and faithfully, surely in the *Ars*

---

21. See, e.g., Ignatius, *To the Romans* 4, and *The Martyrdom of Polycarp* 5-9.

Moriendi. These stories, too, must be tested by the story of Jesus. They fit, frankly, less than comfortably with the story of one who, in contrast to the severity of John the Baptist, was derided as "a glutton and a drunkard" (Matt. 11:19; Luke 7:34).

Still, asceticism is surely no less complicated a phenomenon than martyrdom. On the one hand, if Clement of Alexandria (who was, incidentally, among the first of the early theologians to use "ascetic" positively in connection with the Christian life) can condemn those who sought martyrdom as "hatred to the Creator," the condemnation can easily enough also be turned on certain ascetics. Neither death nor suffering is to be commended or sought. But both may need to be endured for the sake of God's cause in the world. On the other hand, an ascetic impulse runs deep and true in the Christian tradition. It is only when it has been joined to a dualism of body and soul, of matter and spirit, that it is inevitably corrupted.

The Greek term *askeo* originally meant to exercise, to train, to practice (for an athletic event, for example), or to form raw materials into an object of value or beauty. From there it came to have many different meanings and connotations. The idea, although not the term, is used by Paul in 1 Corinthians 9:25, "Athletes exercise self-control in all things; they do it to receive a perishable wreath, but we an imperishable one." (The term *askeo* is used only once in the New Testament, in Acts 24:16, where the NRSV translates it simply, "I do my best always.") However, the New Testament also says "severe treatment of the body" has "no value in checking self-indulgence" (Col. 2:23). And 1 Timothy takes pains (itself an ascetic metaphor) to warn against a false asceticism (4:3-5).

A worthy asceticism practices self-denial and self-control as a spiritual discipline. It looks chiefly not to the self but to God and to the neighbor, trusting God and seeking the neighbor's good.[22] It does not refuse to receive the good gifts of God the creator with thankfulness. Its "otherworldly" orientation is not a matter of taking flight from the world God created and loves; it is rather a matter of unmaking and remaking the world constructed by human sin, a matter of resisting, criticizing, and reshaping that world. A worthy asceticism does not delight in suffering or seek it as a means to transcend the body or the world God gives, but it will endure suffering patiently for the sake of God's cause and the neighbor's good.

22. Calvin, *Institutes* 3.7.4.

A worthy asceticism heeds Paul's warning against "the desires of the flesh" (Gal. 5:16). It knows, however, that Paul's contrast between the flesh and the Spirit was not a contrast between the body and the soul. It was a contrast between a life (of the whole person) submissive to the rule of sin and death and a life (of the whole person) marked by the good future of God. Paul's account of life according to the flesh, for example, included sins like pride as well as lust. And life in the Spirit was an embodied life. There is no place for a dualism of body and soul, or matter and spirit, but there remains a place for asceticism, for when the rule of sin and death alienates us not only from God and our neighbors but also from ourselves, our care for our own bodies can grow disordered and selfish. Then we are blinded to the neighbor's good — and to our own.

The seeds of Christian asceticism were surely in the gospel, but the soil in which it grew up was Greek soil. Some of the Greeks, too, displayed a worthy asceticism, practicing simplicity and frugality as a criticism and an unmaking of the world of pride and greed. But some of them sought suffering, abusing their bodies, which were regarded as holding captive their spirits.[23] And they were followed in both their dualism and their unworthy asceticism by Christian Gnostics, Manicheans, and Marcionites.

Like martyrdom, Christian monasticism has also always been a complex phenomenon. It has displayed sometimes the contemplative ideals of Plato and the renunciation of the world God made and loves. But more often, and especially in its recent history (and in Anglican and Reformed communities as well as Orthodox and Catholic ones), it has displayed hope for God's way and cause in and for the world, resisting the corruption of that world by pride, selfishness, and lust, and responding to the gospel by providing alternative and faithful communities.

We need a worthy asceticism, and we need to remember and tell the stories of worthy ascetics. Again, however, we need to remember and tell not only the stories of the ancient ascetics but also the stories of those who, in more mundane and commonplace ways, still display a worthy asceticism in their dying. A worthy asceticism is not on display by making a good of suffering or by denying oneself relief from pain. It is not on display in withdrawal from community into an Egyptian desert or into a shuttered room. It is on display sometimes in resistance to a medicalized death, controlling the impulse to demand that everything possible be done

23. See E. R. Dodds, *Pagan and Christian in an Age of Anxiety* (New York: Norton, 1970).

to preserve one's life. It is on display sometimes in withdrawal from the world of dying that is shaped by an idolatrous confidence in technology, as if technology were the faithful savior in the face of death, and by an idolatrous desire for survival, as if life were some "second god."[24] It is on display sometimes in a withdrawal from medicalized death *to* community and to the tasks of community that yet remain to us. Such stories of a worthy asceticism need to be told and celebrated if we are to unmake the world of medicalized death and remake practices of faithful dying.

John Garvey tells such a story of his father's dying in his fine little book *Death and the Rest of Our Life*.[25] He had cancer, but by the time it was diagnosed it had spread to his bones and liver. His doctor told him he was dying. When John and his wife arrived at the hospital, they kissed John's father, and he responded to their affection by saying, "Well, so far dying's not so bad." He wanted to die at home and not in the hospital. So John and his wife took him home, set up a hospital bed in his bedroom and a comfortable recliner in the living room. His father was in good spirits. He was not afraid of dying, but he was worried about the pain. The doctor assured him the pain could be controlled and was good to his word. "He had no hesitation about asking for help, and he didn't need to be in control." He spent his last waking days delighting in his family and in their love. They remembered together the good times and the hard times. One evening when the family was gathered there was a moment of silence and his father's eyes were closed. They thought he was asleep, but then he said, "Keep talking." There were many good-bys to be said, many thanks to be said, and many blessings to be given. When John and his wife had to return to their own home, John told his father how grateful he was for his father's love. His father smiled and said, "You're a great son. God bless you." Garvey reports that in his final years his father "had to learn to surrender everything, and he did it gracefully, if not easily." His wife had died two years earlier, after fifty-seven years of marriage. He lost the ability to read because of macular degeneration. He lost his driver's license and the sense of independence that provided. "Finally, he lost what he would once have thought of as his dignity, but he moved beyond that notion. The night before I left, he asked me to help him to the bathroom and wait while he settled himself onto the toilet. . . . He could never have done this before, this

24. Karl Barth, *Church Dogmatics* III/4 (Edinburgh: T. & T. Clark, 1961), p. 392.
25. John Garvey, *Death and the Rest of Our Life* (Grand Rapids: Eerdmans, 2005), pp. 11-19.

nakedness before a child of his, asking for that kind of help; but he had never died before." His father died with other family present, not commending any of his losses but at peace with them, ready to let himself go into the hands of a God whom he trusted. As John's sister Joan said later, "He taught us how to die."

Jon Walton tells such a story of a woman he visited in the hospital. The woman had been hospitalized with severe stomach pain. Walton was her pastor, and he knew she would appreciate hearing some psalms read. After he finished reading Scripture, the woman reported that the doctor had visited her a little earlier and given her the awaited diagnosis. It was lymphoma, the doctor said, "rather advanced." The woman was thankful for the good care she was getting in the hospital, "clean sheets, nurses to attend her, food prepared and served, and the visits of her son and pastors," but she hoped, she said, to go home to spend her last days there.

> She smiled and went on. "I wish you'd been here earlier. The doctor came to see me with three handsome young interns in tow. They told me their names and each one checked me over, and then the doctor said to me, 'Maybe you would like to share with these young men something that they should know as doctors, especially in light of your faith, and what I've just told you.'"
>
> She said, "I hardly knew what to say. It seemed like it was so important. Here I was in this bed and I was supposed to say something that these young doctors could remember. I didn't think I had anything to say, so I just said, 'Somehow I trust that whatever happens to me I will be in God's hands, and that gives me hope. Whatever happens, I will be all right.'"
>
> And then she looked at me and said, "I wish you'd been here. You would have said it so much better than I could."
>
> And I looked at her and I said, "No, I couldn't. I couldn't have said it any better at all."

Walton told that story in a sermon,[26] but without such stories, however they are told, without somebody witnessing them and telling them, we will find it hard to die well and faithfully. When we tell such stories, we may be well reminded of that great "cloud of witnesses" (Heb. 12:1) who

---

26. Jon M. Walton, "Thanks at All Times," a sermon preached at First Presbyterian Church, New York, November 23, 2008; cited by Long, *Accompany Them with Singing*, pp. 112-13.

died in the faith. To remember the saints is to practice "the communion of the saints." We do well to remember them and to give thanks "for all the saints who from their labors rest." In remembering them, it may be that "steals on the ear the distant triumph song, and hearts are brave again and arms are strong." In remembering them we may learn again to hope for God's final triumph over death — for ourselves, to be sure, and for the creation, but also for them — for that "yet more glorious day [when] the saints triumphant rise in bright array."[27]

The Practice of Catechesis

Ars Moriendi included, as we have observed, a little catechism for the dying. It was probably to be read (and memorized) before one got to the time of dying. The church's formation of character and community for dying well and faithfully and for caring for the dying must surely begin long before the time of dying. That formation may take place quite naturally as the church gathers in response to the call of God, reads Scripture together, prays together, celebrates baptism and Eucharist together. It may take place quite naturally in the way the church honors practices of mourning and comforting and conducts funerals. But in its loyalty to God and to the cause of God, the church owns a responsibility to teach, to catechize, its members concerning the meaning of worship, the meaning of Scripture, the significance of the practices of prayer and the sacraments, and the practice of dying well and caring well for the dying.

So let there be a class now and again on death and resurrection, on dying and care for the dying. Let doctors and nurses who are members of the congregation gather now and then for mutual instruction and encouragement in their vocation as servants of a risen Lord who acknowledge the limits of their art and their own limits. Let there be an antidote for the culture's denial of death by the frank acknowledgment of death in the church. Let there be some training not only in praise but also in lament. Let there be the formation of caregiving groups to visit the sick and care for the dying. Compassion for the dying is still the best way to learn good habits for one's own dying. Let those who care in the name of Christ and those who comfort tell the stories of the deaths they have witnessed. Let them help us all to remember the stories of those deaths that were a witness (a *martus*)

27. William W. How, "For All the Saints."

to the goodness of God's gift of life, to the possibility of living faithfully even while dying, and to a Christian confidence in God's faithfulness. And let there be occasions for the community to come together to talk and think and pray about their own mortality in the context of the community's faith.[28]

The Practice of Advance Directives

The church's responsibility for catechesis might prompt the adoption of the creation of advance directives as a Christian practice, to be performed in the context of the church as a community of moral discourse and discernment. At the very least, to adopt such a practice could provide one occasion for the community to talk and think and pray about mortality in the context of the community's faith.[29]

We began this book with an account of the medicalization of death in mid-twentieth-century America. While we praised physicians for their skill and care in preserving life, we also joined the chorus of voices that complained about the reduction of death to a medical event. We took note of various responses to medicalization before turning to the church and its

---

28. There are some resources available to nurture such conversation, instruction, and formation. Notable among them is the ecumenical "tool kit" prepared by the Duke Institute on Care at the End of Life, David Brooks, ed., *The Unbroken Circle: A Toolkit for Congregations around Illness, End of Life, and Grief* (Durham, N.C.: Duke Institute on Care at the End of Life, 2009); it is available at the Web site of the institute, http://www.iceol.duke.edu/resources/toolkit.html. Some congregations have prepared "end of life" brochures, providing the congregation's perspective on death, its guidelines for funerals, its resources for mourning and comforting, and the like. One such congregation is Saint Matthias Episcopal Church in Waukesha, Wisconsin. Their brochure is entitled "Last Things: A Parish Resource for the Time of Death." It may be found as appendix 1 in Cynthia Cohen et al., *Faithful Living, Faithful Dying: Anglican Reflections on End of Life Care* (Harrisburg, Pa.: Morehouse, 2000). That thoughtful volume is the work of the End of Life Task Force of the General Convention of the Episcopal Church. Other denominations, too, have prepared study guides to nurture conversation about end-of-life issues.

29. Among the resources available to help congregations undertake such a practice there is the "tool kit" prepared by the Duke Institute on Care at the End of Life mentioned in the previous note, Brooks, *The Unbroken Circle*, pp. 70-75. The Center for Practical Bioethics (Kansas City, Mo.) has prepared a workbook called *Caring Conversations* that could be adapted for congregational use (available at www.PracticalBioethics.org). And there is the *Five Wishes* brochure that could be used by congregations adopting this practice (available at www.agingwithdignity.org/5wishes.html).

resources for dying well and faithfully. One of those responses was the effort of standard bioethics to limit medicalization by insisting on the autonomy of the patient. It was the patient who was dying, after all. It was the patient's body that had been reduced to a battleground for doctors to do battle against death. Standard bioethics, many court cases, and much legislation have insisted on the patient's right to refuse treatment. Of course, patients were sometimes incompetent to make decisions for themselves as they lay dying. So, standard bioethics and much legislation attempted to extend that autonomy by authorizing advance directives of various sorts. ("Living wills" give instructions concerning a person's wishes for treatment at the end of life; other documents assign durable power of attorney for health care decisions to a trusted friend or family member when and if one became unable to make them for oneself.) We noted also, however, that according to the SUPPORT study, all that effort had little effect on medicalization. The problem, we suggested, was not that the emphasis on autonomy and patients' rights was wrong, but that it was so minimal.

We complained in that context that it is not enough simply to decide who should decide; we also need to raise the substantive moral questions about what should be decided and about the virtues that should mark the one who decides. Indeed, the stress on autonomy and control can risk a kind of agnosticism about what should be decided, treating a decision as right simply because it is freely made. We complained that this myopic focus on the rights of the patient has not provided — and cannot provide — an alternative to a medicalized dying. Moreover, this emphasis on autonomy and independence and control of one's own life and body displays to all who face death just how much our society despises the weakness and withering, the dependence and lack of control, that frequently accompany death. It makes us loath to die — and loath to face our own dying. So, few prepare the advance directives that the law allows. And when they face death, they frequently adopt the default position of the culture, imagining that death is an enemy to be overcome by the greater powers of medicine. And so patients fall back to the perspective of the Baconian project, adopting as their own the very perspective that had led to the medicalization of death. It is no longer always the doctors who insist on doing "everything possible" to resist death; it is now sometimes the patients or their agents. Finally, we complained that the ironic result of the procedural protections of patient autonomy in living will legislation and advance directives is that they can make it harder to die. Medicalized death remains the default position, and if someone has no advance directive, the assumption is too often that everything and anything medical is authorized and must be performed.

To that catalogue of complaints we now add one more. Senator Danforth's Patient Self-Determination Act (1991) was a well-intentioned effort to insist that patients entering the hospital have the opportunity to prepare an advance directive. Senator Danforth had hoped that such legislation would push the conversation "upstream." He hoped it would encourage prudent physicians to converse with their patients about dying and about advance directives *before* their patients were admitted to a hospital or a nursing home. That hope has gone largely unfulfilled. At any rate, a person entering the hospital is now certain to be asked, "Do you have an advance directive?" And if the reply is "no," the follow-up question is likely to be, "Do you want one?" And if the reply is still "no," it will not be regarded as an opening for a conversation about dying but as an opportunity to get a document signed affirming that the hospital has observed the requirements of the Patient Self-Determination Act. Patients are sometimes "Danforthed" in a way as perfunctory and routine as the way alleged criminals are sometimes "Mirandized." But who can blame a patient for refusing the opportunity the hospital must provide? The admitting lobby is not the best place to prepare an advance directive. Nor is when you enter the hospital the best time (although it would be a good time to review one). Nor are strangers, even that kind and thoughtful receptionist in the admitting office, the best persons to help do one.

The church could be — and should be — such a place. A series of lessons on the art of dying well and faithfully could be the time. And the community of friends who share a death at the center of their common life could be the people. It is not my claim that such a time and place and conversation will suddenly render advance directives a sufficient instrument to resist a medicalized dying and to assure dying well and faithfully. But it is my claim that advance directives might be rendered a more effective instrument against medicalized dying than they are now. It is not my claim that such a time and place and conversation will eliminate all the problems with advance directives. But it is my claim that they can help to remedy some of them. In this context respect for the dying patient and her rights is not denied, but it is also not regarded as sufficient. In this context a conversation could be nurtured not only about who should decide but also about what should be decided. In this context a conversation about the virtues important to the one who decides could be sustained. In this context there could be resistance both to the reduction of dying persons to their pathologies and to the reduction of dying persons to their capacities for agency. In this context there could be resistance to reducing covenants to contracts. Here one may hope for a recognition that we are created and redeemed as embodied, communal, and spiritual creatures. Here one may hope for a recognition that we are dependent creatures, dependent upon God and upon each other. Here one may hope for an alternative imagination concerning death and dying, a recognition that we are limited, finite, mortal creatures, and that as real and awful as death is, at the limits of our lives, God can still be trusted. When God raised Jesus from the dead, God vindicated both Jesus and God's own faithfulness. Here one may hope for a recognition that, without celebrating death or aiming at it, our own survival is not the law of our being. Here we may acknowledge that with faith, hope, love, patience, and humility we may refuse those treatments that might prolong our days but only at great risk of rendering them unfit for the simple pleasures of embodied and communal creatures of God or for the tasks, great or small, of discipleship. Then the last act of discipleship, of following Jesus, may be to let ourselves go into the faithful hands of God, trusting that the final triumph over death will be a divine victory, not a technological one.

To be sure, an invitation by the church to participate in such an event may be met with some resistance. People who go to church regularly might still say, "I don't want to talk about it. I don't want to think about it. It's too depressing." But here the response could be, "Haven't you noticed that we talk about a death fairly often in church? Haven't you been baptized into Christ's death in hope of a resurrection like his? Haven't you taken the cup at Eucharist that is our sharing in the death of Christ? How can you now refuse to think about and talk about death? How can you now refuse to think about and talk about and pray about how to live well and faithfully while you are dying?"

If churches were to adopt this practice of helping members to prepare advance directives, and if they set the conversation about them in the context of Christian convictions, they would find, I think, an opportunity for continuing catechesis, for instruction in the faith, for the formation of members. Preparing an advance directive could become an occasion for prudent and prayerful consideration of the gifts and limits of mortal life. The advance directive could be not just a legal instrument to assure our "autonomy" and "control" even at the end of our life, but a spiritual testament to our willingness to acknowledge the limits of our "autonomy" and "control" as well as the limits of our lives. It could be a testament to our readiness, at those limits and in situations that are out of our "control," to entrust ourselves both to God and to our caregivers. It could be the occasion not just for identifying some medical conditions that might prompt a refusal of further efforts to cure but also for identifying ourselves as among those who trust God to win the victory over death, who therefore need not fear death or use all our resources against it, who would live as well and as faithfully as possible even when we are dying, who would live and die in ways that nurture love and peace. Perhaps in the context of the church, advance directives could become a more effective instrument against medicalized death. But surely, and more importantly, such a program might better prepare members of the church to die well and faithfully. Such a program could help the church to take dying back from medicine.

At the very least, those who participated in such a program in the context of the church would have an opportunity for a richly human conversation. The preparation of an advance directive in the context of the church's catechesis should, of course, only be the beginning of conversations. The church, even if its pastor were named durable power of attorney for health care, should encourage continuing conversations with family members about the advance directive. Such conversations might help to minimize family quarrels about decisions concerning health care at the end of life. And such conversations are likely not to be found morbid and frightening but rich and memorable.

Several years ago my mother and father had asked me to accept durable power of attorney for their health care should they become incompetent. (They wisely put durable power of attorney for other matters in the hands of another child of theirs.) I accepted, but I asked for a little conversation about the circumstances that, in their view, should prompt me to refuse treatments that might prolong their lives. So, one evening my mother, my father, my wife Phyllis, and I sat around their table for this "little conversation." I told them that I was honored by the trust they had expressed in me by their request but also that I found the responsibility a little daunting. I wanted to know when they thought I should refuse a treatment that might prolong their life and why. My mother was the first to speak. "Well, you know, Allen, let me go when I get to be a burden." I almost blurted out, "Mom, you've been a burden for about as long as I can remember." Instead, I swallowed that impulse and said instead, "Mom, I have been a burden to you for a long time now; you can be a burden to us for a little while."

I think she liked the reply, but we had not made much headway toward my objectives for this little conversation. So, I proposed a scenario or two, but the scenarios were as vague as the scenarios in any living will. Still, they asked questions that helped me a little. They asked whether they would be able to talk with the grandkids if they came to visit. They asked whether they would be able to pray. They asked how much some treatments would cost. They asked whether some treatments would be likely to succeed and whether they would be painful. I did not know the answers to most of their questions. The scenarios were, of course, unavoidably vague. But I assured them that a doctor would probably have answers to some of these questions when and if they or I needed answers.

Along the way, however, some things did get clarified. They both told me that if it was a scarce technology that someone else also needed, I should refuse it. I said I did not know if I could refuse it for them in such a case, a response for which I was gently chided. It was clear that they both were unwilling to undertake "heroic measures" to extend their days if the extra days or months were likely to be spent in pain or coma. They would welcome some extra days to complete some tasks there might be, to say good-by, to have a little fun with the family maybe, but otherwise I should "let them go into the hands of God."

This also, however, became clear that night: I would not always be ready to "let them go" when they were ready. So finally, my father said, "OK, Allen, you have power of attorney, but let Phyllis make the decision." I remember thinking it was an odd remark. Phyllis loved them, too, and was probably going to be no more ready than I to "let them go." Maybe Dad simply thought that because Phyllis was a nurse, she would be better at that sort of decision. Perhaps he (accurately enough) thought his son's wife had more common sense than his son had. I do not know because I did not follow up on the remark. But maybe he was suggesting that I could be a little more carefree about the responsibility I had so conscientiously assumed. Maybe he was saying that if I were simply to talk to some others and then make a decision about health care for Mom or Dad that I thought fit their lives and their faith, I would have done the best I could. Something he said later makes me think that was exactly what he meant. Toward the end of our conversation that night he said this: "Don't worry about it. Anything you decide will be fine with us." That remark, made long before he was dying, was already his taking care of me trying to take care of him.

One other thing became clear that night: we cared about each other. It's not that it wasn't clear before, but talking with my parents about their death allowed us to say some things that had gone too frequently unsaid, things like "Thanks" and "I love you." That part of the conversation was finally the really important part.

As it turned out, both of my parents died many years after that "little conversation." In neither case did I need to exercise the durable power of attorney, but I cherish the memory of that night and that conversation. They each died well and faithfully, as they had lived. They had opportunities to say good-by, to bless the kids and the grandkids and the great-grandkids, and they took them. They each died, with the help of good palliative care and hospice, without great or extended pain. They each died a little sooner than they would have if everything medically possible had been done. I remember that Mother was a little disappointed that her son, the theologian, did not know more than he did about exactly what happens when one dies, but she was quite content to trust the faithfulness of God, and she looked forward to that day on which God's grace would make all things new, even her.

The Practice of Discourse and Discernment

Whether churches adopt a practice of helping members to prepare advance directives or not, they are and are called to be communities of moral discourse, deliberation, and discernment in memory of Jesus[30] — also about death and dying. Each of these calls for a brief comment.

First, churches are and are called to be communities of moral *discourse.* Members of Christian churches do and should talk together about death and about dying. There should be no fear in these communities to talk of death. There should be no silence and no denial. Perhaps William F. May put it best. "The Lord of the church is not ruler of a surface kingdom. His dominion is nothing if it does not go at least six feet deep. The church affirms the one Lord who went down into the grave, fought a battle with the power of death, and by his own death brought death to an end. For this reason, the church must be unafraid to speak of death."[31] They talk together about the death of Jesus, of course. How can they not? But they also

30. See further Allen Verhey, *Remembering Jesus: Christian Community, Scripture, and the Moral Life* (Grand Rapids: Eerdmans, 2002), pp. 34-48.

31. William F. May, "The Sacral Power of Death in Contemporary Experience," in *On Moral Medicine: Theological Perspectives in Medical Ethics,* ed. Stephen E. Lammers and Allen Verhey, 2nd ed. (Grand Rapids: Eerdmans, 1998), p. 201.

talk about the deaths of family and friends and about the lingering dying of Helen and their hope that Dan will pull through.

Because they are and are called to be communities of *moral* discourse, they do and should talk inevitably about what they should do in response to the sickness that threatens death, in response to dying, in response to death, in response to grief. What should be done or left undone? The conversations may happen after the worship service or in a Sunday school class or in a session meeting or simply when people happen to meet at the market. But wherever they happen, such moral discourse leads almost inevitably to moral *deliberation.* That is to say, they talk together not only about what should be done but also about *why* it should be done. They give and hear reasons for doing one thing rather than another. The reasons are, of course, of various sorts. There will be appeals to what is customarily done in those parts or in that congregation. There will be appeals to culturally accepted norms. There will be appeals to people's autonomy, what they may have said they wanted or didn't want. There will be appeals to what another regards as "therapeutic" in such circumstances. There will be many different sorts of reasons given. And those different reasons will need to be weighed and tested. Moral deliberation thus leads almost inevitably toward testing the reasons given and heard, challenging them or defending them as good reasons, qualifying them and ordering them. That weighing and testing of reasons requires moral *discernment.* And in these communities, in the churches, the reasons must finally be tested on whether they cohere with the gospel, whether they somehow fit the remembered story of Jesus. This community is, and is called to be, a community of moral discourse, deliberation, and discernment *in memory of Jesus.*

There are, of course, other communities and traditions within which conversations about what should be done and why it should be done occur. There are other communities and traditions within which reasons are tested and weighed. There are, for example, the professional associations to which doctors belong. There are cultural traditions like the one we have called the Baconian project. These communities and traditions, too, shape character and provide some account of the human good and how to achieve it. Indeed, for many of us our participation in those other communities and traditions is finally (but strangely) more determinative for our decisions than our membership in the church. Nevertheless, churches can and sometimes do test and qualify these other traditions, call for the reformation of character and conduct, and provide their own account of the human good and the ways to serve it. The churches should nurture and sustain moral discourse and deliberation in the service of discernment of a way of life — and a way of dying — that is "worthy of the gospel of Christ." The churches should resist simply adopting the perspective of other associations and traditions without testing them by their memory of Jesus. The church remains a distinctive community of discourse, deliberation, and discernment by remembering Jesus and by transforming questions of character and conduct into the question of how its people may live the story they still love to tell — even as they lie dying.

This book is not a substitute for that discernment. It attempts, rather, simply to contribute to that communal discernment by asking how the story of Jesus might nurture and sustain the practices of dying well and faithfully and of caring well and faithfully for the dying. Because those practices will be congruent with and informed by other practices of the churches, this chapter has been an effort to examine some of those other practices and the ways in which they may form our dying and our caring for the dying.

Moral Ambiguity and the "Not Yet" Character of Our Existence

Christian churches that faithfully engage in the practices of moral discourse, deliberation, and discernment in memory of Jesus do not escape the moral ambiguities encountered by the dying and those who care for them. Reading Scripture and attending to God in prayer are important practices, but they do not rescue us from moral ambiguity or provide simple answers to some of the hard questions faced by the dying and by their caregivers. When Christian churches, however, faithfully perform these practices, when they remember Jesus, they become communities that form people who can be trusted in the midst of moral ambiguity and who have the courage to make the morally ambiguous decision.

Ambiguities arise in part simply because in this sad world, not yet God's good future, one part of what we recognize to be the cause of God seems to conflict with another part of what we know to be the cause of God. In such cases our loyalty to God and to the cause of God does not resolve the conflict. But we may and should at least recognize the conflict and appreciate the ambiguity.

For Christians the significance of suffering and dying is determined by the story of Scripture, stories of creation and fall and redemption, stories of a cross and of an empty tomb. But the significance is complex; there is a certain dialectic in the dispositions toward suffering and dying in the story of Scripture, and it can give rise to unavoidable ambiguity.

On the one hand, life and its flourishing belong to the creative and redemptive cause of God. The signs of it are breath and a blessing, a rainbow and God's own sanction, a commandment and, finally, an empty tomb. Therefore, life and its flourishing will be recognized and celebrated as goods, as goods against which we may not turn without turning against the cause of God. They are to be received with thanksgiving and used with gratitude. Acts that aim at death and suffering do not fit this story, do not cohere with devotion to the cause of God or with gratitude for the gifts of God.

On the other hand, life and its flourishing are not the ultimate goods. They are not "second gods."[32] Jesus walked a path steadily and courageously that led to his suffering and to his death. Therefore, Christians may not live as though either survival or ease were the law of their being. Sometimes life must be risked, let go, given up. And sometimes suffering must be risked or shared for the sake of God's cause in the world. The refusal ever to let die and the attempt to eliminate suffering altogether are not signals of faithfulness but of idolatry. And if life and its flourishing are not the ultimate goods, neither are death and suffering the ultimate evils. They need not be feared finally, for death and suffering are not as strong as the promise of God. One need not use all one's resources against them. One need only act with integrity in the face of them.

This dialectic is captured in the distinctions between killing and allowing to die and between choosing suffering and patiently bearing it. So far, so good — there is not much ambiguity there.[33] Because there was

---

32. Barth, *Church Dogmatics* III/4, p. 392.

33. The moral significance of those distinctions, of course, is being challenged — and may be difficult to defend when the story in which they are embedded is denied or ignored. The moral distinctions are hard to defend, for example, in the context of a utilitarian calculus, where the only relevant consideration is outcome, results, consequences. If the consequences are the same, it is hard to see in a utilitarian calculus why the moral evaluation of mercifully allowing one to die and mercifully killing someone ought to be different. Moreover, if the standard for assessing the consequences is the maximization of preference satisfaction, and if anyone (whether arbitrarily or reasonably) prefers death to life in his or her particular circumstances, then it is not hard to see the moral obligation to kill the suicidal (or to inflict pain on the masochist).

The distinctions seem more at home — at least initially — in the context of the sort of moral minimalism that focuses on rights and their correlative duties. In this context, for

breath and a blessing, because there was a rainbow and a commandment, because there was an empty tomb, Christians will not choose death, will not intend death. But because the one who was raised had suffered and died, Christians will acknowledge that there may be goods more weighty than their own survival or ease, goods and duties that determine how they should live, even while they are dying. The distinction fits the story of Scripture and the notions of suffering and dying formed by it, but it does not eliminate all ambiguity. When preserving life means to prolong suffering, the distinction allows dying, but it does not make death a good to be sought. When prolonging suffering for the sake of accomplishing some task that remains, the distinction allows continuing treatment, but it does

---

example, one can distinguish between negative and positive rights, between rights to noninterference and rights to assistance. So one can distinguish the right to life as a negative right not to be killed from the right to life as a positive right to assistance in preserving one's life. And one can also distinguish the right to die as a negative right not to have one's dying interfered with from the right to die as a positive right to assistance in ending one's life. Since rights to noninterference are usually regarded as imposing much more stringent correlative duties than rights to assistance, and since the negative right to life imposes a duty not to kill, one could at least argue that, therefore, there can be no positive right to die and no duty to assist in suicide that would be imposed by such a right. But the distinction quickly loses any force against the background of such moral minimalism. Not only does the right to die seem to extend to suicide, it would also seem to extend to assistance in suicide if a contract had been freely entered. Since the right to life, like any right, is a legitimate claim, and since one may refuse autonomously to make the legitimate claims that are one's own to make, if I refuse to claim my negative right to life, then it is hard to see why killing me would be a violation of that right. So, consensual killing looks morally indistinguishable from consensual allowing to die in this context, too.

See further Gilbert Meilaender, "The Distinction between Killing and Allowing to Die," *Theological Studies*, September 1976, pp. 467-70, and Robert N. Wennberg, *Terminal Choices: Euthanasia, Suicide, and the Right to Die* (Grand Rapids: Eerdmans, 1989), pp. 150-56. The distinction between allowing to die and killing cannot be reduced to the distinction between omission and commission. There are clearly some cases of omission that can only be described as intending the death of the patient, as killing — for example, the failure to treat Baby Doe's esophageal atresia (see Verhey, *Reading the Bible*, pp. 345-58). And I surely do not mean to suggest that the distinction provides an easy formula for resolving hard questions. There are some cases that are hard to classify as allowing to die or as killing. (I will consider the Terri Schiavo case below, but see also Wennberg, pp. 136-42, who cites a case in which a diabetic man with painful and terminal cancer stops taking his insulin. Did the diabetic man allow himself to die or did he kill himself? Still, as Wennberg says, "there is a theologically significant difference between shaping one's dying and creating one's dying" [p. 137], between intending death and foreseeing it, between choosing death and choosing how to live while one is dying.)

not make pain or humiliation or suffering good. Sometimes the choice is not simply right or wrong. Sometimes it will be hard to decide between the good of preserving life and the good of minimizing suffering, to decide whether to preserve life or to allow death, even to decide whether to continue to pray for continuing life or to pray for the strength and virtue to die well and peaceably. Sometimes it will be a tragic choice, a choice when evils have gathered and cannot all be avoided, a choice where goods collide and cannot all be chosen.[34] Such ambiguity is another mark of the not-yet character of our existence, another hard reminder that we still watch and pray for the good future of God in which there will be no evil and in which God will establish peace also among the many disparate goods that belong to God's cause.

Jesus and his resurrection point us beyond tragedy to the good future of God, but here and now tragedy and ambiguity remain. The community of discourse, deliberation, and discernment cannot eliminate the tragedy or the ambiguity. But looking to God will nurture and sustain humility in the face of such decisions, truthfulness about the difficulty and ambiguity of such decisions, gratitude for opportunities within the limits of such decisions to seek and serve God's cause, care for those caught between death and suffering, and respect for their embodied and communal and spiritual integrity. Looking to God will nurture and sustain also a sense of God's forgiveness in the midst of such ambiguity and the courage to make the ambiguous choice we need to make in the confidence of God's good future.

Moral Ambiguity and the Schiavo Case

Sometimes the ambiguity reaches to that distinction between allowing to die and killing. As we have said, that distinction fits the story, and it has been consistently important to moral discernment of the Christian community. But sometimes it is not easy to make that distinction. That ambiguity, for example, surrounds the withdrawal of artificial nutrition and hydration from someone in a persistent vegetative state.[35] It surely was

34. On tragedy, see further Allen Verhey, "Technology and Tragedy: An Evangelical Theology of Care," in *Covenants of Life: Contemporary Medical Ethics in the Light of Paul Ramsey*, ed. Kenneth L. Vaux, Sara Vaux, and Mark Stenberg, Philosophy and Medicine, vol. 77 (Dordrecht: Kluwer, 2002), pp. 127-45.

35. Persistent vegetative state must be distinguished from brain death. In brain death

central in the celebrated case, to give one particular example, of Terri Schiavo.[36] The public and legal quarrel between Terri's husband and her parents captured the attention of the nation. Family quarrels, of course, can be ugly — and uglier still when made public and co-opted by media bioethicists and politicians. Like March Madness, we seemed driven to pick a team and root it on to victory, vanquishing the opponents. But it's time to put the madness behind us. It's time to attend not just to the passion but to the compassion on both sides of this debate. Both sides, after all, claimed to be on Terri's side.

Consider two arguments, both Christian and both "pro-Terri." The first argument: we must provide food and drink for Terri. Terri might not count for much as the world counts, but she surely counts as among "the least of these" in Jesus' parable. "Inasmuch" as you gave food to the hungry or drink to the thirsty, you did it "as unto me" (Matt. 25). To provide food and drink is simply the sort of care one human being owes another, even the least of them. It doesn't matter whether the person is at home or in the hospital or in a hospice. It doesn't matter whether food and drink are provided in a cup or in a bowl, through a straw or a tube.

Moreover, to withhold food and drink is to aim at Terri's death, and that we must not do. We may allow some to die sometimes when they are going to die anyway, but we may not kill them. Finally, even if you regard providing food and drink as medical treatment, it must be regarded as "or-

---

there is an irreversible loss of the capacity of the organism as a whole to function. The sign of it is the lack of any electrical activity in the whole brain, including the brain stem. If a person is brain-dead, the question cannot be, "Should we allow this person to die?" The person in persistent vegetative state is not yet dead, and the question is frequently, "Shall we allow this person to die?" It was the condition endured by Karen Quinlan and Nancy Cruzan as well as Terri Schiavo. Recovery is very rare, especially after three months following a nontraumatic injury and after one year following a traumatic injury. The lack of absolute certainty, of course, serves to make the choice an exceptionally difficult one. On the one hand, the lack of absolute "clinical certainty" joined to the recognition that life is a great good, some argue, requires the conclusion that the morally safest course is to continue life-saving treatment. On the other hand, "moral certainty" does not require absolute "clinical certainty," and some argue that to continue treatment when recovery is so very rare is itself to dishonor the patient, to reduce her to a biological organism, and simply to prolong her (thoroughly medicalized) dying. In cases of disagreement about what is to be done or left undone, limited time trials might provide a basis for conversation and compromise.

36. The remarks about the arguments concerning the death of Terri Schiavo were originally prepared for a conference sponsored by the Duke Institute on Care at the End of Life and later published in *Christian Century* (Allen Verhey, "Necessary Decisions: Taking Sides for Schiavo," *Christian Century,* April 19, 2005, pp. 9-10).

dinary treatment," not "extraordinary treatment." The distinction depends not on whether the treatment is customarily given but on whether the benefits *to the patient* outweigh the burdens of the treatment *to the patient*. To an unconscious patient like Terri, a feeding tube is hardly a burden — and the benefit is life. If we fail to see life as a good, as a benefit to her, we have evidently accepted an unbiblical and Cartesian dualism of body and soul, reduced the self to its powers of rationality and choice and reduced the body to a mere container.

Withholding food and drink may be an effective means to make certain that biologically tenacious patients die when their life is a burden *to us,* but it should be classified with other means of making certain people die, like blowing their brains out. Don't do it! Don't allow it!

I hope you find this argument compelling. I have tried to present it as well as I briefly could, but there is a second "pro-Terri" argument that I hope you also find compelling.

We must withdraw artificial nutrition and hydration from Terri. Nasal-gastric tubes, J-tubes, and IVs are medical procedures, and the same standards that apply to the withholding or withdrawing of other medical procedures should apply also to artificial nutrition and hydration. Those standards must start from the recognition that caring for Terri requires respect for her integrity. Legally this is reflected in the right of competent patients to refuse medical treatment. Christians regard life as a good, to be sure, but not as "a second god." Remembering Jesus and following him, we can hardly make our own survival the law of our being. Christians may refuse medical care that another may live. They may refuse those procedures that may lengthen their days but do nothing to make those days more apt for their tasks of reconciliation, fellowship, or just plain fun with the family.

It is not shocking that Terri, or any other Christian, would have suggested that she would refuse artificial nutrition and hydration if she were in a persistent vegetative state, and that decision must finally be honored if we would respect Terri's Christian integrity. If there were no evidence of such a decision, or very uncertain evidence, then others would have to weigh the burdens and benefits of these medical procedures to Terri. Then we still may and still should withdraw artificial nutrition and hydration. Terri is in a persistent vegetative state with no hope of recovery. If we consider the preservation of her biological life a benefit to her, we have evidently accepted an unbiblical vitalism, reduced her to her body and her body to mere organism.

Moreover, although withdrawing artificial nutrition and hydration may have death as a consequence, death is not intended but accepted. To insist that artificial nutrition and hydration be continued is to make Terri a prisoner of medical technology and should be classified with other imprisonments without due process. Don't do it! Don't allow it!

There they are: two Christian arguments, two "pro-Terri" arguments. What shall we say about them? First, simply that they were not new or original. They can be tracked not just for the thirty days or so before the feeding tubes were removed from Terri but for at least thirty years among both Catholic and Protestant moral theologians.

Second, these two quite different positions share important areas of agreement. They agree that there is an important moral distinction between killing and allowing to die. They disagree, of course, on whether to describe withdrawing "food and drink" (or "artificial nutrition and hydration") as more like killing or more like letting die. Both use the language of "ordinary" and "extraordinary" to insist on the moral importance of weighing the burdens and benefits of the treatment *to Terri*. They disagree, however, about how to describe and weigh the benefits and burdens. And both insist that Terri is to be treated and cared for as an embodied self. They disagree, however, about whether the greater risk is that she will be reduced to her capacities for rational choice or that she will be reduced to biological organism.

Third, the disagreements suggest the importance of perspective, of how we see and describe what's going on. Do we see a refusal to give food and drink or a withdrawal of medical technology? Do we see an embodied self reduced to capacities for rational agency or reduced to biological organism? It's not easy to say what is *the right way to see* (or to say) what's going on. Short of an agreement about what should be decided, we ask, "Who should decide?" And short of an agreement about how to describe the case, we ask, "Who should decide how to describe what's going on?" But now it gets tricky, because how we see matters here, too. If what we see is the refusal to provide food and drink, and if that leads us to describe the case as killing, then killing is not a choice for *anyone* to make. To allow the procedural question "Who should decide?" now seems dangerously close to a license to kill. Of course, the question looks innocent and reasonable when we don't see the case in that way. But how to see and describe the case is precisely what is at stake. So we enter a regress, "Who should decide who should decide what's going on?"

The answer to that question in our culture has frequently been the courts. The courts allocate choice-making powers to some and render others choiceless. Sometimes there is no alternative. Sometimes as a last resort, we must simply decide who should decide. But we should not rush to the last resort.[37] The obligation is not just to decide who should decide but to listen to each other and to consider our own need for "corrective vision."

The lessons, I think, are two. First, continue the conversation. The courts too often put a stop to the conversation by simply deciding who should decide. Because the patient is the one who should decide, it has become a commonplace to urge people to prepare an advance directive. Earlier we urged churches to help people prepare such advance directives. But I'm not sure that helps as much as is commonly supposed — unless they are done in conversation with one's community.

One context for continuing this conversation must be the churches. Churches need to be communities of moral discourse and discernment. There in memory of Jesus Christians learn that life is a great gift but that death is not the greatest evil. They learn that we need not use all our resources against death, that the victory over death is finally a divine victory, not a technological victory. They learn, moreover, to talk together, to give and hear reasons, and to test them together against the story of Jesus. By listening to the stories of Scripture and to the stories of Christian physicians and nurses and families that care for the dying, we may yet learn together a wisdom that can correct our vision.

The second lesson is this: appreciate ambiguity. There are situations where there are no right answers, no good answers, situations where goods collide and cannot all be chosen, where evils gather and cannot all be avoided. There may be situations — and I think there are — in which it is morally appropriate to withhold medical procedures (including procedures for nutrition and hydration), but that does not make death a good. That, of course, discloses my greater sympathy with the second "pro-Terri" argument. The first "pro-Terri" argument, however, may at least warn me — and us — against the possibility of slipping into a readiness to regard Terri as the burden and to justify this way (or others) of eliminating *our* burdens by making certain that biologically tenacious patients die. The ambiguity remains, but it need not paralyze us. It should not become an

37. See Robert Burt, *Taking Care of Strangers: The Rule of Law in Doctor-Patient Relations* (New York: Free Press, 1979), pp. 124-43. Burt proposes that courts refrain from allocating choice-making powers initially. They should rather require a conversation in which the participants attempt to come to a consensus, to a compromise. If they fail, then it may be necessary to decide who will decide, but the courts then could decide in part on the basis of consulting a verbatim of the conversation to see who participated in good faith in the conversation.

occasion for quarrels and pretentious claims that I alone care for Terri and for people in similar condition. Rather it should be an occasion for continuing the conversation, for listening carefully and charitably to the recommendations of another, for prayer, for a readiness to look for areas of agreement and to accept a compromise (perhaps something like a time-limited trial). Looking to God rather than to technology as the basis of our hope, we may find the courage to make a necessary but necessarily ambiguous decision.

Miracles and Eschatological Realism

The ambiguities reach further than the distinctions between choosing death and accepting death, between intending suffering and enduring it. They reach into our existence between the times, our life and dying during this interval between Christ's resurrection and the final resurrection, our care for people when it is both "already" and "not yet" God's good future. It shows up from time to time when we are looking for a miracle to save our own life or the life of a loved one. Earlier, when we considered the practice of prayer, we called attention to some worries about "praying for a miracle," but because of the importance of this question to many and because of the ambiguities surrounding it, we revisit it briefly here.

We have an eschatological hope, and we believe that the future power of God can and does already make its power felt, sometimes in quite mundane ways and sometimes in surprising and unpredictable ways. When people pray to God for healing, they pray in accord with what we know of the cause of God. God intends life, not death. God intends human flourishing, including the human flourishing we call "health," not pain and suffering. They pray then for a little foretaste of God's good future. Properly so. We may lament the threat of death, and call God to God's own faithfulness. The psalmists of Israel surely did. But when the doctors report that there is little hope for recovery, sometimes Christians say, "I know it looks bad, but God has worked miracles before. Didn't Jesus raise Lazarus? Didn't he heal that woman doctors couldn't heal? We should keep Sam alive and hope for a miracle." Now, perhaps Calvin thought that the age of miracles was past,[38] but I don't. God's good future still breaks into the

---

38. Calvin's suspicion of miracles was in no small part a reaction to the excesses of the stories of miracles involving the cult of relics and visits to shrines in the late Middle Ages. He

present. God's cause still makes its power felt, sometimes in quite ordinary ways and sometimes in ways we cannot explain.

The hope for a miracle is sometimes ridiculed in a hospital, and the ridicule sometimes intimidates the believer into giving up this hope (but with an uneasy conscience) and sometimes causes the believer who refuses to be intimidated to dig in his or her heels and refuse to listen to talk of "futility." It would be better by far both for the dying and for those who keep company with the dying if the church considered the ambiguity of such an expectation long before such prayers were needed.

Without denying the reality of miracles, we should admit that the expectation of a miracle can be deeply ambiguous and, well, unfaithful. In one of his delightful "letters to Ellen,"[39] Gil Meilaender tried to imagine a world in which God regularly intervened to perform the miracles his people might request. He failed. "I can't even imagine it," he said. "For it would be a world without any order or regularity. We could depend on nothing, since we'd never know when God would be cutting the cards again. I don't disbelieve in miracles, but almost by definition, they have to be rare. Otherwise life becomes impossible." He goes on to say that to expect God to work miracles whenever we ask, although it sounds pious, "doesn't really take God seriously." God is not "a magician at our beck and call. And the course of the world should not be rearranged every time we want things different. That notion is, if you think about it, the ultimate in narcissism — as if I were the center of the universe. To take God seriously is to leave the center to him."

We have an eschatological hope, to be sure, a hope that God's good future is breaking into our present time, but that hope must be accompanied by an eschatological realism, by the acknowledgment that it is not yet God's good future. That realism requires also the acknowledgment that it is God who must finally bring that future, not our technology and not even our prayers. Without that eschatological realism in response to suffering and dying, we are always at risk of temptations to triumphalism. And the triumphalism that sometimes attends the expectation of a miracle can prompt a denial of death. Against triumphalism the Gospels tied the

would have no part of what he regarded as a superstitious and magical religious devotion, and he reduced miracles to a confirmation of the truth of the gospel. Accordingly, when the church became established, miracles ceased. Against Calvin I take miracles to be God's good future breaking into the present.

39. Gilbert Meilaender, *Letters to Ellen* (Grand Rapids: Eerdmans, 1996), pp. 47-49. The citations are from p. 48.

memory of Jesus as the risen one to the cross. No memory of Jesus may neglect or ignore the cross. We live — and suffer and die — under the sign of it. It is not yet, still not yet, God's good future. Apart from the story of the cross the church is always at risk of distorting the gospel into a Pollyanna triumphalism and then of self-deceptively ignoring or denying the sad truth about our world or the sad truth about the person we love.

The expectation of a miracle is ironically parallel to the triumphalism of a culture shaped by the Baconian project. Our culture is always at risk of trumpeting the good news of some medical breakthrough and then ignoring the sad truth that there is no medical technology to rescue the human condition from mortality or vulnerability to suffering. Because the culture lacks an eschatological realism, it is at risk of extravagant (and idolatrous) expectations of medicine, tempted to regard the physician as a medical wizard whose magic will deliver us from death and suffering. And when our expectation of a miracle lacks an eschatological realism, it is tempted to regard the prayers of the righteous no less magically, to make God an idol, to forget that we are God's servants, not God ours.

The parallel is rendered still more ironic when we continue treatment in the expectation of a miracle, as though the miracle we expect were contingent upon the technology. And the final irony is the result that the expectation of a miracle can serve rather than resist the medicalization of death.

The expectation of a miracle can be deeply ambiguous and, indeed, unfaithful when it is used as a conversation stopper. But the conversation should continue. A good and faithful dying and good and faithful care for the dying require consideration of the comfort of the embodied person threatened by death, the tasks that may remain to this communal self. It requires consideration of the strain on the person's body and the strain on the person's family and the strain on the community's resources with expensive treatments. It is not more faithful but less to set aside such considerations by insisting that treatment be continued while we wait for a miracle. Of course, it may be the case that treatment should be continued. But that decision must be reached in a process of discernment that attends to all these considerations while attending to God, not by attending to God as an *alternative* to attending prayerfully to all these other things.

Finally, the expectation of a miracle can be ambiguous because it can blind us to the miracles around us, however mundane they may seem. When people face dying with courage, the good future of God makes its power felt. When they are ready to let themselves go into God's hands,

God's good future has made its power felt. When at the limits of our lives and at the end of them people trust God, then the eschatological hope is present. When in their dependence they trust God and find others who are trustworthy to care for them, God's future has broken in. When there is forgiveness and reconciliation, God's good future makes its power felt. When there is love, even the love that mourns, that is the mark of God's good future. These are all miracles in their way, even if we do not find them inexplicable.

CHAPTER SIXTEEN

The Practice of Care

*"Truly I tell you, just as you did it to one of the least of these . . . ,
you did it to me."*

Matthew 25:40

It is not good to die alone. That was hardly the discovery of the fifteenth
century. From the beginning the Christian church has been formed by its
memory of Jesus to visit the sick, to be present to the suffering, and to care
for the dying. Jesus died in solidarity with humanity. He made the human
cry of lament his own cry. He identified himself especially with those who
do not count for much as the world counts, with those the world regards as
"the least of these," with those it would shun and ignore. Perhaps the impulse to shun and ignore them comes because of some worry about the
contagion of suffering or perhaps it is simply because they are reminders
of the common human vulnerability to suffering and death. But in memory of Jesus, "the least of these" are given a privileged position. Because of
Christ's identification with them, to care for them is to care for Christ and
to abandon them is to abandon Christ.

The conclusion is unavoidable given Jesus' parable of the last judgment (Matt. 25:31-46). Matthew brings his account of watchfulness to a climactic conclusion with this parable.[1] When the Son of Man comes in his

---

1. Matthew adopts Mark's chapter about watchfulness (cf. Mark 13:1-37 and Matt.

glory, the story goes, he invites some to enter the kingdom — because, as he said, "I was hungry and you gave me food, I was thirsty and you gave me something to drink, I was a stranger and you welcomed me, . . . I was sick and you took care of me. . . ." Those who heard him were surprised, shocked, by the words. "When?" they asked. "We were watching for you, waiting for you, but when, Lord, did we care for you?" And the Son of Man answered them, "Inasmuch as you cared for one of the least of these, you cared for me."

The parable is eloquent testimony that watchfulness takes the shape of care for the sick and dying. It has provided an elegant reminder to the community that the presence of God is mediated to them through those in need, including the sick and dying. Remembering Jesus' suffering and death, Christians saw in the sick, in their weakness and vulnerability, in their hurt and loneliness, the very image of their Lord. And they discerned in their care for them (or in their abandoning them) an image of their care for Christ himself (or for their abandoning Christ himself).[2] That "inasmuch," that solidarity of the sick and dying with the crucified Christ, shaped the community from the very beginning. In memory of Jesus the Christian community turned toward the sick, not against them, caring for them in their suffering and attending to them in their dying, practicing hospitality to them rather than ostracizing them from community. In the plague of the third century in Alexandria, for example, Christians distinguished themselves by their heroic care for the sick while the pagans of the city abandoned the sick, deserted their friends, and "cast them out into the roads half-dead."[3] By the ministry of Christians, some of the sick were healed, but many of those who cared for the sick died — their deaths a witness *(martus)* to this memory of Jesus and to their hope in Jesus. Down through the centuries the memory of Jesus echoed in the care of the sick — in the heroism of Alexandrian Christians, in the founding of hospitals, in the sense of vocation of many a Christian doctor and nurse, and in the

---

25:1-44), but he adds to it a collection of parables about watchfulness (Matt. 25:45–26:46), a collection that climaxes in the parable of judgment (Matt. 26:31-46).

2. See, for example, the *Rule of St. Benedict,* chapter 36, where Matt. 25:31-45 is explicitly cited in its instruction to care for the sick "as if it were Christ himself who was served."

3. From a letter of Dionysius, bishop of Alexandria, quoted in Eusebius, *Ecclesiastical History* 7.20, trans. Christian Frederick Cruse (Grand Rapids: Baker, 1966), p. 293. The remark about those "half-dead" is a reminder of the Jewish traveler attended to by the Good Samaritan (Luke 10:30). The Alexandrian Christians followed Jesus' command to "do likewise" (Luke 10:37).

simple practice of visiting the sick and dying in Christian communities. In memory of Jesus the sick have been accorded a preferential position, and in memory of Jesus care for them has been regarded as a duty of Christian community.

And it was not just the church that was formed by this memory of Jesus. According to Henry Sigerist, in memory of Jesus the position of the sick was fundamentally changed; the sick were ascribed "a preferential position." It was, he said, "the most revolutionary and decisive change" in the tradition of medicine.[4] Caregivers may still stand there stuttering and sputtering, "Do you mean to say that that was you, Lord? She certainly had a rough time of it, and she was you, even so? Do you really mean to say that that broken body was your spiritual presence?" And the answer is always yes, and that answer always calls for a kind of reverence in response, a reverence that inspires care.

This reverence and care prompted Francis Bacon to seek to preserve the lives even of those who had been regarded as "overmastered by disease." That old category, he insisted, licensed neglect and inattention and

---

4. Henry E. Sigerist, *Civilization and Disease* (Ithaca, N.Y.: Cornell University Press, 1943), pp. 69-70. It is noteworthy, moreover, that because care for the sick was required by the gospel, the church required competence and diligence of physicians. The medieval penitential literature, for example, required physicians to confess incompetence and negligence. Darrel Amundsen's survey of the penitential literature prompted by the decree of Lateran IV (1215), which required annual confession by all Catholics, reveals that physicians were expected to confess incompetence and negligence. Both rashness and excessive caution were regarded as sins if patients were harmed (or not helped). By requiring competence, the duty of care nurtured medical learning and training, but also restrained it and ordered it, for exposing a patient (especially a poor patient) to unnecessary risk for the sake of an experiment was also mentioned. See Darrel W. Amundsen, "Casuistry and Professional Obligations: The Regulation of Physicians by the Court of Conscience in the Late Middle Ages," in his *Medicine, Society, and Faith in the Ancient and Medieval Worlds* (Baltimore: Johns Hopkins University Press, 1996), pp. 248-88. The same literature made it clear, however, as we have seen, that although care for the sick included competent medical care, it could not be reduced to "medical" care. The Fourth Lateran Council (1215) had also decreed that "physicians of the body . . . admonish [the sick] to call for the physician of souls" to make confession. (See R. J. Schroeder, *Disciplinary Decrees of the General Councils* [St. Louis: Herder, 1957], p. 236.) At the very least, the decree stood as a reminder that, although physical health and life are great goods, they are not the greatest goods. They are great goods, gifts of God the creator and part of the cause of God the redeemer, but they are not "second gods." Life and health may be the goals of "physicians of the body," but those who would remember and follow one who endured suffering and death for the sake of God's cause will hardly count them the law of their being (Karl Barth, *Church Dogmatics* III/4 [Edinburgh: T. & T. Clark, 1961], p. 342).

exempted ignorance from discredit. The old category did not require medicine to learn how to care for those it identified as "overmastered by disease." Care was required; neglect and inattention were prohibited. Thus began the commendable efforts to find a cure for those who had been regarded as incurable. Thus began the Baconian project. We have celebrated the successes of the Baconian project, but we have also rued the failures of those successes. It issued finally in the medicalization of death. It led to the denial of death, to the denial that anyone is dying, in spite of the obvious fact that some of us — and finally all of us — are overmastered by trauma or disease. The singular focus on cure pushed care to the margins. The power of the biomedical view of the body led, ironically, to the neglect of patients as persons, to inattention to their stories, and to ignorance of their embodied and communal life as they lay dying.

In response to medicalized death, that same "inasmuch" now requires medicine to recover a practice of care as the context for (and limit for) its efforts to cure. And the same "inasmuch" also requires the Christian community to recover its own practices of care as the context for (and limit for) medicine.

To insist on care in response to the medicalization of death is to insist on care for patients as embodied and communal and spiritual selves. Care will not, like the patients' rights movement, simply insist in Cartesian fashion that the patient is also an agent. Care will not set the mind (or the will) simply over and over against the body. It will not simply demand respect for a patient's autonomy while the body remains manipulable nature. A practice of care with reverence will not be satisfied either with that technical expert who reduces the sick to manipulable nature or with that moral expert who reduces the patient to capacities for choice. The practice of care with reverence will be attentive to the suffering of patients. Patients suffer, after all, neither as ghostly minds nor as biological organisms but as whole persons.[5]

The parable is eloquent testimony that watchfulness calls for care, but it is also an elegant reminder of the humility appropriate to caregivers, both medical caregivers and congregational caregivers. It gives no warrant for any messianic pretensions. If any have a claim to being messiah in this parable, it is "the least of these," including the sick and dying. The caregiver is not messiah. A watchful medicine will not deny the not-yet charac-

5. Eric J. Cassell, "Recognizing Suffering," *Hastings Center Report* 21, no. 3 (May-June 1991): 24-31.

ter of its medicine, not to itself and not to its patients. It will not deny that some are dying; it will not withhold that truth from patients or pretend that the chances of recovery are better than they are. It will not hesitate to instruct the dying to attend to the tasks of dying well. And a watchful community will not deny the not-yet character of its existence, not to itself and not to the sick and dying in the congregation. On the contrary, a watchful medicine and a watchful community will sustain and nurture truthfulness about our finitude, about our own limits. Humility, after all, finds its twin in truthfulness.

To be reminded that one is not the messiah is not insulting; it is liberating. It is to be freed by watchfulness and its humility for a more care-free care. A watchful medicine need not bear that finally intolerable burden of being messiah; a watchful community need not substitute anxiously for a finally powerless God. Watchful caregivers need not panic in the presence of suffering and dying.[6] They can simply "be there" with and for the sick and dying, present to them. When there are no words, when the suffering is mute, a watchful caregiver can "be there" with a silent readiness to listen — and that silent presence can help a patient to find words to express the hurt. And when the dying person finds those words, a watchful caregiver can "be there," ready to join her voice to his in com-plaintive lament — and that "expressive compassion" can help a patient to find meaning and to begin to construct the next chapter of a life, even if it will be the last chapter.[7] Watchfulness can nurture and sustain a more carefree care, and bring calm to chaos.

Neither a watchful medicine nor a watchful community can finally deliver us from death. Only God can do that. But the response of reverence and care can provide a little foretaste of God's victory. Without denying death, it will not celebrate it either. It will respond to the threats of death with care and with confidence that death will not have the last word.

Death threatens, as we have said, alienation from our bodies. A watchful medicine will care — and meet that threat by medical attention

6. William F. May, *The Physician's Covenant: Images of the Healer in Medical Ethics* (Philadelphia: Westminster, 1983), p. 60.

7. Warren Reich, "Speaking of Suffering: A Moral Account of Compassion," *Soundings* 72, no. 1 (Spring 1989): 83-108, pp. 93-97, describes a progress from "mute suffering" (and a silent compassion) to "expressive suffering" (and an expressive compassion) to the reconstruction of an identity and integrity with it. See also Margaret E. Mohrmann, *Medicine as Ministry: Reflections on Suffering, Ethics, and Hope* (Cleveland: Pilgrim Press, 1995), pp. 75-88.

to embodied selves, relieving pain and nurturing the strength of patients to exercise self-control and responsibility. A watchful community, too, will care — and meet that threat by attention to the delights of one's flesh, to the music he likes and to the flowers she loves, to his environment and to her dining (no less than to her diet), and by the human touch that signals compassion.

Death, we said, threatens alienation from our communities. A watchful medicine will care — and meet the threat by hospitality not only to patients but to those whom patients love and by whom they are loved, by making those visiting the sick and dying comfortable and welcome, by ministering to those who can only stand and wait, for in such hospitality medicine cares for the patient, too. A watchful community, too, will care — and meet the threat by visiting the sick and the dying, by doing what it can to help with the tasks of dying well and faithfully. It will practice presence, a presence that allows the dying person to recover her voice, even if only in lament. It will practice a presence that helps the dying person to write the final chapter of his life in a way that fits his loyalty to God and to the cause of God, in a way that fits his faithful participation in the community, and in a way that fits his own integrity. It will practice a presence that displays and assures the dying that they have not been and will not be abandoned. And it will pray.

And death, we said, threatens alienation from God. A watchful medicine will care, attentive to the dying as a religious self. A watchful community, too, will care — and meet that threat with the assurance of God's love, from which not even death can separate us. It does not meet this threat by trying to dispense God, by trying to provide God in pleasant little doses, convenient tablets, say, designed to make God easier to swallow. Care is not undertaken as though God were not present to those threatened by death unless someone produces God. It is undertaken as a sign of a divine love that is always present and as a signal of a human hope that is already real.

A watchful medicine, it needs finally to be said again, requires a watchful community.[8] A watchful community will not abandon the sick or the suffering to medicine, nor will it abandon caregivers to their technology. A watchful community will call the sick and suffering to the virtues of dying well, to faith and hope and love, to patience and humility and "let-

---

8. Stanley Hauerwas, *Suffering Presence: Theological Reflections on Medicine, the Mentally Handicapped, and the Church* (Notre Dame, Ind.: University of Notre Dame Press, 1986), pp. 63-83.

ting go." It will comfort them in their lament, and encourage them to the courage of their comfort. And a watchful community will call caregivers to understand their work as a calling, indeed as a "holy calling,"[9] a form of discipleship of the suffering and saving Christ, a vocation in which and through which they can serve the cause of God, rejoicing sometimes in some little token of God's good future they are able to bring, lamenting sometimes with a patient that it is still not yet God's good future.

This attention to the dying patient as embodied, communal, and spiritual reflects, of course, the wisdom of the hospice movement. That is hardly accidental; the hospice movement, as we have said, was born out of the Christian convictions of Dame Cicely Saunders. The hospice movement remains a place in which Christian doctors, nurses, chaplains, social workers, and volunteers — as well as the dying — can find a home. The worries we expressed earlier about the hospice movement remain, but they are worries prompted by the failures of its successes. Its success in alleviating pain has created the danger that it may medicalize the suffering that attends dying, reducing it to the pain that drugs can manage. Its success in winning inclusion in the health care delivery system has put at risk the sense of vocation that inspired Cicely Saunders. Its increasing professionalization has substituted contractual relationships of expert and client for the relationships of covenant and community that Cicely Saunders envisioned. And its success in the context of religiously pluralistic societies prompted it to adopt a generic spirituality as a substitute for the robust Christian faith of its founder. Still, I commend hospice care for those who are dying — and for those Christians who are dying. I only insist that the church not surrender its responsibility for caring to hospice. Let hospice care be set in the context of the church's care.

The church, formed by its practices and by its faith in God, can provide responses to suffering that do not simply manage it by drugs for pain. The church has a vocation to care for its members, a vocation captured in Jesus' parable of the last judgment (Matt. 25:31-46). The church can provide a covenanted community of care, not experts but friends. The church does not speak the language of generic spirituality; it speaks the native language of the Christian believer. The church can keep faith with — and sometimes for — the dying person. It knows the source and the object of

---

9. Walter Rauschenbusch, "For Doctors and Nurses" (1909), reprinted in Stephen E. Lammers and Allen Verhey, eds., *On Moral Medicine: Theological Perspectives in Medical Ethics* (Grand Rapids: Eerdmans, 1987), p. 5.

Christian hope, and it can speak of it. It knows that love is already the rule of God, and it can nurture it. It is trained in patience, looking for the good future of God. It knows its neediness, knows that there is no boasting before God, and it can nurture humility. And because it trusts God, it knows and teaches that the tightfisted anxiety that thinks our security and our lives are in our own hands is folly.

The church will, of course, partner with medicine, grateful like Jesus ben Sirach for the gifts of God that bring relief and sometimes preserve life. It will, however, not worship at technology's altar or surrender dying to medicine. It will minister to the health care professionals in the congregation, listening attentively to them, allowing them an honest recognition of their own neediness, their own "flesh," and calling them to discipleship of the saving and compassionate Christ.

It will partner also with hospice, grateful for the skill and knowledge of hospice workers, but it will not surrender to the "experts" its responsibility to teach its members how to die well and faithfully or its responsibility to care well for the dying. It will commend those in the congregation who work to provide hospice care at the end of life, listen to their stories and to their struggles, and nurture their compassion with care for the caregivers.

It will partner also with the dying. How can it not? For it is partner first of all and fundamentally with Christ, who died in solidarity with our human flesh, in solidarity with all who suffer and die. In solidarity with Christ, the church will partner with any and all who are vulnerable to death. It will make a place for lament and proclaim God's victory. It will offer instruction concerning dying well and help with discernment in the contexts of ambiguity. It will not abandon them to technology or to those experts who know how to use it. It will provide the gifts of God for the people of God, even as they lie dying. (Moreover, neither dying well nor caring well for the dying comes simply by wishing for it at the end of life. Both are learned behaviors. The virtues are habits, not simply summoned when they would be useful. Perhaps the best way to learn to die well and faithfully is to participate in practices of compassionate care for the dying. It is a point that the *Ars Moriendi* tradition regularly made. Presence to and compassion for the dying can be instructive about what things to do and what things to leave undone as we lie dying ourselves.)

Then we may signal together another and better destiny, that death is not the last word, and that God's good future makes its power felt not where the dying cling desperately to life, nor where the dying are deliberately killed, but where dying is faced with courage and accompanied by care. Then, without celebrating death, we may signal together a faithful response both to the medicalized death of the mid–twentieth century and to the threats of death since the Fall.

CHAPTER SEVENTEEN

Last Words

"Best of all, God is with us."

The last words of John Wesley

Joe Sandwich is a character in Peter De Vries' novel *The Vale of Laughter,*[1] and he is indeed a character. Early on we discover that he has a hobby of collecting, not stamps or coins, but funny names. There are Justin Case, Miles Long, Brighton Early, O. B. Still, and so on. He is always on the lookout for them, searching the telephone directory for them. So it comes as no shock when we read later that he names his own son Ham.

The story starts, however, when Joe is a teenager. His own father is sick, recovering from a heart attack, and Joe and his mother take turns sitting with him. Joe's father, a typical De Vries character, regards himself as an urbane unbeliever in an otherwise pious household. Having been reminded of his mortality, he begins to worry about what his last words should be. He reads *How They Went,* a collection, with commentary, of the last words of famous people. It told, for example, that when Thoreau was asked whether he had made his peace with God, he retorted, "We have never quarreled" (p. 10). It seems an obsession to Joe, but to his father it is important. And to Joe's impatient question about what difference it

---

1. Peter De Vries, *The Vale of Laughter* (New York: Bantam Books, 1968); page references are included in parentheses.

makes, his father replies, "A lot of difference. It's a statement. It characterizes a man, and it's something to leave behind for others to remember him by. . . . A sort of summing up" (p. 11).

Joe sees no reasonable motive for his father's concern about his last words "except the desire to strut your stuff to the end" (p. 14). What escapes Joe, however, is clear enough to the reader. Joe's father wants indeed to "strut his stuff," if not to the end, at least at the end. He wants his dying to give some definitive expression to his identity as the urbane unbeliever, unfettered finally by the piety of his good wife.

Then his father announces a new worry about his last words: "What if a man goes in the middle of the night and says something there's nobody to hear?" (p. 13). In an effort "to cheer him up," Joe replies to that worry, "It might be completely trite and worthless, and lucky nobody did hear it" (p. 14). Unsurprisingly, that remark fails to soothe his father. Joe gives this new worry a little further thought and suggests the following remedy. His father should decide what he would like his last words to be, tell Joe, and when he dies, Joe will tell the others that he had said those very words just before his death. But his father does not like Joe's suggestion. "That would be cheating," his father says (p. 14). "It would be too contrived. Not extemporaneous" (p. 15). This prompts Joe to return to his claims that his father is obsessing about his last words and that they are not that important. He reminds his father — a little impatiently — that *How They Went* had attributed more than one set of last words to Thoreau. Besides that remark about not having quarreled with God, it also reported that when a visitor suggested a conversation about the afterlife, Thoreau had said, "One world at a time, please," and then he died. A third account claimed that his last words as he sank into unconsciousness just before his death were "Moose" and "Indians." "What's so great about that?" Joe demands (p. 15).

I find myself on Joe's side in this little family quarrel. Joe's father is attaching too much importance to his last words. But let's admit that Joe's father has a point. Last words can give a definitive expression to one's identity, and there have been some memorable ones. When Rabbi Akiba died as a result of being tortured by the Romans, while his flesh was still being raked, he recited the Shema, "Hear, O Israel, the Lord our God is one." Those were his last words, a testimony both to his loyalty to God and to God's faithfulness to the covenant. The last words of John Wesley, "Best of all, God is with us," spoke of his confidence in God's presence in spite of death. The last public words of Dr. Martin Luther King Jr. summed up his life:

Well, I don't know what will happen now. We've got some difficult days ahead. But it really doesn't matter with me now. Because I've been to the mountain top. I won't mind. Like anybody, I would like to live a long life. Longevity has its place. But I'm not concerned about that now. I just want to do God's will. And He's allowed me to go up to the mountain. And I've looked over, and I've seen the promised land. I may not get there with you, but I want you to know tonight that we as a people will get to the promised land. So I'm happy tonight. I'm not worried about anything. I'm not fearing any man. Mine eyes have seen the glory of the coming of the Lord.[2]

We should add to this list, of course, the last words of Jesus on the cross, the most famous of all last words, words that we examined earlier when we considered the death of Jesus as paradigmatic for a Christian's dying well and faithfully. I admit, moreover, that I have given some thought to what I would like my last words to be (maybe "shalom," maybe "thanks," or "I love you, I love you all," but I will be satisfied with a whisper of hope, "O Lord God, you know"). I acknowledge, however, that my last sounds are as likely to be a whimper as to be a coherent and pious thought. That itself is surely one reason to prefer Joe's side of this quarrel. His father put too much stress on his last words.

It seems Peter De Vries took Joe's side of the argument, too. On the night Joe's father died, Joe was sitting with him again. He was convalescing from another heart attack. That night, during a sudden thunderstorm, there was a great flash of lightning accompanied by a violent crash of thunder. Joe's father yelled, "Jesus H. Christ," and promptly died (p. 20). When Joe reported these final words to his pious mother, he omitted the middle initial, turning the exclamation into an invocation. His pious mother took great solace in the fact that "he made his peace at the end" (p. 20). Surely De Vries is poking fun at the ways American culture in the mid–twentieth century cared little for the integrity of the dying person, and was only concerned not to inconvenience the survivors too much. Still, it is hard to escape the impression that he agrees that "last words" are a slender reed upon which to hang one's desire to give a definitive disclosure on one's identity. Joe's father relied too much on what his last words would be.

2. Martin Luther King Jr., Memphis, Tennessee, April 3, 1968 (from back cover of King, *Why We Can't Wait* [New York: New American Library, Signet Book, 1964; as reissued in 1968]).

Christians — as well as urbane unbelievers like Joe's father — who want to make their dying a definitive disclosure of their identity would be wise to attend less to what last words they say and more to the way they write the last chapter of their lives. Let it be a faithful and well-lived final chapter. Let it be marked by the confidence that, although death remains an enemy, God has already defeated it and will accomplish the renewal of the cosmos and the redemption of our bodies. Let the last chapter (at least) be formed by the paradigmatic significance of Christ's dying. Let it be marked by faith, hope, and love, by patience, humility, and generosity.

There are words to be said, of course. There are the familiar words of the church, words from Scripture and from creed. There are words to be addressed to God in the simple attentiveness of prayer, words of confession and gratitude, words of lament and hope. There are the words to be said to spouses and parents and children, said to friends and to enemies, grateful words as simple as "Thank you," affectionate words as simple as "I love you," and reconciling words like "Please forgive me," and in response to a request for forgiveness, "Of course, I forgive you," as difficult as those words sometimes are. Such words take some time, of course. They take something like a chapter, not just a few sentences at the end.

Of course, some do not have that time. Some still die suddenly, of a heart attack, from an auto accident, by violence, or in some other way. Although the stories of medicalized dying prompted many to say they would prefer the sudden death, the sudden death is not a good way to die, not for the dying person and not for those left to grieve without the opportunity to have said good-by. It provides no opportunity for dying well and faithfully, no opportunity for speaking and hearing words of faith and community, no opportunity for gestures of affection and reconciliation.

Many of us, however, will have time. The advances of medicine in the twentieth century that led to medicalized dying have also provided more time between diagnosis and death. First, penicillin and other antibiotics were effective against the quick death threatened by infectious diseases. Then, the advances of medicine effectively reduced the number of sudden deaths by heart attack or trauma. Most people today die of chronic diseases, congestive heart failure, kidney failure, lung failure, Alzheimer's disease, Parkinson's disease, Lou Gehrig's disease (ALS), and the like. Medicine has not succeeded in defeating death, and it will not. It has, however, frequently made dying a longer process. It has given us time. When that time is spent in the denial of death, when biological survival becomes the law of our being, when we surrender the last chapter of our lives to the medical experts, then we will have a medicalized dying. (And doubtless, a medicalized dying takes a long time.) But the time between diagnosis and death is also an opportunity to write the last chapter of our lives well and faithfully. We may not live quite as long if we attend to tasks besides staying alive, but while life is a great good, it is not the greatest good. We have duties that outweigh our own survival. The paradigmatic Christ is pretty clear about that. The gift of a little more time should not prompt us to demand more and more time as though death were the enemy to be defeated by the greater powers of medicine. It should prompt us to take the opportunity to write a final chapter that displays confidence in God and loyalty to God's cause and the affection and reconciliation that belong to God's cause.

In another (and the best) of Peter De Vries' novels, *The Blood of the Lamb*,[3] Don Wanderhope, lapsed Calvinist, and his skeptical Jewish friend Stein are on the roof terrace of Westminster Hospital, where their daughters are both being treated for leukemia back when, not so long ago, leukemia usually brought death in its wake. They look down to the street, where the church of St. Catharine could be seen directly across from the research wing of the hospital. "Quite a juxtaposition," Wanderhope says. "Science versus religion." Stein snorts and replies cynically, "We get about as much from one as the other" (p. 177). Stein did not believe in God and had little confidence in medicine. When Wanderhope points out that at least medical research had made a little progress against leukemia, Stein responds, "So death by leukemia is now a local instead of an express. Same run, only a few more stops. But that's medicine, the art of prolonging disease." Wanderhope laughs at the image, but replies incredulously, "Why would anybody want to prolong it?" To that inquiry Stein has a ready response: "In order to postpone grief" (pp. 178-79).

That's the path to the denial of death and to a medicalized dying. Instead we may give thanks not only for the successes of medicine against the childhood leukemia that took the lives of precious children of people like Wanderhope and Stein but also for a little time to write the last chapter. Instead we may be grateful for medicine's skill not "in order to postpone grief" but in order to accomplish the tasks that attend our dying. Instead of "science versus religion," it is time for a new partnership.[4] That partner-

---

3. Peter De Vries, *The Blood of the Lamb* (New York: Little, Brown, Popular Library Edition, 1961). The citations in parentheses are from this edition. In the reprint by University of Chicago Press, 2005, the citations are from pp. 181, 182-83.

4. On this "partnership" see especially David H. Smith, *Partnership with the Dying:*

ship will require a new (and ancient) imagination, capable of acknowledging that death is an enemy, of acknowledging as well the limits of the powers of medicine, of celebrating God's victory over "the last enemy," and of living grateful and faithful lives even as we are dying.

Of course, the time medicine gives is not always accompanied by the capacities to perform the tasks that attend our dying. Alzheimer's disease, for example, can diminish our capacities for these tasks. The diagnosis usually comes, however, before the disease or the treatment for it or the pain that attends it robs us of the capacities to die well and faithfully. And even when our own capacities are diminished or absent, even when we cannot or do not display serenity, let the church be there, refusing to surrender dying to medicine, present to its dying member, keeping faith with her or him, sometimes keeping faith for him or her. Dying well always — and especially in these cases — takes a community. The Christian community, formed by the Spirit, will be the *paraklete* for its members, the comforter and the advocate. To be the advocate will not mean always demanding that "everything" be done to keep the patient alive nor always acquiescing in the recommendation of a physician that something more be tried.

This partnership and this advocacy will require discernment and will not be empty of ambiguity. We have already suggested that conversations about medical care at the end of life can and should take place in the context of the Christian community and long before one faces such decisions. If the church is not to surrender dying to medicine or abandon the dying person to technology and the experts who know how to use it, then the church must also be prepared to be a community of discernment in memory of Jesus also when a member of the community does face them.

Perhaps something like the Quaker tradition of Clearness Committees should become a part of Christian practice with respect to medical decisions near the end of life. The Clearness Committee, committed to confidentiality, to keeping faith with the person, does not tell the person what to do, but does assist that person in making decisions about difficult issues. In the Quaker tradition the assumption is that each has an Inner Teacher, which is not simply identical to the voice of our conscience but is rather

Where Medicine and Ministry Should Meet (Lanham, Md.: Rowman and Littlefield, 2005), and Abigail Rian Evans, "Healing in the Midst of Dying: A Collaborative Approach to End-of-Life Care," in *Living Well and Dying Faithfully: Christian Perspectives on End-of-Life Care,* ed. John Swinton and Richard Payne (Grand Rapids: Eerdmans, 2009), pp. 165-87.

the presence of the Holy Spirit to us, guiding and strengthening us for the challenge.[5] The Spirit, of course, teaches us by reminding us of what Jesus said and did (John 14:26). The Spirit nurtures discernment and creates a community of discernment precisely in memory of Jesus.

Whether there be something like a Clearness Committee or not, let the church and its memory of Jesus be present. Let the paradigmatic significance of Jesus' death be rehearsed again. Let there be reminders that life is a great good, but not the greatest good, that our own survival may not become the law of our being. That's the path to a medicalized dying. Let there be reminders that death is an enemy, but an enemy already defeated not by medicine but by the power and faithfulness of God displayed in raising Jesus from the dead. Let there be assurances of the resurrection. Let there be invitations to follow Jesus also in a faithful dying. Let there be prayers.

There are words to be said in the context of this process of discernment, too, of course, conversations to be had, questions to ask. Prayer does not work like magic for hard decisions either. It is not that we pray rather than think hard about what we ought to do. It is rather that we attend carefully to the relevant considerations in ways that are attentive also to God. To look to God is not to look away. When an illness that threatens death is diagnosed, there are questions to be asked of one's doctor: What's the exact diagnosis? How certain are you of the diagnosis? What is the range of ways that this disease affects those who suffer from it? What is likely to happen if the disease goes untreated? What are the treatment options? What are the chances of success with these different options? What are the costs and burdens of the different treatment options? Are some more likely than others to render the last chapter of my life less apt for the tasks of affection, reconciliation, and just plain fun with the family? What are the real chances of success? And how would you measure it? Just in terms of my biological survival or also in terms of what that survival would be like? Asking such questions early makes it easier to return to them. To some questions the answer may well be "I don't know." That is at least an honest answer, and it is important in such conversation to insist on honesty and candor.

5. See Parker Palmer, "The Clearness Committee: A Communal Approach to Discernment," Center for Courage and Renewal, 2006, www.couragerenewal.org. See also Karen Scheib, " 'Make Love Your Aim': Ecclesial Practices of Care at the End of Life," in *Living Well and Dying Faithfully*, pp. 30-56, who suggests Clearness Committees and who alerted me to the Parker Palmer essay.

There might be more to this conversation with your doctor than just your questions and the doctor's answers. You might report that your image of death is not that it is the great enemy to be defeated by the greater powers of medicine but the enemy already defeated by the resurrection of Jesus from the dead. You might report that you do not have extravagant expectations of medicine's powers but are grateful for the care and skill of physicians and nurses. You might report that you regard life as a great good but not as the greatest good, that your own survival is not the law of your being, that you will therefore make thankful use of medicine but refuse treatments that might provide more days or months of life but only at the cost of rendering that time unfruitful for the task of dying well and faithfully or for the goods that outweigh survival. If you have prepared advance directives in the context of the church's faith and hope, you should share them with him. You should inquire whether there is the possibility of a partnership as you begin to write what may be the final chapter of your life. (The problems of continuity of care in major medical centers may require that such conversations take place with more than one doctor.)

Honesty and candor are essential ingredients of such a partnership. But they can be elusive. There is nothing dishonest about a physician asking, "Do you want me to do CPR on your father?" And for an otherwise healthy person who had suffered a heart attack it would surely make sense (and probably not be asked). But if the father is an old man suffering his way to death with cancer, it might be more honest to ask, "Shall we crack some of his ribs as he lies dying?" To the family the question "Shall I do CPR?" is like the question "Shall I do everything I can for your father?" It's hard to say no. It's one reason earlier conversations and decisions and a partnership are so important. For truth is finally tested not just by whether our words fit the facts but by whether our words and deeds fit the "troth" we have pledged.

Conversations should also be had with pastors and community, with family and friends — and with enemies. Family members should be informed and consulted about the medical decisions you face; family quarrels about such matters are not uncommon when that has not happened. But some conversations are more important than "an organ recital" (as Bill May said somewhere). There are words of affection to be said, words of gratitude. Words of reconciliation are sometimes necessary, requests for forgiveness and assurances of forgiveness. The last chapter is no time to be holding a grudge. There are testimonies of faith and hope to be spoken. There are requests to be made for the care of those you leave behind, and yes, instructions to be given concerning your stuff. And in all your words and deeds, display some faith and some faithfulness, some hope in the God who raised Jesus from the dead and promises redemption for the cosmos and for these bodies, some love for your family and friends and enemies, some patience with those who would care for you, some humility, acknowledging your neediness and graciously receiving the care of others, and some generosity. Attend to God. Take courage and comfort from the promises of God, vindicated and assured when God raised Jesus from the dead. Attend to all things as related to God. Give thanks for God's good but fragile gifts of your community and your body. Take time for the delights of community — and for the delights of the flesh. Lament and give thanks. Be at peace.

To use some famous last words about this book: "It is finished." The last word, of course, does not belong to this book. The last word belongs to God. Thanks be to God!

Subject and Name Index

162, 167, 170, 200, 233, 234, 237, 239, 240, 268, 284, 323, 336, 337
Miracles, 9, 13, 14, 21, 22, 25, 29n.9, 70, 310, 311, 316-17, 319-20, 373-76; of Jesus, 211, 223-24, 319-20
Mitford, Jessica, 344, 345
Moll, Rob, 174n.1
Monasticism, 127, 353
Moore, George Foot, 189
Moore-Keish, Martha, 307n.14
Moral ambiguity, 324, 365-73
Moral discourse, 299, 357, 363-65, 372
Mortal(ity), xi, 7, 12, 20, 31, 35, 37, 55, 75, 149, 154, 160, 179-80, 181, 182, 192, 209, 224, 256, 257, 262, 263, 269, 296, 306, 310, 311, 316, 317, 318, 323-24, 326, 357, 360, 375, 386
Mother Nature, 56, 57, 288
Mourning: practice of, 6, 15, 101n.19, 145, 184, 200, 206, 265, 268-69, 280, 299, 326, 327, 331, 333-44, 345, 347-50, 356, 376. *See also* Grief
Mystical theology, 85, 86, 106, 159, 217n.2

Nature: control of, 12, 30-32, 34, 35, 37, 40, 49, 56, 149, 263, 311, 388; distrust of, 37; as enemy, 12, 19, 37, 56, 58; untamed, 13
Neoplatonism, 105
Nephesh, 183, 191-93, 220, 250, 262, 262n.8
"New Learning," 29-32
Niebuhr, H. Richard, 147n.18, 257n.3, 275
Nygren, Anders, 273n.15

O'Connor, Flannery, "Revelation," 284
O'Connor, Mary Catherine, 86n.17, 92n.6, 120n.13, 129n.20, 158, 170
Olson-Getty, Dayna, 318-19
Otto, Rudolf, 139
"Overmastered by Disease," 27, 28, 31, 38, 43, 49, 61, 63, 137, 149, 173, 379, 380

Pain, relief from, 60, 62, 63, 64, 67, 253, 276, 312, 318, 319, 353, 354, 363, 382, 383. *See also* Palliative medicine
Palliative medicine, 41, 62, 63, 64, 66, 67, 287, 289, 363. *See also* Pain, relief from
Pantheism, 56, 57
Parousia, 178n.3, 201, 203, 204
Paternalism, 45
Patience, 99-101, 120, 122-25, 127, 129, 137, 145, 150-52, 155, 199, 217, 256, 261, 270, 278-83, 293, 287, 319, 320, 326, 328, 352, 360, 382, 284, 389, 394. *See also* Impatience
Patient rights, 23, 42, 43-49, 77
Patient Self-Determination Act, 47, 359
Paul, Saint, 93, 99-104, 107, 113, 119, 122, 127, 149, 151, 194, 195, 200-210, 247n.35, 264, 265, 270, 274n.15, 277, 278, 281, 282, 287, 291, 292, 326, 329, 330, 352, 353
Persistent vegetative state, 368, 368n.35, 370
Petition(s), 13, 162, 255, 305, 315-16, 317, 320, 321, 324. *See also* Prayer(s)
Phaedo, 2, 220
Physician authority, 45, 48
Piety, 140, 244, 303-7, 387
Pius XII, 45
Plague, 12, 79-83, 85, 86, 88, 93, 101n.19, 102, 138, 158, 167n.9, 378. *See also* Black Death
Plato, 2, 5, 15n.4, 35n.24, 105n.27, 106, 271n.12, 273, 282, 297, 353
Platonism, 12, 101n.19, 105-8, 174, 183, 191, 201, 203, 204, 206, 218, 220, 223n.9, 225, 243, 250, 272n.12, 289, 347n.16
Plotinus, 106, 272
Polkinghorne, John, 212
Polycarp, 351
Pontius Pilate, 69, 197, 264
Popular psychology, 53, 71
"Pornography of Death," 15, 50, 67
Positivism, 57
Powerlessness, 16, 27, 44, 228, 257, 311, 314

Scripture Index